The Lives of University Hospitals of Cleveland

THE LIVES OF UNIVERSITY HOSPITALS OF CLEVELAND

The 125-Year Evolution of an Academic Medical Center

MARK GOTTLIEB

Wilson Street Press   *Cleveland, Ohio*

Published by Wilson Street Press

Library of Congress Catalog Card No.: 91-66654
ISBN: 0-940601-06-0

Text design, editing, and production coordination by
Kathleen Mills Editorial & Production Services

Printed in the United States of America

Contents

Illustrations follow pages 118 and 222

Acknowledgments

In the course of researching and writing this book I have incurred innumerable debts of gratitude to a very large group of people. Time, now, to begin settling up.

To James A. Block, president and chief executive officer of University Hospitals of Cleveland, I owe my sincere thanks for giving me the opportunity to pursue the fascinating subject of the medical center's history.

I am also deeply indebted to former UHC chief of staff L. Douglas Lenkoski, former UHC president Scott R. Inkley, UHC senior vice president M. Orry Jacobs, and UHC chief of staff David R. Bickers, all of whom served on the editorial committee overseeing my work. I thank them for the time and effort they devoted to the project, for their helpful comments, criticisms, and suggestions, for their unflagging enthusiasm and good humor, and for their friendship.

A number of individuals graciously submitted to lengthy interviews during my research. I extend thanks to Nathan Berger, Jonathon Bishop, James A. Block, George Crile, Jr., Carl Doershuk, Avroy Fanaroff, Edward Halloran, Kingsbury Heiple, Herman Hellerstein, Scott R. Inkley, L. Douglas Lenkoski, Adel Mahmoud, John Mannix, Herbert Meltzer, Roland Newman, Nancy Pierce, Tracy Rabold, Dennis Rusch, William T. Speck, Christine Straub, Elden C. Weckesser, and Peter Whitehouse.

For their assistance in ways too numerous to delineate here, I also wish to thank Gail Allore, Cynthia Cover, Ingrid Ebner, James Edmonson, Ellen Gambrill, John J. Gargus, Patsy Gerstner, Dennis Harrison, Tom Hinson, Glen Jenkins, Bruce Latimer, Catharine M. Lewis, Diana Lounsbury, Nancy McCann, William C. McCoy, Jr., Sylvia Morrison, Amelia S. Osborne, William M. Osborne, Jr., Kermit J. Pike, Jill Pope, Michele Scheufler, Ann Sindelar, Jill Tatem, Diana Tittle, Elizabeth Vollstadt, and Ross, Mary, and Joey.

To Debra Pearman and Gerard Shorb, from The Johns Hopkins Medical Institutions, my sincere appreciation for the timely assistance that was so kindly offered to a total stranger who called one day from out of the blue. And I am especially indebted to Kathleen M. Mills, whose editorial skills and judgment are without parallel.

Lastly, I wish to offer my warmest thanks to the doctors, nurses, respiratory therapists, technicians, and staff of the Neonatal Intensive Care Unit of Rainbow Babies and Childrens Hospital. These dedicated and hard-working individuals gave me a crash course in the ways of the NICU, not only providing me with detailed explanations of many of the complex procedures that are performed daily in the unit, but also cheerfully answering what must have seemed to them to be an endless series of questions. It was a privilege to have watched them at their work.

Foreword

This is the story of a great health-care institution—its beginnings one hundred and twenty-five years ago as a voluntary charity hospital for the care of the sick poor, its early alliance with what was then known as the Medical Department of Western Reserve College, and its evolution into the modern academic medical center that we know today. It is also the story of the institution's successive boards of trustees, men and women imbued with a sense of responsibility for their community and the desire to maintain the highest standards of patient care, medical education, and medical research. Above all, it is the story of farsighted, dedicated individuals who have made lasting contributions not only to the life of the institution but to medicine and health care as well.

It is not, however, a history of tranquil progress. Given all of the problems that have plagued the component hospitals of the medical center over the years—from leaky nineteenth-century roofs to debilitating twentieth-century financial depressions—their mere survival is itself a wonder. And not all of the players in this drama could be described as entirely self-effacing. Gustav Weber, for example, was a first-class surgeon but a tyrannical leader, and his long-running feud with Dudley P. Allen, another celebrated surgeon, ultimately precipitated his own downfall. Allen's academic credentials, patrician background, and ties by blood and marriage to influential Clevelanders gave him easy access to the board of trustees, access that he did not hesitate to use. Yet Allen, too, would eventually be outmaneuvered, this time by a former farmboy named George Crile, who was even more adept at political machinations than his two predecessors.

If there were personality conflicts along the way, however, there were also extraordinary contributions to academic medicine, beginning shortly after the founding of the tiny Wilson Street Hospital in 1866. The most notable achievement, of course, came in 1952, with the brilliant curriculum reform instituted by Joseph T. Wearn, who was both director of the Department of Medicine and dean of the medical school. The Wearn revolution fundamentally changed for the better the way that medicine was taught, and University Hospitals and its affiliated medical school have been viewed as educational innovators ever since.

In its first hundred and twenty-five years, University Hospitals of Cleveland has gained prestige both nationally and internationally. It has been and continues to be an asset of inestimable value to its community, an established institution that will endure as long as academic medical centers exist.

—Robert H. Ebert, M.D.

Robert H. Ebert, M.D., former director of the Department of Medicine of University Hospitals of Cleveland, is the Caroline Shields Walker Professor of Medicine, Emeritus, and former Dean of the Faculty of Medicine of Harvard University.

The Lives of
University Hospitals
of Cleveland

Prologue

Barely five seconds after his decidedly early entry into the world, a baby boy so small that he looks less like a human infant than an oddly shaped lump of clay is about to meet a group of total strangers who will, for the foreseeable future, constitute his immediate family and closest friends.

It is late in the evening of Thanksgiving Day when Baby J is taken from his mother at the moment of his birth. Wrapped loosely in a pair of blankets, he is carried out of an operating room on the second floor of University MacDonald Womens Hospital, which is but one of the component facilities of the medical center group known as University Hospitals of Cleveland. From the OR, which is used for Caesarean-section deliveries and deliveries of what are termed "high-risk" pregnancies, Baby J is whisked around a corner and into a specially equipped treatment room, where now the group of strangers—doctors and nurses from the Neonatal Intensive Care Unit of Rainbow Babies and Childrens Hospital, the pediatric unit of University Hospitals—are setting to work on what will be their sole concern for the next few hectic minutes: breathing life into the minuscule frame of a very tiny and very sick baby boy.

Baby J is a preemie, a child born some three months prematurely after less than twenty-seven weeks of gestation. Stretched out as he is now on a special warming bed in the treatment room, he presents a disquieting sight. Not yet ten seconds old, he is already *in extremis*, and it does not require a trained eye to see that his hold on life is tenuous at best. In length he measures little more than twelve inches. His pupils are fixed and dilated, he is not breathing on his own, and he makes no sounds or spontaneous movements. His entire body is limp, and his skin has taken on a decidedly bluish tint.

Earlier in the day, Baby J's mother had suffered a partial abruption, the premature detachment of the placenta from the uterine wall. The abruption had interrupted the baby's supply of blood, a desperate situation that required immediate intervention if the child were to be saved. Emergency surgery—a "crash C-section," as it is known in hospital parlance—was ordered and performed.

As the surgery had begun, one of the senior residents on duty in the Neonatal Intensive Care Unit was alerted to the impending arrival of a new patient. The senior resident and one of the junior residents on duty in the NICU (pronounced "Nick-You") both dropped everything and hurried through a door at the far end of the unit. They ran the length of a corridor that connects Rainbow to the second-floor Labor and Delivery area of MacDonald, which is most often referred to by its longtime nickname, Mac House. At the end of the corridor—a distance of about twelve running strides—they were buzzed through two locked swinging doors that opened onto the lobby area of Labor and Delivery. Once inside, the senior resident went directly to the treatment room while the junior ran to the OR, where in a matter of seconds he donned a sterile jumpsuit, hat, mask, shoe covers, and gloves.

At the same time, the message "Mac House nurse to Labor and Delivery, stat" was being announced over the NICU's public address system. ("Mac House nurse," in this instance, refers to the NICU nurse whose duty during her work shift includes assisting in the treatment of high-risk infants delivered next door. "Stat" means immediately.) The Mac House nurse and a NICU respiratory therapist followed the same drill as the residents, charging out of the unit, down the corridor, and into Labor and Delivery. Entering the specially designed treatment room they began to prepare the equipment and medications that have become the standard tools of the trade for resuscitating sick preemies. The room is kept stocked with ample supplies of sterile gloves and gowns, syringes, intravenous microinfusion pumps, an assortment of medications, endotracheal tubes of various diameters, Ambu bags for manually forcing air into an infant's lungs, clamps, gauze—everything from computerized heart-rate monitors to rolls of common adhesive tape. By the time the junior resident arrived with Baby J in his arms, the room—and everyone in it—was prepared for work.

The tiny infant, silent and inert, is positioned with his head at the foot of a warmer bed, a small adjustable platform on wheels that serves multiple duty as a bassinet, a source of heat for the by-now very chilly patient, and an easily accessible work table for the NICU doctors and nurses. Indeed, the baby on the warming table is now the focus of attention of a group of six. At the foot of the table, hovering over the infant's head, is the senior resident. To his left is the junior resident, to his right the nurse from the NICU. Also on the right, a step or so back from the semi-circle, is the respiratory therapist, waiting to provide his services. Behind them all is another physician who has been in the NICU doing advanced research in neonatology on a postdoctoral fellowship. If a postdoc is in the unit at the time of a high-risk delivery of an infant younger than thirty weeks gestation, he or she will accompany the residents to the treatment room. Occasionally, the NICU's attending physician, one of a group of senior neonatologists who share overall responsibility for the unit, will also be there. A nurse from MacDonald, the same one who had been in the OR at Baby J's delivery, is also present, sitting at a small desk and taking notes on the procedures performed, the medications administered, and all the numbers—from heart rate to the time of day—that will be called out to her by the team members as they work. Sometimes—at the birth of twins, for example—the treatment room is so crowded that working there has been compared to changing clothes in a phone booth.

Baby J is now rubbed briskly with a warm blanket, both to clean him and to stimulate what little breathing he might be capable of on his own. The senior resident immediately grabs a laryngoscope, a device that resembles a small flashlight, and attaches a long thin blade to one end. He tilts back the newborn's head and begins ever so slowly to slide the blade into Baby J's mouth and down into his now-open airway, preparing a path for the endotracheal tube. "Trache" tubes can be inserted more easily when they are chilled and therefore slightly stiff, which is why the NICU nurse has already prepared a few of different sizes, putting them on ice in a blue plastic tray. The tray seems oddly incongruous in the setting because it looks very much like a banana-split boat.

The resident manages to insert the trache tube on the first try, which is no small feat considering the dimensions of his patient. With the tube positioned precisely at a point just above the branching of the infant's bronchial tubes, the respiratory therapist attaches an Ambu bag to a fitting on the trache tube and begins to squeeze air into the infant's lungs.

Baby J is now one minute old, and it is time for the first of his three Apgar tests, visual examinations of the child that are performed by the junior and senior residents as they attend to their other duties. They evaluate the infant's physical status, looking at his skin color, heart rate, response to stimulation, muscle tone, and respiratory effort. They then perform a fast mental calculation to score each category with either zero, one, or two, to a maximum total score of ten. Baby J's first Apgar score totals only two.

The NICU nurse grasps the baby's umbilical cord between the thumb and first two fingers of her right hand. She keeps the resident informed of the pulse she detects in the cord's arteries by tapping out the rate with the forefinger of her free hand. An antibiotic ointment is administered to the baby's eyes to prevent possible infection, and he receives an injection of Vitamin K in his tiny upper leg to bolster his blood-clotting mechanisms. (The two procedures are known in NICU shorthand as "eyes and thighs.") Blood samples are taken to determine the concentration of various gases and other components.

Because Baby J's organs and life systems are so immature, the relatively minor stresses that a full-term baby usually shrugs off could prove fatal to him. He faces the possibility of a whole catalogue of ailments, syndromes, diseases, and disasters, any one of which might be life-threatening. There are other, hidden dangers as well: the NICU doctors and nurses do not yet know whether he has been born addicted to cocaine—a phenomenon seen increasingly in the unit—or if he is already infected with the virus that produces Acquired Immune Deficiency Syndrome, the dreaded AIDS.

At this stage in Baby J's life, time is his enemy; only after he is stabilized and comfortably ensconced in the NICU will the passage of every minute increase his slim chances for survival. Despite the need for haste, however, the work of the medical team proceeds in a businesslike, almost routine way, without histrionics. The NICU nurse does most of the talking, calling out cryptic bits of information—"IV in...two milligrams sodium bicarb...heart rate twenty"—to the nurse from Mac House, who notes each item on Baby J's chart under the heading "D.O.L. #1," the first day of life.

With the respiratory therapist doing his breathing for him, Baby J begins to gain color, his fingers and toes becoming sufficiently perfused with oxygenated blood to bring up a rosier hue. His heart rate increases to one hundred beats per minute in response to the manual ventilation he is receiving, a good sign. Now he is placed on a scale, and his weight is determined to be seven hundred and eighty grams, less than one and three-quarter pounds, or about the same weight as a fully grown guinea pig. Skin hangs in folds from his underdeveloped frame. His fingers are the thickness of matchsticks, and his head is the size and color of an overripe peach. But he is beginning to stabilize.

The medical team attaches probes to Baby J's chest so that the computer monitor can track his heart rate, respiration, and body temperature automatically and continuously. The respiratory therapist continues to bag the infant even as he is wheeled out of the treatment room, down along the hallway, through more swinging doors, and into one of the NICU's seven nursery areas—the artificial womb in which he will be allowed to mature and develop. His trache tube is hooked up to an automatic jet ventilator machine that will provide him with "breaths" of pure oxygen for as long as he needs them. If he follows the form of other preemies, he will need them for quite some time. He will also almost certainly develop jaundice, and he will probably lose up to fifteen percent of his already minimal body weight in the first week of his life—if he makes it even that far. For the moment, however, he is home.

§

Rainbow's current NICU is a direct descendant of the hospital's original "premature nursery," which was created in 1952. The old unit, on the seventh floor, had become cramped and overcrowded over the years, as more and more babies were brought in to receive the benefits of a rapidly evolving and growingly important branch of medical care. The new unit, opened in 1988 in a four-story addition to the old Rainbow building, is by contrast a spacious, pleasant place, decorated with wallpaper of muted pastels sporting cheerful images of teddy bears and rocking horses. But it is something else, as well: yet another reminder of the phenomenal progress in the care of high-risk babies that has been made in the past three decades—more progress, in fact, than in all the rest of human history. There are thirty-eight beds available in the unit, the basic division being six beds to a nursery. As often as not, the NICU runs toward a full house.

With Baby J's warming bed rolled into his assigned space in one of the nurseries, the medical team returns to the everyday business of the unit. In a few hours it will be time for rounds, when two attendings lead the unit's young doctors through the nurseries, stopping at each incubator, warming bed, and crib to check on the progress and discuss the future of each of the tiny patients. On any given day the patient census can offer a wide range of cases to study, quality teaching material for the month's crop of interns and residents.

House officers rotate through the unit every thirty days as part of their clinical experience after graduation from medical school. Each month a new group of a dozen or so interns and junior and senior residents—most of them looking dismayingly young—are given responsibility for the daily care of the NICU's tiny patients. Their work is overseen by the unit's postdoctoral fellows and by the attending physicians, who are full-time members of the Division of Neonatology, a subspecialty of Pediatrics, as well as associate and assistant professors in the School of Medicine of neighboring Case Western Reserve University.

In the NICU there is very little of the squalling and yowling normally associated with a nursery, primarily because intubated babies do not cry —they can't—and even those who are breathing on their own generally do not have the energy to spare. The most commonly heard sounds in the NICU are the piercing shrieks of monitor alarms, alerting the nurses to some change in a baby's breathing, heart rate, or temperature. Alarms sound almost continuously, although most reflect only minor and transitory incongruities. Nevertheless, the nurses check out every one.

There are some one hundred and thirty nurses available for duty in the NICU, more than in any other unit in University Hospitals. Working eight- and twelve-hour shifts—days, nights, weekends, holidays—each nurse manages the care of two or at most three infants per shift, administering medications ordered by the doctors, drawing blood samples, recording body temperatures, cleaning, holding, cuddling, stroking, and talking to their tiny charges. The system employed in the NICU is called primary nursing; each infant is assigned a primary nurse who is responsible for creating and constantly updating a care plan for her patient. The primary nurse is the person in the NICU who knows her baby the best, who learns, for example, that a particular infant may squirm and fidget and clearly show discomfort when turned to rest on his right side but will quiet down immediately and rest comfortably when turned on his left side. All such observations and helpful bits of information she includes in her care plan, so that the rotating house medical staff and the other nurses who take care of the child when the primary is off duty will have the benefit of her accumulated wisdom even when she is not there.

Once rounds begin today, it quickly becomes obvious that a good number of the patients are low-birth-weight babies with no particular problems, who have been brought into the NICU purely as a precautionary measure. Known in the parlance of the unit as "NICU Rockets," they will stay for a day or two or perhaps just a few hours following birth, until the doctors are assured that they can safely be sent upstairs to "7 West," the step-down unit for NICU alumni that is located on Rainbow's seventh floor, in the same space that once housed the old NICU. There are also some "Growers and Gainers" in the unit today, babies who have successfully negotiated one crisis or another, have stabilized nicely, and are putting on weight. Barring complications, they too will soon be moving up to 7 West.

There are the hard cases too, of course. In one nursery a little girl of angelic mien sleeps quietly on a warming bed, by all appearances a perfectly normal child. A hand-lettered sign taped to her bed, however, reveals that she has been born with osteogenesis fragilus, a rare condition in which the bones are so brittle that any but the gentlest touch will produce fractures. Her prognosis is bleak.

Elsewhere in the unit there are babies suffering from the effects of hypoxia, asphyxia, sepsis, hydrocephalus, congenital defects of the heart, the lungs, the brain—the list goes on and on. There are full-term babies receiving treatment for various afflictions. There are children over a year old with chronic disorders, seeming freakishly large—almost Brobdingnagian—in relation to the tiny preemies. One strapping boy of thirteen months, who has spent all but two weeks of his life in the NICU, is having a seizure in his crib, a daily occurrence.

Ironically, some of the sickest babies in the NICU will spend the shortest amount of time there. Infants with severe respiratory ailments are candidates for a new procedure called Extracorporeal Membrane Oxygenation—ECMO, for short—which is, in effect, a heart-lung bypass. ECMO allows diseased or damaged lungs to rest and recover without additional damage to their delicate tissues. Because it is so new a technique, ECMO is a last resort. But for a dying child, as short a stint as three days on the bypass can produce near-miraculous results. At the moment, ECMO is the newest and most exciting addition to the NICU's arsenal of treatments and therapies.

As sick as he is, Baby J is not a candidate for ECMO. Although he is too weak to breathe on his own and his lungs cannot extract sufficient oxygen from room air to keep him from asphyxiating, he can be sustained by the pulsing breaths delivered through the jet ventilator. There is, however, a hidden danger in the very treatment that supports his life. Neonatologists have found that too much pure oxygen administered in a preemie's first weeks can produce a condition called retinopathy, and retinopathy can leave a child completely blind. Baby J finds himself trapped within a terrible irony: the one form of treatment that can keep him alive carries with it the possibility of devastating consequences. From the start, therefore, the NICU doctors and nurses will attempt to reduce the amount of oxygen and increase the amount of room air Baby J receives through his endotracheal tube. In fact, the entry that will appear most often in his chart over the coming weeks will be the same four-word phrase: "Continue weaning from vent."

Retinopathy represents just one of the many unanticipated dilemmas inherent in modern medicine: often, doing good on one front can produce harm on another. The same is true not just of various other clinical treatments and procedures but also of medicine itself, particularly medicine as it is practiced in major hospitals and academic medical centers. Physicians can now achieve more beneficial results for patients than ever before, but those results usually come at a price that is also higher than ever before, a potentially crippling blow to families facing huge medical bills, as well as a growing drain on the nation's economy.

Just one floor up from the NICU is the office of the Division of Neonatology, home base for the unit's full-time staff of attending physicians and fellows. A fairly nondescript area of secretaries' desks, file cabinets, chest-high room dividers, and commercial-grade carpeting, the division headquarters could at first glance be mistaken for the offices of a thriving small business. In some respects, of course, that is exactly what it is: one asset in a vast service conglomerate called University Hospitals of Cleveland. Neonatology is, after all, just one division within the Department of Pediatrics in Rainbow Babies and Childrens Hospital, and Rainbow is just one of the five hospitals—including MacDonald; Lakeside Hospital and Hanna House (for general medicine and surgery); and University Psychiatric Center in Hanna Pavilion—that, along with a host of outpatient centers and supporting services in various buildings along Adelbert, Abington, and Cornell Roads in Cleveland's University Circle area, constitute the medical center. Indeed, University Hospitals is and has been for years a huge and complex corporation, with an annual operating budget in the neighborhood of $250 million.

Since the middle of the twentieth century the delivery of medical care in hospital settings has more and more come to be perceived as a business, and with good reason. Sophisticated new equipment and procedures, vast employment rolls, skyrocketing costs—all have combined to alter the public's perception of medicine, from the "art of healing" to simply another vast commercial enterprise. With the cost of medical care now consuming some twelve percent of the gross national product, the prevalent use of the term health-care "industry" is not entirely inappropriate.

Nowhere can the changes in medicine be seen more clearly than in a place like Rainbow's NICU, where the background noise is less the soothing hum of human voices than a cacophony of electronically generated beeps and squeals, and where the price of a single day's care can run into thousands of dollars. But the NICU is also a place in which babies who until just recently would have become infant-mortality statistics can be given a chance to live, and it is within that reality that the vast gap between the past and the present seems suddenly not quite so wide. The Neonatal Intensive Care Unit embodies much that is new in the practice of medicine, but it also retains older, more fundamental values.

Nurses in the NICU often note that there is a curious sameness to the facial expressions of parents when they enter the unit to visit their babies for the first time. Actually, it is the absence of expression, a blank stare that conveys not only deep concern about a gravely ill child but also the effect produced by the sheer overwhelming incomprehensibility of modern medicine as it is arrayed in the NICU. In time, however, the parents usually discover a simple truth: all of the shrieking computer monitors, all of the machines pumping oxygen into tiny lungs and circulating blood through tiny bodies, do not really represent a radical change from traditional care-giving efforts. The apparatus may be different, but the basic concept is still the same.

Since the founding of the facility that was its first predecessor, barely a year after the end of the American Civil War, University Hospitals of Cleveland has continued to pursue that basic concept: its core mission has always been to provide the best available medical care to the people of its community, even when, as has so often been the case, a prospective patient does not have the means to pay for that care. As the institution evolved over the years it would include in its mission the education of young doctors and the search for new and better methods of treating the sick. For a century and a quarter those fundamental tenets have been maintained, not only through years of substantive growth but through periods of severe, near-fatal crises as well.

It is a legacy passed along by the founders of the individual institutions that came together in 1926 under the standard of University Hos-

pitals. And because it was nurtured and sustained by succeeding generations of trustees, administrators, physicians, nurses, researchers, teachers,
students, technicians, cooks, laundresses, and maintenance workers, a
simple idea conceived one hundred and twenty-five years ago would in
time be embodied in a medical institution acclaimed for its pioneering
work in such areas as cardiac surgery, cystic fibrosis research, orthopedic
surgery, child and infant care, and the education of aspiring young doctors; an institution that early in its life was honored as one of the two
best medical centers east of the Mississippi; an institution so respected
and appreciated by the community it served that once, in the 1920s, the
citizens of Cleveland raised $8 million in five days to ensure its continued
growth and success.

Which is not to imply that every individual associated with University
Hospitals over the years has been a candidate for sainthood. The proponents and early supporters of the institution—most of them from the
wealthiest and most powerful families in Cleveland—did indeed give
generously of their time, effort, and money to establish and maintain a
place of care for those in need. But their charitable motivations were, by
and large, tempered with a liberal dose of religious bigotry, and they had
no qualms about imposing their own moral standards on those they were
helping, exercising a near-Calvinist stewardship over the charity cases of
the hospitals' wards.

The hospitals have seen physicians whose accomplishments and abiding humanity seemed to invest them with a preternatural glow of goodness, like one pediatrician whose untimely death at the age of forty-eight
was headline news that sent the entire city into mourning. But there have
also been men like the cofounder of Cleveland's first medical school, an
irascible egomaniac who once peppered a personal enemy with a load of
birdshot, then treated the victim for his wounds and demanded to be
paid for his services.

It could easily be argued, however, that no institution in Cleveland has
had so profound an effect on the lives of so many Clevelanders. Over the
past one hundred and twenty-five years, millions of individuals have received state-of-the-art treatment of illness or injury; thousands of young
physicians, nurses, and technicians have received firsthand training and
experience in their crafts; and untold numbers have benefited from the
advances and breakthroughs that have come out of the hospital's laboratories. The medical center has provided jobs for tens of thousands—it is
now one of the city's largest private employers—and it continues to make

a substantial impact on the economies of the city and the region as a whole. It also performs more uncompensated care for the poor than any other private hospital in Ohio.

Although the full array of medical technology in use at University Hospitals resembles an arsenal of high-tech weaponry, the institution traces its origins to a time when the physician's black bag contained a limited assortment of crude instruments, along with such popular "medications" as arsenic and pure mercury. How, then, did the medical center become what it is today? How did a makeshift operation of donated beds and homemade bandages transform itself into a mammoth health-care delivery system?

In many respects, the evolution of the hospital from a single, sparsely furnished wood-frame house to a giant complex of brick, mortar, and sophisticated equipment follows the evolution of medicine itself. Over the years the growing capabilities of medical science pushed and prodded the institution to grow into new and larger responsibilities. But to understand fully the evolution of University Hospitals it is also necessary to understand the nature and effect of the *other* forces that have shaped it over time. Individual efforts, local, national, and world events, demographics, greed, ego, even pure chance—all have played roles in steering the medical center to its present course. It is these less obvious forces that must be seen in context to understand the true nature of the institution as it stands today.

Of course, delving into the medical center's past also reveals answers to many of the mysteries inherent in the place. Why, for example, should a hospital building located some four miles from the shore of Lake Erie carry the name "Lakeside"? Or why, in a Cleveland suburb nearly five miles east of the present Rainbow Babies and Childrens Hospital, is there a quiet, tree-shaded street called "Rainbow Road"?

But perhaps the greatest mystery is simply the unlikely biography of the medical center itself. How did an institution that began life as a sickly infant and barely survived a troubled adolescence manage to achieve a stable maturity in which it represents the highest standards of health-care delivery? Or, to put it another way, how, from those humble origins, could University Hospitals have reached the point that it might be able to offer hope to a baby boy weighing less than two pounds at birth—the hope that one day, after months of care and treatment and nurturing, he might, perhaps, be sent home with his parents, to get on with the business of growing up?

CHAPTER ONE

Principal Concerns

As with so many innovations of lasting value, University Hospitals of Cleveland came into being as a direct result of that least valuable of human endeavors: war.

The concept of a private, nonsectarian charity hospital for Cleveland—a general hospital supported not by public funds but by the donations of individual supporters and by modest fees charged to those patients who could afford them—had been in the air for some time before October of 1865, but it was not until then that the first informal steps were taken to implement the idea. Just six months after the end of the Civil War, a small group of prominent Clevelanders met in a room in the city's courthouse to discuss the possibility of creating a new hospital, a facility to which all citizens, especially the poorest, could come for care and treatment of illness or injury. To the nearly two dozen men and women who met at the courthouse on the evening of Monday, October 23rd, the need for such an institution was abundantly clear: Cleveland was thriving, growing, and flexing new-found muscles, but for many of its inhabitants it was most decidedly a town without pity.

Founded in 1796, Cleveland in its earliest years was less a village than a loose collection of log cabins, pioneer homes built from the area's seemingly inexhaustible supply of virgin timber. Because of its ideal location on the south shore of Lake Erie, at the mouth of the tortuous Cuyahoga River, the little outpost had the potential to become a great port city and nexus of transportation in the Northwest Territory. Yet even as late as 1830 the "city" was still a hamlet of modest proportions, populated by little more than a thousand adventurous souls, most of them hardy transplants from New England. Then, in just one generation, Cleveland's population exploded to over forty thousand. By 1860 it was the twenty-first-largest city in the United States and still growing, a boom town well on its way to becoming one of the most powerful cities west of the Alleghenies.

Cleveland evolved first into a great mercantile center—the commissary to an entire region—thanks primarily to the 1832 completion of the Ohio and Erie Canal. In the ensuing four decades, especially during the war years 1861 to 1865, it transformed itself into a manufacturing powerhouse. In 1860, for example, there were no iron foundries or forges in the city. By 1864, spurred by demand for war materiel, there were twenty-one, employing some three thousand individuals. Soon oil-refining, steel-making, and related industries began to produce immense wealth for men with names like Rockefeller, Hanna, Stone, and Mather. And as was true of the majority of Clevelanders for many years, the city's leading families of the time were virtually all Anglo-Saxon in heritage and Protestant in religious affiliation.

Beginning in the late 1820s, however, employment opportunities on the construction of the canal had drawn a host of Irish-Catholic immigrants to the city. By the mid-1860s, the population of Cleveland had grown to nearly ninety thousand, and of these some ten thousand were Irish-born immigrants, with many more who were native-born of Irish parents. The bulk of the Irish in Cleveland were unskilled or semiskilled laborers; most of them were quite poor, and to live in poverty then was to live in almost medieval squalor. But the impact on the city of its Irish-Catholic population would be felt in many ways, not the least of which was as an indirect motivating factor behind the creation of a new general hospital for Cleveland in 1865.

Despite the brisk pace of growth and change in those years, the city retained much of its early bucolic temperament. Even as the factories and refineries that had grown up along the river spewed great plumes of acrid smoke into the air—the very symbol of progress—a citizen could still be arrested and fined $5 for the offense of "furious driving." And editors of the daily papers could be so desperate for local news that they considered virtually any event sufficiently interesting to merit coverage, including so scintillating an item as: "A couple of mules, standing in front of Murch's saloon, ran away yesterday, but were caught before any damage was done."

Of course, if one of those runaway mules had trampled an innocent bystander in the streets, it was likely that the hapless victim would have been carried back to his own home for treatment, rather than to a hospital. The value of professional medical care at the time—not just in

Cleveland but throughout the world—was at best minimal, because so little was understood about the nature of the human body and the diseases and injuries with which it was afflicted. Health care was, for the most part, delivered at home by relatives, and that care consisted primarily of bed rest and nutritious food, with traditional healing practices called upon when applicable. If a doctor were even involved in the process it was *he* who would travel to the patient; hospitals were few and far between, and they provided little more in the way of care (and often less) than could be obtained at home.

Practitioners themselves were a motley bunch, their loyalties divided among a number of different systems and approaches to medicine. There were Allopaths, the ancestors of modern medical doctors, and there were Homeopaths, followers of a system devised at the turn of the nineteenth century by a German physician named Hahnemann. (The Homeopaths believed that a given condition could be cured by administering extremely small doses of an ultradiluted drug, the same drug which, in a healthy person, would induce symptoms like those of the condition being treated.) There were also Eclectics, Thomsonians, herbalists, and dozens more, some practicing a "science" that they had somehow found delineated in the Bible, others just making it all up as they went along.

By far the most common form of medical care was self-administered, usually treatments derived from folk wisdom and experience that were complemented by doses or applications of any of an infinite array of pills, salves, tonics, nostrums, cure-alls, and elixirs offered for sale by self-styled doctors, professors, experts, and the occasional free-lance "genius." With no uniform method of licensing medical practitioners and virtually no governmental control of the thriving "drug" industry, any engaging entrepreneur with a soothing manner and an active imagination could hang out his shingle and claim to be a healer heaven-sent. Newspapers of the period felt no compunction about accepting advertisements from such wonderworkers as a Cleveland physician named Gibson, who billed himself as "Professor of Electropathy and Medicine" and who guaranteed cures for "seminal weakness, impotency and gleet." For mail-order advice or pharmaceuticals, the ailing patient could choose from among thousands of quacks and quackeries, including "Dr. Seelye's Liquid Catarrh Remedy," "Dr. Bigelow's Guide to Health for Ladies and Gentlemen," "Coe's Dyspepsia Cure" or "Dr. Duponco's Golden Periodical Pills for Females."

When home remedies failed, or when the sick had no family and nowhere else to turn, the last resort was to enter a hospital. The better institutions around the country provided what amounted to an extension of home care, a relatively clean environment in which the old bed-rest-and-good-food treatment was augmented by the attentions of sympathetic doctors and nurses. Such an exemplary institution could do little harm to the patient, which in itself was no small achievement. The worst hospitals, on the other hand, were foul, dark, crowded hellholes from which few patients left except on the horizontal.

Cleveland's first hospital, for example, was little more than a shack, a good-sized log cabin erected during the War of 1812 by one Captain Stanton Sholes to treat sick and wounded soldiers and sailors evacuated to Cleveland from Detroit. The Military Hospital, as it was designated, was located on the lakefront, not far from the mouth of the Cuyahoga River. The hospital was abandoned immediately after the war, and although no record of the disposition of its patients exists, it is doubtful that many were particularly uplifted by their stay there. For the next twenty years Cleveland had no hospital at all; the people of the city simply continued to rely on home care and on the ministrations of a succession of practitioners who wandered into town and offered their services.

In 1837, when the population of Cleveland proper had grown to about six thousand, an epidemic of cholera was the impetus for the creation of a badly needed municipal health-care facility. City Hospital was built that year with public funds on Clinton Street (later East 14th Street), but its location—contiguous with the Erie Street Cemetery—would prove to be wholly appropriate. Within a short time the hospital degenerated into little more than an almshouse, a place in which the destitute sick were sent not to be cured but, in effect, to die. The reputation of City Hospital —as with similar institutions in cities around the country—would have a lasting effect on the poor of those communities. Well into the twentieth century many people still held the belief that entering a hospital was tantamount to signing one's own death warrant.

In the same year that Cleveland created its municipal hospital, the United States Congress appropriated funds to build a medical facility for the merchant seamen of the Great Lakes fleets. The Marine Hospital, which did not accept its first patients until 1847, was also erected on the lakefront, at what would later be Lakeside Avenue between East 9th and East 12th Streets. With the opening of the Marine Hospital, Cleveland had the dubious distinction of possessing two facilities for health-care delivery, neither of which was of any real value to the community. Both hospitals were administered by public entities, but only one—the pigsty City Hospital—was open to the general public. It would be eight more years before the advent of a truly effective facility, the new City Infirmary, which was built in 1855 at the corner of Scranton and Valentine Streets to supplant the decrepit almshouse on East 14th.

Despite the problematic stature of its two hospitals, Cleveland did have a full-fledged medical school of high repute as early as 1843. Founded by four disgruntled faculty members from the failing Willoughby Medical College—actually the "medical department" of the nearby Willoughby University of Lake Erie, an institution established in 1834 some twenty miles east of Cleveland—the Cleveland Medical College was itself started as a department of Western Reserve College, then located in the township of Hudson. Unlike the dozens of proprietary and unaffiliated medical schools around the country, which churned out hundreds of unqualified "doctors" each year, the Cleveland Medical College could grant a legitimate Doctor of Medicine degree, one of the reasons it was a success from the start. The school grew quickly, thanks in part to the imprimatur of Western Reserve and in part to the reputation of its faculty, especially its four founders.

John Delamater, Jared P. Kirtland, John Cassels, and Horace A. Ackley were all respected practitioners and excellent teachers, particularly Delamater, whose lectures were once described by Dr. Oliver Wendell Holmes (father of the Supreme Court justice) as being "lucid as the water of a mountain stream." Men of reason and substance, the founders were also polymathic in the scope of their interests and pursuits. Kirtland, for example, maintained a lifelong interest in horticulture and zoology and was a founder of the Cleveland Academy of Natural Science, later known as the Cleveland Museum of Natural History. Cassels, who would eventually be named dean of the medical school, was also a prominent chemist and widely known geologist, and it was in the latter role that he would make his most important contribution to medicine.

In the summer of 1846, Cassels was commissioned by the Dead River Silver & Copper Mining Company of Cleveland to explore and perform a geologic survey of the Lake Superior country of upper Michigan. Some months later, in an address to the members of Kirtland's Academy of Natural Science, Cassels described the region he had visited as being blessed with an abundance of clean water, marine life, and what he called "unequalled metalliferous deposits," a claim that most Clevelanders received with incredulity. But Cassels had indeed found evidence of vast, untapped reserves of iron ore, and he had been perspicacious enough to, as he said, take "squatter's possession" of a square mile of ore-rich land, a spot to which he had been guided by an Indian in a birch-bark canoe.

Cassels's discoveries paved the way for the development of Cleveland's iron and steel industries, and they would prove to be the foundation upon which many a Cleveland family's fortune was built. In ensuing years, of course, many of those families would contribute a portion of that wealth to their home city, in the form of philanthropies that encompassed education, the arts, social welfare, and especially medicine. John Cassels had set off for Michigan with the sole purpose of surveying a hitherto unexplored region, but in the process he unwittingly secured the future of both his own medical school and the precursors of University Hospitals.

Each of the school's founders left professional and personal legacies worthy of emulation and respect. (It was once said of Delamater, for example, that he was "so well and favorably known that every man would take off his hat at the mention of his name"). Of the four, however, one in particular would be remembered as the first example of a remarkable breed of physician-teacher-investigator, later versions of which would turn up again and again in Cleveland's medical community.

Horace Ackley was a tall, lean, and imposing figure, a profane man of fierce demeanor with a hair-trigger temper, the strength and endurance of an ox, a limitless capacity for strong drink, and an abiding obsession over the timely payment of the fees he charged for his services. A mass of contradictions, he was a "Type A" personality in a "Type B" world, and so forceful and aggressive a character that he actually inspired fear in some of his patients, who nonetheless continued to seek him out because of his proven abilities and outstanding professional reputation. Stephen A. Douglas once traveled all the way from Illinois to put himself in Ackley's capable hands, although the great orator found the experience something less than pleasant. (After a series of operations on his throat, the future presidential candidate wrote to a friend to describe Ackley's apparent "delight" in "running probings down the windpipe and cutting off palates and snipping tonsils and all such amusements. I confess that I do not enjoy the fun quite as well as he seems to....")

Above all, Ackley was an accomplished and innovative medical practitioner, a surgeon of rare skills for the time and a challenging teacher who was adored by his students, through whom his influence on the practice of surgery would be felt for more than a generation after his death. Often called the pioneer surgeon of northern Ohio, Ackley was eulogized as "a thorough Napoleon in the field of surgery, his use of the knife being as skillful as it was dashing." He was also accused of being willfully ignorant of established medical procedure, one critic going so far as to doubt whether Ackley had "ever read a book through in his life." Yet unlike most of his colleagues, who feared and usually rejected new ideas, Ackley embraced progress. In January of 1847, for example, he became the first surgeon in the region to use ether anesthesia, an act of considerable courage at the time considering the fact that the first public demonstration of the technique's effectiveness (by William Morton of Boston) had taken place just three months before.

It was Ackley who had convinced Delamater, Kirtland, and Cassels to leave the Willoughby school and join him in starting a new medical college in Cleveland. And it was also Ackley who led the defense of the medical school when it was attacked by unruly mobs of Clevelanders, which was a fairly common occurrence at the time. Crowds of angry townsfolk, knowing full well that the school had no legal means of obtaining cadavers for anatomy classes, routinely laid siege to the building, hoping to break in and find evidence of body-snatching, not to mention the odd deceased relative. (As late as 1866, a local newspaper noted with shame that city council was still forced to order "an efficient night watch be placed in the various cemeteries of the city" when the medical school was in session.) On such occasions Ackley would arm himself and his students, shout his defiance of the mob, and hold off the rabble at gunpoint.

The same man who cried openly when one grateful patient, a little girl, kissed him on the cheek, was also capable of emptying a shotgun at a farmer who had killed his hunting dog, then treating the man's wounds and demanding payment of his usual fee. When a patient whom Ackley had treated for a dislocated thumb balked at his charge of $10, the good doctor promptly re-dislocated the man's thumb and told him to find someone who would do the job cheaper. Yet he also once rode to Toledo and spent two weeks working without pay and virtually without rest to care for the victims of a cholera epidemic.

Horace Ackley died in April 1859 of what was termed "bilious pneumonia"; just forty-nine, his final years had seen an acceleration of what was termed "the irregularity of his habits," a delicate way to describe his heavy drinking. On his deathbed, his last words were, if somewhat inappropriate for the moment, entirely characteristic: knowing that he was mortally ill, he pronounced himself "a goner," then asked a friend to see to the "collection of certain debts" that were owed him.

Horace Ackley was the archetype of a long line of Cleveland physicians who would prove exceptionally skilled in the practice of their craft and relentless in their pursuit of new knowledge. Some would change the face of medicine, not only in their home city but around the world. Although none of the later firebrands was quite so frenzied a character as the original, all would have recognized in Ackley the curious blend of drive, ambition, intelligence, and eccentricity that they shared. Each was afflicted with an insatiable curiosity; each held the unshakable conviction that he and he alone was always right; and each displayed the sort of courage—both personal and professional—that springs from overweening faith in one's convictions. They were inventors, explorers, craftsmen, and autocrats, and they would raise egotism to an art form. But they would also expand the boundaries of medical science, continually challenging the limits of the possible.

§

By the outbreak of the Civil War in April 1861, Cleveland had a third health-care facility, the Cleveland Homeopathic Hospital, which had been founded in 1856 by a local practitioner named Seth R. Beckwith. Underwritten to a large extent by the local railroads, which contracted for the care of their sick and injured employees, the Homeopath hospital began as a modest, twenty-bed affair on what would later be Lakeside Avenue. In ensuing years it moved to more spacious quarters in the center of town, especially after some of the more prosperous and prominent residents of Cleveland—a group that included the petroleum king, John D. Rockefeller, among others—chose Homeopaths as their personal physicians. Indeed, Homeopathic medicine was so widely accepted in the city that a Homeopathic medical college, only the second in the nation at the time, had been founded in Cleveland some years before.

But the decade of the 1860s marked the advent of Cleveland's boom years as a rapidly growing commercial and industrial dynamo, and if the flush times brought with them a healthy glow of prosperity for many, they also created a serious social-welfare problem with which the city and its three hospitals were unprepared to cope. Beginning in 1861, wartime production demands fueled the growth of business and industry and, concomitantly, the size of the labor force. With the sudden surge in population—particularly of unskilled workers and their families, who more often than not lived and worked under wretched conditions and were therefore more prone to disease and injury—the city's health-care services were strained to the breaking point. Adding to the muddle was a wholly unexpected development: a trickle of displaced and destitute war refugees from the South, who wandered into town homeless, penniless, undernourished, and often ill.

The trickle of refugees had become a steady stream by 1863, when a group of churchwomen—the Ladies Aid Society of Cleveland's First Presbyterian Church (known informally as the Old Stone Church)—created the "Home for Friendless Strangers." Less a hospital than a temporary shelter or way station, the Home was really nothing more than a rented house at the corner of what would later be Lakeside Avenue and East 9th Street. Supported by small individual donations and occasional contributions from the Protestant churches of the city, the "Home for the Friendless," as it was also sometimes known, was staffed by volunteers from the Ladies Aid Society, who by 1865 had provided bed, board, and what then passed for medical attention to hundreds of indigent and desperate people. As the immediate need for a refugee shelter diminished at the conclusion of the war, the Home was eventually closed, but not before the women of the Ladies Aid Society had learned a number of valuable lessons in facility management. They were lessons that would soon be put to good use when the women turned their attention to a much more ambitious undertaking—the creation of a full-fledged hospital.

Even before the closing of the Home for Friendless Strangers, however, yet another Cleveland hospital was opening its doors. On October 5, 1865, dedication ceremonies for St. Vincent's Charity Hospital were attended by a diverse crowd of several hundred local dignitaries, politicians, and well-wishers from the community. Conceived and built by Louis Amadeus Rappe, first bishop of the Cleveland Catholic Diocese, St. Vincent's was a two-story structure on what was then Perry Street (later East 22nd Street). Dr. Gustav C. E. Weber, a respected surgeon and teacher, was in charge of the hospital, which was staffed by nurses from the Sisters of Charity of St. Augustine and attended by a handful of local doctors and surgeons, all of whom donated their services.

Bishop Rappe had arrived in Cleveland in 1847 and had immediately recognized the community's need for more hospital beds, particularly for his flock, the growing underclass of Irish and German immigrant workers. In 1852 he opened a tiny "hospital" called St. Joseph's—on Monroe Street in the neighboring community of Ohio City—which was also managed by the Sisters of Charity. The facility proved so unacceptably small that it was eventually converted into an orphanage, so in 1863 Rappe began a fund-raising campaign to build a real hospital. He buttonholed every family of substance in town—which meant, of course, every *Protestant* family—with great success, promoting the new facility as a charity hospital in which patients of all religious affiliations would be treated equally and without discrimination. He even convinced Cleveland City Council to underwrite the yearly cost of some twenty beds for indigents.

"I ran from door to door, store to store," Rappe recalled gratefully at the dedication-day assemblage, "and I saw greenbacks fall into my hands like leaves in autumn." Among the other speakers at the ceremony that day, however, Henry B. Payne, a prominent attorney and local politician, would follow his praise of the new hospital by excoriating the city's Protestant churches for not launching similar efforts. And Probate Judge Daniel R. Tilden told the crowd that although his ancestors "were Puritans, and they hated the Catholics a little worse than the devil," he believed that "no such noble work [as St. Vincent's] could or would have been put through by the Protestant Church...."

Just four days later—on the same day that St. Vincent's officially admitted its first patient—an unsigned "communication" written by what was described as "one of our most estimable ladies" was printed in the Cleveland *Leader*. Under the heading "Protestant Home and Hospital," the letter was, in effect, a call to arms from an anonymous member of the Ladies Aid Society, clearly a veteran of the Home for the Friendless.

"The practical working of 'The Home' has made so manifest the necessity of some hospital of a Protestant character for indigent sick in our midst," she wrote, "that it is impossible for its managers to shut their eyes to this important development.... The experience of the war has given us unlimited faith in the good works which might be called into exercise by the claims of a hospital. Surely there are amongst us Protestant angels of mercy who would gladly spend and be spent in such a holy and noble undertaking!"

The writer pointed to the example set by other cities, where "clerks and employees of different grades, reared in Protestant homes" are not "thrown in sickness upon such tender mercies as a hotel or boarding house can furnish." Rather, they find in Protestant charity hospitals "the loving care of a home, with such surroundings and influences as prove, not unfrequently, a life-long elevation to the character." She concluded her letter with a question that could as easily have been read as a challenge: "Might not the experiment be made of continuing the [Home for the Friendless] with a hospital...?"

The publication of the letter had two immediate effects. The first, unfortunately, was to provide *Leader* publisher and editor Edwin Cowles with an opportunity to pen another of the anti-Catholic editorials he so dearly loved. Cowles, who was something of an eccentric (he was said to have carried a loaded gun at all times, and he enjoyed shooting target practice in his own office), for years used his newspaper as a forum for virulent screeds against the "Popish Church." The occasion of the "estimable lady's" letter gave him the chance to write a piece in which he endorsed the idea of a Protestant hospital because it would mean that Protestant patients need not rely on St. Vincent's, which he referred to as "simply a Roman Catholic institution" whose "fundamental object" was to convert unbelievers to Catholicism.

The letter's second effect, however, was to galvanize to action nearly two dozen of the leading members of the city's Protestant community, many of whom were themselves officers of the Home for Friendless Strangers. Two weeks later—on the evening of Monday, October 23, 1865 —a "considerable number of gentlemen and ladies," as the *Leader* reported, met in a room of the city's courthouse to "consider the propriety and expediency of organizing an association for the purchase or erection of such a hospital as will answer the demands of the city."

§

The men and women who came together to discuss the possibility of creating a new hospital for Cleveland were wise enough to understand that, no matter how heartily they favored the idea, they still knew next to nothing about the myriad pragmatic details of initiating such a project. Where, for example, would the hospital be located? Would they have to build a new structure to house it, or could they purchase an existing building? How would the hospital be organized, who would be in charge, and what could they expect in the way of annual operating costs? After mulling over these obvious but fundamentally important questions, the founders concluded their first organizational meeting in a way that even then was already a proven and time-honored method: they appointed a committee.

Actually, they appointed three committees, the first two of which were to study and report back on the three basic issues—site, cost, and organization—that had been raised during the meeting. Leander M. Hubby, president of the Cleveland, Columbus & Cincinnati Railroad, chaired the site committee, whose membership included attorney William J. Boardman, the *Leader*'s Edwin Cowles, and Philo Chamberlain, president of the Northern Transportation Company, a Great Lakes steamship concern. Determining the cost and organization of the proposed hospital were Joseph Perkins, son of one of the original settlers of the Western Reserve, insurance company president Stillman Witt, and lumber mill operator Arthur Quinn. The third committee, consisting of local banker Hinman Hurlbut, attorney Samuel Williamson, Jr., and John D. Rockefeller, was asked to examine the statutory regulation of hospitals and prepare the documents necessary for the creation of such an institution.

During that first meeting, however, the founders made a special point of noting that, in the words of prominent bridge and railroad builder Amasa Stone, Jr., "A city of the population of Cleveland...needs and by all means should have a charity hospital." Although Stone's remark seemed to ignore the fact that the city already possessed a health-care facility for the poor in the shape of Bishop Rappe's recently opened St. Vincent's, it was not the result of a failure of memory. In truth, it was the first of what would prove to be numerous taunts and slaps—some thinly veiled, some quite blatant—aimed at Bishop Rappe and St. Vincent's, an institution that some members of the Protestant community perceived less as a health-care facility than a hotbed of Papist proselytism, as well as a "charity" hospital in name only. Ultimately, Protestant and Catholic partisans would wage a lengthy war of words on this subject, debating publicly in the pages of the *Leader* in a contretemps fueled by the bigoted editorializing of the paper's publisher and editor, Edwin Cowles.

Not surprisingly, the *Leader* gave prominent coverage to the first meeting of the hospital's founders, devoting almost an entire column to the story. The evening *Plain Dealer*, however, virtually ignored the gathering, giving it but scant mention in a two-sentence item. In ensuing months the *Plain Dealer* continued to give short shrift to news of the impending Protestant charity hospital, in part because the paper—whose editorial policy supported the Democratic Party and whose natural constituency was

Cleveland's immigrant community—had nothing to gain by providing lengthy coverage of a project initiated by a group that was predominately Republican, Protestant, and native-born. The Republican *Leader*, on the other hand, was a virtual house organ of Cleveland's Protestant elite, and the fact that its editor was a member of the new hospital's organizing body guaranteed ample and glowing coverage for the fledgling institution. (The two newspapers also held no great affection for each other: The *Leader* once editorialized that the *Plain Dealer* was "guilty of willful slander" and showed "brazen mendacity," while the *Plain Dealer* had once called the *Leader*'s politics "pestilential" and on one occasion referred to the morning daily as "the damnedest, meanest paper in Ohio.")

It was another seven months before the committees were prepared to make their reports, but on May 14, 1866, the whole group at last convened again, deciding unanimously that the founding of a hospital was indeed a worthwhile and feasible endeavor. They elected a board of trustees for an organization whose goal was to create an institution "for the reception, care and medical treatment of sick and disabled persons," an institution to be called "Cleveland City Hospital." Among the trustees elected were Boardman; merchant A.C. Blossom; insurance company president Martin B. Scott; George A. Stanley, who was in the oil and candle business; iron and steel producer Henry Chisholm; Cuyahoga Steam Furnace Company president William B. Castle, who had served as Cleveland's mayor in 1855; and salesman George W. Whitney. Yet another committee—consisting of the Reverend Julius H. Rylance, rector of St. Paul's Episcopal Church; Dr. John Wheeler, one of Cleveland's first Homeopathic practitioners; Dr. John S. Newberry, a local physician and well-known naturalist; and Dr. Charles A. Terry, professor of obstetrics in the Medical Department of Western Reserve College—was appointed to formulate a written statement that delineated "the necessity of the hospital, the proper kind of building and the use to which it is to be applied." One week later, on May 21, 1866, the group formally incorporated as the "Cleveland City Hospital Society."

The Rylance committee completed its work by the end of that same month and immediately issued its report. Characteristically, the *Plain Dealer* ignored the news while the *Leader* gave it bold play, reprinting the report in its entirety under the headlines "CLEVELAND CITY HOSPITAL/ REPORT OF THE COMMITTEE/Cleveland Needs a Free Hospital." A remarkable document, the Rylance report not only provided a solid rationale for creating what was by then being called a "free public hospital," but it also managed to camouflage a number of disparaging comments about St. Vincent's amidst the flowery phraseology of mid-nineteenth century literary style.

"Among the most splendid of public or private munificences which are the pride of states or cities," the report began, "there are few more imposing and more blessed than the hospitals." Urban charities, it continued, had been devised to "meet in the fullest manner the wants of the three elements of humanity—the soul, the mind and the body," and although Cleveland had many free churches and free schools, "of free hospitals she has...*none which deserve the name* [emphasis added]." Free hospitals were "the natural fruit of our refined and Christian civilization," institutions "whose doors are open to all the victims of accident or disease, where not only all the resources of art and science are invoked for their relief, but thoughtful kindness anticipates their every want, and woman's gentle ministrations reach and heal even the wounds of the spirit." Noting the city's rapidly growing population, the report estimated that each year some one thousand Clevelanders received "no adequate medical or surgical care," despite the existence of "a hospital established under the auspices of the Roman Catholic Church, which...is not a free hospital and from which, should none be excluded by the act of those who control it, many would be withheld by their own preferences or prejudices...whether right or wrong...."

The conclusions of the report were obvious: there should be a new hospital, and it should be "free to all..., the most needy being considered the most worthy." ("How noble the charity," wrote Rylance, "that offers to the poor and homeless all the appliances for comfort and recovery that wealth can procure....") It would also be "wise and merciful" to accommodate "those taken sick while in service in the different families in the city" by offering asylum to "this class" at the expense of their employers. As to other paying patients, provisions would be made to ensure "special apartments and special attendance for an adequate compensation," although "it should not be forgotten that our hospital is a charity, and not a speculation."

The committee strongly recommended that the new hospital be "emancipated from all political and even official influence." It would be "a city hospital only in name, if even that," operated "under the supervision and control of our best men." The new hospital would also be "so organized and managed that our best women should give it the benefit of their sympathy and care, and the purifying and elevating influence of their presence." And although "a healthful and beautiful location" boasting "ample and beautiful grounds" would be the "first material consideration," the details could be worked out at a later date, "when a sufficient endowment fund is secured...."

Two weeks before the release of the Rylance report, a *Leader* editorial noted that the task of creating the new Protestant hospital "promises to be prosecuted with vigor," and so it must have seemed at the time. But the decision to hold back on the project until a suitable endowment could be raised—a precaution that had been suggested at the first organizational meeting by both Joseph Perkins and Amasa Stone, Jr.—delayed substantive progress for months. The founders' caution was due in part to the ingrained conservatism of what was essentially a group of displaced Connecticut Yankees, but it was also a response to the example of St. Vincent's, which, more than a year after its opening, still faced past-due bills amounting to some $20,000, nearly thirty percent of the cost of its construction. In addition, many of the supporters of the new hospital had earlier made large contributions to St. Vincent's building fund, and they may well have been feeling a bit pinched by the time the Cleveland City Hospital Society was ready to begin soliciting donations. Indeed, the philanthropic resources of the community were clearly strained, and new solicitations by the trustees of a proposed new Homeopathic hospital, as well as the continuing fund-raising efforts of Bishop Rappe, only added to the pressure. The public-relations value of the latter fact, however, was not lost on Edwin Cowles, because for the next two years the chief drumbeater for the Protestant hospital did his best to aid the fund-raising effort and keep alive public interest in the project through a simple expedient: his medium was the *Leader*, and his method was Rappe-bashing.

Having already accused Bishop Rappe of "playing the benevolent dodge shrewdly" to obtain some $30,000 in donations from Protestant contributors, Cowles wondered in print why "the Catholic priests are able to use Protestants in raising [additional] money for their hospital, while the Protestant hospital receives no such support." He published numerous letters to the editor—most of them unsigned—which decried the lack of a hospital in which "a Protestant patient can be treated without being annoyed on his dying bed with having the extreme unction inflicted upon him, as it has been done at St. Vincent's." Other letters urged Protestants to refrain from making donations to St. Vincent's because it discriminated against non-Catholics and because it was one of the institutions "which constitute the means by which a medieval despot across the sea is tightening his hold upon our New World republic." One correspondent asked if Bishop Rappe and the Sisters of Charity might not "do more real good by looking after the squalid misery existing among the members of his church...? They have a large field in that direction, as all our businessmen will testify, who are annoyed daily by a crowd of beggars, nineteen out of twenty of whom are Catholics...." And another Cowles editorial found it "a curious fact...that in this city where two-thirds of the population, nine-tenths of the wealth and ninety-nine hundredths of the intelligence are Protestant, the only hospital should be a Catholic one."

Additional anti-Rappe sentiments were also expressed by the faculty of the Medical Department of Western Reserve College, who felt the bishop had reneged on a promise—made during the initial solicitation of funds for St. Vincent's—that they would hold and control teaching privileges at the hospital. Rappe had instead brought in Gustav Weber as St. Vincent's chief of staff, and Weber, a former Western Reserve faculty member who had been dismissed from his position in May of 1863, promptly excluded his erstwhile colleagues and started his own private medical school within the hospital.

Meanwhile, as local Homeopathic physicians attempted to start *their* own hospital, they called on many of the same benefactors who could be expected to contribute to the City Hospital Society. Referring to their proposed facility as the "Cleveland Protestant Hospital" or the "Protestant City Hospital," the Homeopaths and their supporters held a number of open meetings on the subject beginning in 1867, and by the following year they were seriously attempting to secure a building in which to house the institution. But the apparent duplication of effort on the part of two groups of Protestants, each intent on opening its own hospital, precluded any real progress for either.

A compromise was clearly needed, and it came early in 1868, when a portion of the physicians and supporters from the Homeopathic camp agreed to throw in their lot with the Cleveland City Hospital Society, believing that together they could raise sufficient funds to purchase a suitable structure to house both Homeopathic and Allopathic physicians. On April 16th, the coalition made a down payment of $1,000 toward the total purchase price of a two-story frame house on the lakefront. Located at 83 Wilson Street (later known as Davenport Street, one block north of Lakeside Avenue and just east of 14th Street), the former residence would serve as the first home of the city's newest hospital.

Three weeks later, the Wilson Street Hospital Association was organized as an unincorporated subsidiary of the Cleveland City Hospital Society. Hinman Hurlbut was elected president of the association, whose board of trustees included Peter Thatcher, a principal of bridge builders McNairy, Claflen & Company; carriage manufacturer Jacob Lowman, member of a pioneer Cleveland family; paint and varnish dealer and importer Truman Dunham; oil refiner Morris B. Clark, a former partner of John D. Rockefeller when the latter was in the produce business; Frederick W. Pelton, treasurer of Buckeye Mutual Insurance Company; Theodore S. Lindsay, an officer of the Cleveland & Toledo Railroad; Mrs. Stillman Witt, wife of the president of the Sun Insurance Company; Mrs. George B. Senter, whose husband was a wholesale wine and liquor dealer; Mrs. Samuel L. Mather, wife of the founder of the Cleveland Iron Mining Company; Mrs. S.F. Lester, wife of a prominent commission merchant; and Mrs. Samuel H. Crowl, whose husband was one of the city's major lumber dealers. Allopath and Homeopath supporters were represented roughly equally on the board, and a six-member medical staff—also evenly divided between the two systems—was appointed. As the *Leader* so undiplomatically noted, "A general city hospital, established by Protestant funds and controlled by Protestant hands, is about to be opened...."

The total cost of the Wilson Street house was $9,000, far less than the amount needed to erect a new building, but a substantial sum nonetheless. Refurbishing the old house and equipping it as a hospital required further expenditures, so to minimize actual cash outlays the association combined its continuing efforts to raise an endowment with requests for donations of household furniture, bedding, kitchen utensils, foodstuffs—any items that could be put to good use in the new hospital. A "Board of Managers," composed almost entirely of the women members of the board and the wives and daughters of the founders and supporters, was created to pursue such donations, as well as to oversee maintenance of the building and grounds.

The Board of Managers also proved ingenious in staging a variety of fund-raising events over the years, the first of which they mounted in June. The "festival of music and food," as the first fund-raiser was called, was a lighthearted means to a serious end, and the board's members relied on the businesslike method of appointing committees to organize and manage the event—a strategy that led to the creation of such curiously named bodies as the "Committee on Ice Cream and Cake," the "Committee on Flowers, Decorations and Music," and even the "Committee on Strawberries."

On July 23, 1868, the fully outfitted Wilson Street Hospital opened its doors at last, admitting the first of what would be more than one hundred patients to be cared for in the institution's first year of operation. The imposing old frame house accommodated twenty cases at a time, with multiple-bed "wards" in the larger rooms and single-bed private quarters for paying patients. Unfortunately, no record of the first year's activities survived, but it would be safe to assume that the cases admitted to the Wilson Street Hospital in 1868 represented a typical cross section of the diseases, injuries, ailments, and conditions to which most poor urban dwellers were susceptible at the time. These ranged from broken bones, dropsy, and the effects of a mule-kick in the head to ulcerations, malnutrition, cancer, and raging infections of every description.

Widely accepted treatments for nearly all disorders were routinely prescribed by physicians of the day, but more often than not their value was questionable, to say the least. The better practitioners, particularly those who had received at least a portion of their training in Europe, where new ideas were more readily adopted, tried their best to deal with illnesses the true causes of which they understood only vaguely if at all. Often, though, hospital patients who were discharged as "cured" had been helped less by the doctors' efforts than by the regimen of bed rest and nutritious food that allowed the body's natural healing mechanisms to work. Pasteur's Germ Theory and Lister's antiseptic surgical technique were so new at the time that few American physicians accepted or applied them in practice. There was only a minimal understanding of bodily systems, and the word "bacteriology" had yet to be coined.

Physicians were indeed closing in on the actual causes of disease, but it would be years before the face of medicine was changed by the great leaps of understanding that swept away the old, misguided concepts like so much dust. For the moment, the average hospital physician still moved from patient to patient without first washing his hands. Puzzled then by the onset of new infections in his patients, he ascribed them to "the influence of contagious miasmata," mysterious elements in foul air. In surgery, as one standard teaching text of the time had it, wielding the knife "with rapidity" was "of the first advantage," and to prepare for an operation, a surgeon's "immediate precautions" were to "see that the table is solid and of a conventional height" and ensure a "sufficient supply of sponges and of basins." If the impending operation were likely to be "attended by much hemorrhage, a tray filled with sand or sawdust should be provided, in order to catch the blood."

Treatments for specific ailments were as often based on guesswork as fact, and most had little if any therapeutic value. Bleeding was still recommended to "lessen the supply of blood" to an inflamed organ and "abate the force with which the blood reaches it," and leeches were a part of every good doctor's arsenal. (When confronted with young hydrocephalic patients, physicians were taught to apply leeches "to the crown of the head rather than to the temples, where they dangle about the eyes and terrify the child....") For cases of violent inflammation or high fever, a powerful purgative was recommended as "an expedient...which should scarcely ever be omitted." Often physicians unwittingly committed pharmacological mayhem on their patients by prescribing ample doses of such widely accepted remedies as mercury, opium, arsenic, sugar of lead, oil of turpentine, belladonna, "electricity and galvanism," prussic acid, strychnine, ammonia, and even tobacco juice.

Ironically, the Homeopathic method of treating illness—the administration of extremely diluted doses of "medications"—often appeared to be more productive than Allopathic methods, simply because dilution of the substances introduced into the body reduced their toxicity and allowed the patient to recover from his illness without also having to recover from his treatment. At the Wilson Street Hospital, for example, Homeopaths were not only accepted as effective physicians by most patients, but were actively sought out, particularly by the *paying* patients, many of whom favored the system and who, like Marcus A. Hanna and John D. Rockefeller, were staunch supporters.

But the "success" of the Homeopaths who were practicing cheek-by-jowl with their Allopathic cousins at Wilson Street soon produced its own variety of inflammation. Several of the city's Allopathic and Homeopathic physicians had predicted from the start that the experiment of allowing representatives from each school to practice in the same building would lead to conflict. At first the critics appeared to have been proved wrong, because the new hospital seemed to run smoothly. But the compromise that had initially brought together the Allopaths and the Homeopaths in the Wilson Street Hospital—the agreement that each would have "equal representation in the management" of the facility—had been nothing more than a marriage of convenience to facilitate fund raising. And the domestic strife that inevitably ensued eventually precipitated the institution's first crisis.

Before long, arguments and disagreements arose between proponents of each system, and by the end of the hospital's first year of operation, full-scale internecine warfare had broken out. As the bitter struggle intensified, it quickly became obvious that no compromise could be effected, and the trustees of the hospital decided to take drastic action. On September 1, 1869, having been open for little more than a year, the Wilson Street Hospital was summarily closed, its patients either discharged or transferred to other facilities.

Hospital president Hinman Hurlbut then took the extraordinary step of using his own funds to buy out the Homeopaths' interest in the hospital. The first in a long line of "saints" who over the years would rescue the hospital in times of financial crisis, Hurlbut purchased all of the Homeopaths' equipment as well as their shares in the ownership of the building. He then donated the lot to the Wilson Street Hospital Association.

The building reopened on November 4th as a purely Allopathic hospital, and two of the Allopaths who had been on the original Wilson Street staff were given full responsibility for management of the facility. Alleyn Maynard, who had earned his medical degree at the University of Edinburgh and was one of the most respected physicians in Cleveland, and Henry Kirke Cushing, a second-generation member of what would become perhaps the most famous medical family in the country, were asked to lead the young hospital in the coming months.

For a short time after the departure of the Homeopaths, the proportion of paying and charity cases in the hospital remained roughly equal, as it had been since the building opened its doors. In ensuing years, however, the number and percentage of indigent cases began to rise steadily, in part because more and more of the poor came to trust the new hospital, but also because when the Homeopaths left Wilson Street, many of their paying patients followed. Most of the Homeopath physicians, their patients, and their supporters on the board of trustees opted to go to the Cleveland Homeopathic Protestant Hospital (precursor of the later Huron Road Hospital), which had been opened on a shoestring budget in October of 1868 and was desperately looking for additional patronage. For the Wilson Street Hospital, the price of peace was the loss of many of its paying patients, which was one of the reasons the hospital faced recurring operating deficits each year. Only the proceeds from an endless string of fund-raising events, bolstered by the individual donations of Hinman Hurlbut, kept the facility afloat.

By May of 1870, however, the house staff of the hospital was augmented by a number of visiting and consulting physicians, all of whom provided services to the poor on a voluntary basis. A house matron and a handful of nurses, few of whom had any real training to speak of, were responsible for most day-to-day functions within the building. That same year, students from the Medical Department of Western Reserve College began to receive clinical training and experience in the new hospital, which gave the appearance of being run on the model of a fairly strict children's camp. The official duties of a house physician, for example, included the collection of fees—in advance—from those patients capable of paying. And the patients themselves were strictly segregated by sex and forbidden to use profanity, to drink, smoke, gamble, or spit on the floor. In fact, those charity cases who were ambulatory or well on the way to recovery were also expected to lend a hand with the cleaning and nursing chores.

Nevertheless, the hospital was filled to overflowing throughout the first half of the 1870s. Even after construction of a ten-bed addition early in the decade, by 1874 the building was so crowded with charity cases that the attic was used as an extra ward and even more beds lined the hallways. The shortage of space was becoming acute when Leonard Case, Jr., a prominent local businessman (and later founder of the Case School of Applied Science), stepped in. Case, who had inherited the better part of his father's vast real estate holdings in Cleveland, donated several acres of lakeshore property to the hospital society, ostensibly as a site on which to erect a new and larger building of its own. Unfortunately, Case's gift coincided with the advent of the nationwide depression that followed the great bank panic of 1873. Construction of a new facility was, therefore, postponed indefinitely.

With ample land but insufficient funds to actually build on it, the hospital's trustees then began to consider the possibility of further additions to the Wilson Street house. They went so far as to have plans drawn up for the construction of two new wings before deciding that the cost of the improvements would be prohibitive. In desperation they turned their attention to finding a larger, existing structure to buy or lease, and soon they returned to an old idea that had been rejected years before. Ironically, the solution to their problem was located only a few blocks away.

The United States Marine Hospital, which had opened in 1847, was still being operated by the federal government as a refuge for injured and disabled Great Lakes sailors, but for some years it had been functioning at well under its capacity. A handsome and stately structure set on five acres of lakefront property, the Marine Hospital was a three-story building of stone and brick that boasted small colonnades on each floor and was topped with an ornamental cupola. Although the layout of rooms was not particularly conducive to the efficient operation of a health-care facility—not to mention the fact that patients had to be carried from floor to floor—the hospital could accommodate seventy or more beds, and it had always proved itself to be entirely adequate for its purpose. It was also a well-known institution in town, and several local practitioners had at various times served lucrative appointments there as "physician and surgeon" (including, in 1853, the notorious Horace Ackley). During the Civil War, a section of the building had been assigned to the use of Cleveland's Soldiers' Aid Society, and the faculty of the Cleveland Medical College had provided free care to returning invalid fighting men, a group that even included two veterans of the battle between the *Monitor* and the *Merrimac*. Of course, the medical faculty's gesture, while laudatory, was not wholly charitable: the physicians also used the wounded soldiers as prime teaching material for their students, a practice of long standing.

By 1874, having fallen into disrepair, the structure was expensive to maintain and in dire need of extensive rehabilitation. Despite the condition of the building, however, the City of Cleveland attempted to lease the facility that year for use as a new city hospital, an effort that ultimately failed due to a minor legal technicality. The following year, the federal government proved more receptive to an arrangement proposed by the Wilson Street trustees, who had always coveted the building anyway. (The Marine Hospital had actually been the first choice for a home for the still-embryonic Protestant hospital; it was suggested as early as 1866 in an Edwin Cowles editorial, when a then-current rumor had it that the government was planning to close the facility.) For the nominal rent of $1 a year, to be paid to the United States Treasury Department, the trustees could move their entire operation into the Marine Hospital building. The only proviso was that they would also take responsibility for the care of the sailors there, and even then they were allotted reimbursement for each patient at a rate of fifty-four cents a day. The deal was struck on September 21, 1875, when the Cleveland City Hospital Society—the corporate body in charge of the Wilson Street Hospital—signed a twenty-year lease on its new home.

Resurrecting the name that the founders had originally intended for their institution, the trustees scheduled an October 1st opening for what was to be called "Cleveland City Hospital." The task of repairing the thirty-year-old Marine Hospital building and preparing it for its new tenants dragged on for some time, however, and it was two months before all of the patients from the cramped old house on Wilson Street could be settled into the refurbished facility. But on December 8, 1875, Cleveland's newest hospital opened its doors at last. And on that same date, the Wilson Street Hospital—the embodiment of the efforts of so many dedicated individuals—simply ceased to exist.

CHAPTER TWO

Saints and Sinners

With the abandonment of their original home on Wilson Street and subsequent move into the more spacious quarters of the former Marine Hospital building, the staff and visiting physicians of the newly renamed Cleveland City Hospital gained two distinct assets. They now had seventy patient beds rather than the wholly inadequate thirty of the old building, with enough additional space to more than double the bed capacity in emergencies or during city-wide epidemics. And they inherited the marine facility's sailor patients, many of whom were afflicted with challenging diseases and conditions that constituted fresh opportunities for the doctors to hone their skills, as well as dramatic new teaching material for the students of the Cleveland Medical College, who continued to receive part of their clinical training in the "new" hospital.

The more mundane cases in the old Wilson Street building had usually ranged from abscesses and bronchitis to ulcers and varicose veins, with a sampling of somewhat less prosaic afflictions in between. Typhoid fever, for example, appeared fairly regularly—one consequence of the poor state of Cleveland's sanitation system—as did tuberculosis, leukorrhea, hysteria, frostbite, lead poisoning, and a range of ailments that were listed under the generic catchall, "debility." Limb amputations were not uncommon procedures at the old hospital, and the doctors were occasionally called upon to repair the butchery inflicted on women who had sought out remedial measures from one of the free-lance abortionists who operated *sub rosa* in the city. Given the state of medical science at the time, it was remarkable that more than ninety percent of the general patients of the period left the hospital labeled as either "cured, relieved or discharged." Of course, just how the Wilson Street physicians defined "cured" and "relieved" is problematic.

Medicine at the time was indeed capable of providing useful treat-

ments to more complaints than it had been even twenty years before, but
the list of notable exceptions to its effectiveness was still painfully long.
Tetanus, gangrene, and even diarrhea, for example, continued to be mor-
tal afflictions, and no human being in the history of the species had ever
yet survived the bite of a rabid dog. Perhaps the era's most dramatic
example of medicine's failings would occur in 1881, when a man named
Charles Guiteau attempted to assassinate President James A. Garfield.
Garfield actually lived for eighty days following the shooting, but in that
time he was poked, prodded, and probed repeatedly by physicians who
did not even bother to wash their hands, let alone their instruments,
before examining the wounded chief executive. Subsequently, the assassin
Guiteau argued with some justification at his trial that he had not, in fact,
killed the President. "The doctors did that," Guiteau contended. "I simply
shot at him."

No member of the medical staff of the Wilson Street Hospital, however, was ever subjected to the sort of negative publicity that could
accrue from the mishandling of so well-known a patient as the President.
Indeed, their patients were, by and large, among the least-known individuals in Cleveland, and the cases the physicians addressed were remarkable only for their sameness. After the move to the Marine Hospital
building, however, the Great Lakes sailors whose care became the responsibility of the staff of the newly named City Hospital added a measure
of spice to an otherwise humble stew of common ailments.

Sailors, being sailors, could always be counted on to increase the
hospital's annual year-end tally of noteworthy venereal diseases treated
(twenty-seven instances of syphilis in 1877 alone, including eight in the
tertiary stage). There were also numerous cases of delirium tremens and
the brutal abrasions, concussions, fractures, knife wounds, and bullet
holes that tend to proliferate among serious brawlers. Of course, patients
similarly indisposed occasionally appeared among the hospital's general
population as well. Indeed, it was probably the taint of moral turpitude
associated with such cases that prompted the line in the narrative portion
of one hospital annual report of the time that mentioned the "relief" that
had been furnished not just for patients' "bodily ailments" but also for
their spiritual suffering, relief that "has, perhaps, saved them from future
crimes and wrongdoings."

Such virtuous sentiments were often expressed in the hospital's annual
reports, which were used not only to provide a genuine accounting of the
number of patients treated, the nature of their ailments, and even their

national origins, but also to communicate the precepts, parables, and pontifications of the trustees. Seeing themselves as both conservators of the hospital and as stewards of its patients—their flock, as it were—the trustees expected the institution to dole out moral suasion along with medical care, and that attitude was reflected in their yearly communications to the hospital's supporters. Thus, the author of the 1876 report could write enthusiastically that "our hearts have been lifted up to the Divine helper and healer of men, in whose name and for whose sake we minister...."

It was more than mere coincidence that for years the board held its annual meetings not in the hospital itself, but in the parlors of local Protestant churches. For the trustees, the hospital was an extension of the church, yet another weapon for good in the unending battle against the evils which resulted from—or, as some had it, *bred*—lives of poverty. In light of such standards, it was not surprising that the annual reports also categorized charity patients by their occupations, and that one such category would be denominated with the weighted term "Loafer." Nor would there be any question but that the hospital reserved the right to refuse treatment to persons deemed morally unfit, as happened to one pregnant Irish girl at the time, who was summarily tossed out because, as her patient record noted, she was found to be "of ill repute."

The most important function served by the institution's annual report, however, was as the primary channel through which the trustees could make their case for additional financial contributions from the "friends of the hospital," among whom were numbered all individuals who had previously made donations of any sort as well as those who, in the opinion of the trustees, should have seen it as their duty to do so. Hamstrung to an extent by its very name—some people assumed that a "Cleveland *City* Hospital" must be publicly funded, when in fact it was privately supported, with only minimal financial aid coming from the city —the hospital pursued a precarious hand-to-mouth existence year after year, and was forced to rely on innumerable fund-raising sales, balls, art shows, and entertainments to supplement the meager revenues generated by its still fairly small number of paying patients.

The Board of Managers canvassed unceasingly for contributions of food, clothing, and services, as well as for individual and corporate subscriptions to underwrite the costs of charity beds. To justify these continual requests for donations, the trustees used the annual report to highlight the "good works" of the hospital; it was the perfect vehicle through which to disseminate appeals that were carefully crafted to inspire a level of guilt sufficient to force readers to open their pocketbooks. And for a while, at least, the appeals tended to work. In fact, a list of donors for any given year in the 1870s read like an abbreviated Who's Who of the industrial, commercial, legal, and banking elite of the city.

By the early 1880s, however, the hospital was annually providing care to nearly four hundred general patients and some two hundred sailors, and the increased activity only served to accelerate the process of deterioration that had begun to take its toll on the structure when it was still known as the U.S. Marine Hospital. (A classic early example of a government building project, the Marine Hospital was so poorly constructed that repairs in its first two decades cost the federal treasury roughly $1,000 a year [some $40,000 in modern dollars] over and above normal maintenance, just to keep the doors open.) The trustees were, therefore, perennially strapped for cash to cover the cost of maintenance and repairs. During the decade, thousands of dollars were spent on new sewer pipes, a heating system, painting, replastering, and the like, although some of the work was financed by specific donations from the hospital's original saint, Hinman Hurlbut.

Substantial sums were spent to build an amphitheater for teaching purposes and a tiny pathology laboratory. There were also rising annual operating costs to contend with, including the salaries of the "House Physician and Surgeon," his assistants, and the matron and her small cadre of nurses, as well as laundresses, a cook, an engineer, and the rest of the support staff. Even before Hurlbut's death in 1884, therefore, fiscal concerns had become the principal preoccupation of many of the hospital's supporters. The demise of the institution's most prominent and generous trustee only exacerbated the problems for the remaining members of the board. Indeed, as the hospital took on more and more charity patients and thus assumed an ever-growing financial burden, the board's annual reports began to reflect a sentiment previously unknown to, or at least unexpressed by, the trustees: a sense of bitterness.

Having carried the torch on their own for nearly twenty years, the trustees were apparently growing weary and somewhat disillusioned, and they let their feelings be known in the annual reports. Diatribes against Cleveland City Council, which was waffling on its promise to underwrite part of the cost of treating emergency cases sent to the hospital, began to appear each year like new installments in an ongoing serial. Then, after one patient filed suit against the hospital in 1883—the first malpractice action in the institution's history—a frustrated Dr. Isaac Himes, the board's secretary, slipped out from under the cloak of Christian brotherhood and allowed himself the luxury of using the following year's annual report to let fly at the "ungrateful" member of the hospital's flock. ("When it is considered," wrote Himes, "that any worthless person thrown upon you by sickness or injury may, in Ohio law, bring an expensive defense upon the hospital which receives and the physician who attends, in charity, such individual without any expense to himself and no trouble but a blackmailing agreement with some 'shyster' lawyer, it may be certified that the flame of charity which burns upon a hospital altar must indeed have had its fires kept lighted from the Source of all Goodness.") Even the usual requests for monetary assistance from "friends" of the hospital gradually changed, assuming an almost plaintive tone that fell somewhere between a *cri de coeur* and a pitiful whine, with a touch of desperation thrown in to reinforce the point.

Clearly, the years of financial instability could not continue if the hospital were to maintain its viability. Fortunately, there were two potential solutions to the problem: the hospital could either vastly increase the number of paying patients it admitted by limiting the number of charity cases accepted; or it could concentrate on building long-term endowments, to accumulate a reserve that might be tapped to cover operating shortfalls and the occasional big-ticket repair job. The former option being untenable—the building was already bulging with patients, and to deny admission to charity cases to make room for more of those who could pay was antithetical to the hospital's very reason for being—the latter option became the focus of the trustees' concerted efforts. And to facilitate the hoped-for large donations of cash, the annual reports soon began to include not just the overworked narrative appeals but also specimens of conventional legal instruments with which to record contributions. Donors could simply copy the forms for their own use, filling in the blanks with an appropriate dollar figure. There was even a complete "Form of Bequest" with which the wealthier patrons could painlessly endow a charity bed "in perpetuity" for the sum of $5,000.

By 1886, however, the hospital was treating more than six hundred general patients a year along with nearly three hundred sailors, and the average cost of care per patient had risen to what was considered the astronomical figure of $1.20 a day. The continuing problem of maintenance—$1,500 alone for a new roof, for example—coupled with the knowledge that the lease on the Marine Hospital would expire in 1895, just nine years hence, moved some of the more farsighted trustees to consider the ultimate solution to the hospital's major dilemma: Cleveland City Hospital had to build and hold title to a new home of its own. In 1886, therefore, the annual report included a rousing call to the friends of the hospital, the start of the laborious process of canvassing for and securing sufficient capital funds to finance construction of a wholly new hospital building.

The response to the first year's efforts proved to be less than encouraging, however, which must have been a particularly dispiriting development for the trustees and Board of Managers, among whom were still some veterans of the group of men and women who two decades before had invented the hospital and nursed it through its tenuous first years. After all, what had at the start been a hospital in name only was by then a full-fledged medical institution that provided what for the time was genuinely effective health care to the people of Cleveland. It would seem only natural, then, that Clevelanders should want their hospital to have a larger and more secure home, a building in which to grow and mature and expand its ability to deliver care. Yet just twelve months after the opening of the hospital's capital-funding campaign, the trustees were reduced to outright begging. The 1887 annual report consisted primarily of an account—singularly aggrieved in tone—of the hospital's tribulations, an account that culminated in the pathetic plea, "Will not someone come to our aid...?"

§

If the years in the former Marine Hospital building were among the most discouraging in the hospital's history, in many ways they also proved to be among the most valuable and important. During the two decades of Cleveland City Hospital's residence in the massive old stone structure on the lakefront, the trustees made their first strong commitment to the creation of long-term endowments, a difficult process in the beginning but one that would pay huge dividends in later years. The Marine Hospital also saw the first efforts toward creating an in-house school of nursing, an important addition to the institution's educational capabilities. The second and without doubt most influential of the hospital's saints first became involved with the institution during its years in the leased building. And, of course, it was a time that saw the advent of a host of doctors who would have a long-lasting impact not just on the hospital but on the city as a whole.

The author of the plaintive appeal for aid in the 1887 annual report, for example, was one such physician, a local boy who was himself the son and grandson of medical men and who would be the first surgeon in the hospital's history to be accorded that most modern manifestation of popular acceptance: celebrity. Dudley Peter Allen was a pedigreed practitioner, an Oberlin College and Harvard Medical School graduate who would equal and eventually exceed the prominence of his father, Dudley, and his grandfather Peter, both distinguished pioneer physicians of northern Ohio. And just a few years after Allen's arrival, another luminary appeared: Edward F. Cushing—son of Henry Kirke Cushing, one of the hospital's earliest consulting physicians—who was Cleveland's first great pediatrician and who, in his lifetime, did more to improve the health and welfare of the city's children than any other individual.

Of course, the hospital could boast of a number of respected physicians throughout its first twenty years, among both the house staff of interns and residents and the visiting staff of physicians and surgeons. An inordinately large percentage of the latter had, for example, obtained advanced training in the prestigious schools and hospitals of London, Paris, Edinburgh, Vienna, and Berlin—no small asset, considering that many of the most striking advances in medical care arose from the work of the Europeans, and their discoveries and new techniques more often than not crossed the Atlantic through the medium of returning American physicians. But if they were capable, competent doctors in their time, none of the hospital's early practitioners possessed all the lineaments of celebrity, that delicate balance of ability, self-confidence, and aggressiveness, coupled with a talent for the active promotion, or at least circumspect furtherance, of one's own reputation. Only Edward Cushing, a man who inspired not just high regard but also genuine love from an entire community, managed to achieve celebrity without even trying.

In comparison with the peacocks, swashbucklers, knights-errant, and grand seigneurs of later years, the majority of the institution's early physicians were virtual wallflowers. Proctor Thayer, a respected surgeon who had studied under and later taught beside John Delamater at the Cleveland Medical College and was on the hospital's visiting staff and board of trustees for decades; Henry Kirke Cushing, Edward's father, who specialized in diseases of women and children but whose expertise extended to virtually all areas of medicine; Hunter H. Powell, in charge of the hospital's first pediatric service and also the city's leading obstetrician for more than twenty years; Isaac Himes, visiting physician and surgeon, member of the board of trustees, pioneering pathologist and eventually dean of the Western Reserve College medical school—all were widely known, and their achievements and personal attributes inspired panegyrics by the dozen after their deaths. But they were, by and large, a modest and self-effacing group, gentlemen and gentle men who were more interested in the work at hand than in acquiring prestige, amassing authority, or exercising power.

There was, however, one early physician who could easily have been the hospital's—for that matter, the city's—first true medical superstar. Gustav Carl Erich Weber was a highly skilled surgeon who had practiced in New York for some years before emigrating to Cleveland and joining the faculty of the Medical Department of Western Reserve College in 1856. Born in Europe and trained there and in the United States, he was an able administrator and organizer in addition to being an artist with the knife, a rare combination of abilities that under ordinary circumstances would have made him a valuable commodity for any fledgling hospital. But Weber was a brooding, stiff-necked Teuton with an imperious manner and a raging ego, and he was nearly obsessive in his need to be in charge of any enterprise with which he was involved. He was also shrewd, calculating, and manipulative when trying to get his way—none of which endeared him to his colleagues.

A tyrant and a bully given to infantile temper tantrums and behind-the-scenes intriguing, Weber had actually been relieved of his professorship at the medical school while he was away on a trip to Europe in 1863. The rest of the faculty convened in his absence and voted unanimously to "abolish" his teaching position, primarily because they could not abide the man. Upon his return from Europe, however, Weber, in characteristic fashion, ingratiated himself with Bishop Rappe to become medical director of the new St. Vincent's. There he started his own medical school—the Charity Hospital Medical College—to compete directly with his former colleagues at Western Reserve.

Weber recruited his own faculty from among physicians not allied with either Western Reserve or Cleveland City Hospital, creating, in effect, both a parallel medical establishment in the city and a cadre of lifelong Weber loyalists. A few years later he entered into an affiliation with the University of Wooster, through which his Charity Hospital

Medical College became the medical department of the university. But in 1880, after a serious falling-out with Bishop Richard Gilmour (who had succeeded Rappe in 1872), Weber negotiated a partial union of his own faculty and that of Western Reserve. By 1881 the two schools merged under the name Medical Department of Western Reserve University.* In that same year Weber was officially brought back into the fold of Western Reserve when he was named professor of surgery at the newly constituted medical school, as well as visiting surgeon to the Cleveland City Hospital. And just two years later, in the culmination of a genuinely bizarre comeback, Weber was named dean of the same school from which he had been unceremoniously booted two decades before.

Weber practiced at both Cleveland City Hospital and St. Vincent's for most of the latter half of the nineteenth century, and his work as a surgeon in both institutions was generally considered superb. In the arena of personal relations he may have been a scheming, insufferable popinjay, but professionally he was virtually without peer. Even one of his enemies once admitted to a newspaper reporter that, although there were many good physicians in Cleveland, "compared with Dr. Weber...in experience and ability they count for almost nothing." Indeed, simply to have assembled and led the medical staff of St. Vincent's while at the same time creating a new medical school was an undertaking that few if any of his contemporaries could have managed successfully.

In his practice Weber had been quick to realize the value of Joseph Lister's method of misting the operating room with a continuous spray of carbolic acid to create an "antiseptic" surgical environment. He adopted the revolutionary technique himself in the early 1870s, long before many other surgeons were convinced of its merit. As a teacher he recognized early on the importance of combining clinical experience in hospitals—patients as "teaching material"—with classroom lectures, a fairly advanced point of view at the time. Many of his students adored him, as did most of his patients; for decades he maintained a large private practice among some of the more prosperous families on the city's west side. Weber was also particularly adept at turning on the Old World charm when the spirit moved him, as often happened when presented with the opportunity to coax large contributions from wealthy

---

*It was a premature baptism, since Western Reserve did not incorporate as a university until 1884, two years after its move to Cleveland from its original home in Hudson.

potential donors, either for St. Vincent's or, later, the Medical Department of Western Reserve.

A revealing example of Weber's *modus operandi* was played out one day in March of 1884, just hours after the funeral of Hinman Hurlbut, the longtime benefactor of not only the Cleveland City Hospital but also Western Reserve's medical school. Weber, then dean of the school, had for some time been attempting to convince Hurlbut to include the institution in his will, but Hurlbut's sudden death occurred before such provision could be made. On the evening of the day on which Hurlbut was buried, therefore, Weber paid a call on John Lund Woods, a wealthy local lumber dealer who was also one of Weber's longtime private patients. In the midst of commiserating over the death of their mutual acquaintance, Weber, with great feeling, sighed deeply. "The only friend the [medical] college has we have buried today," he said. Spellbound, Woods replied earnestly, "I will be your friend."

Some months later, in the midst of one of the many intramural feuds that seemed to sprout up around him like poison mushrooms in spring, Weber threatened to resign from the medical school if another faculty member did not apologize for having made a statement that the dean perceived as a personal insult. The rest of the faculty, many of whom had been driven to fits of apoplexy by Weber's high-handed rule, would have been delighted to see him leave. Nonetheless, they realized that his resignation might jeopardize a very large prospective contribution to the school from none other than John Lund Woods, who, since his post-funeral chat the year before, had become the city's most ardent Weber admirer. Under pressure, the faculty wrote a group apology to Weber, "beseeching" him to reconsider. Less than a week later Weber rescinded his resignation. Woods eventually proceeded with his donation, underwriting the entire cost of construction—nearly $250,000—of a new home for the school.

By 1887 the new medical school building was erected at the corner of East 9th Street and St. Clair Avenue, on the same site as its by-then demolished predecessor. The new facility included ample laboratory space and equipment, luxuries that had previously been unknown at the school but which delighted the editors of the *Western Reserve Medical Journal*, who later wrote to the effect that "a modern medical college without laboratories is a stumbling block in the path of progress" and concluded that the school now made available "scientific apparatus for research, without which the physician of today is but a dabbler."

As tradition demanded, upon completion of the new medical school building the faculty commissioned an official rendering of the edifice from a local artist. And lest anyone forget to whom credit was due for the grand new structure, the artist was instructed to include in his engraving more than just a standard view of the building itself. The finished rendering would, therefore, incorporate two small portraits as well: one, in the upper right corner of the picture, delineated the benign profile of the benefactor, John Lund Woods; the other, in the upper left corner, portrayed the scowling, bearded visage of the maximum leader, Dr. Gustav C.E. Weber.

With a majority of the faculty beholden to the dean for their positions, Weber was, in effect, all-powerful within the school. He ran the university's medical department essentially as an old-fashioned proprietary college, an autonomous and self-sustaining entity that happened to be affiliated with Western Reserve for no reason other than that a medical degree conferred by a university was a more attractive inducement to potential students. Weber did not allow university president Hiram C. Haydn to attend medical faculty meetings, nor did he provide the university with accountings of the income or expenses of its nominal "department." In the mixed metaphor of a newspaper writer of the time, the dean was the "high cockalorum of the [medical] faculty," who "ruled the roost with a rod of iron." Of all Weber's misuses of authority, however, the most blatant was his treatment of Dudley P. Allen.

Following his graduation from the Harvard Medical School, Allen had spent three years studying at surgical clinics throughout Europe before returning to Cleveland in 1883. He immediately set up a practice in office space shared with his friend, ophthalmologist Benjamin L. Millikin, and together the two men began to bid on "casualty surgery" contracts, arrangements by which local industrial concerns paid annual fees to physicians for emergency medical services for their employees. The casualty business was one of the ways in which a young doctor could ensure himself a steady flow of income while establishing a private practice, and contracts with mining concerns, manufacturing firms, and particularly railroads—where workers were injured virtually on a daily basis—were avidly pursued.

Additional income as well as prestige could be derived from serving on the faculty of a medical school, and Allen wasted no time in presenting himself to the medical faculty of Western Reserve. In 1883 he was given the position of demonstrator in minor surgery, a low-paying, low-status post that, he believed at the time, would be a stepping stone to a more estimable and more lucrative place on the faculty. By 1888, however, Allen had advanced in the school no further than a nominal promotion to the position of "lecturer" in minor surgery. That year he wrote to the faculty requesting two additional teaching posts: surgical treatment of diseases of the urethra and bladder and operations on the cadaver. Dean Weber, who retained most of the surgical teaching positions for himself and his protégés, responded to Allen's request by simply ignoring it.

Short of stature and physically unintimidating, Allen was not the type to take on Weber in a face-to-face showdown. (Even one of Allen's oldest friends remembered in later years that "Dudley was never rugged.") Instead, he turned for help to university president Hiram Haydn, who was himself anxious to rein in what he considered to be a rogue department. Weber, however, stood firmly opposed to any intervention in the management of "his" school. Allen continued to make waves by attempting to enlist the aid of hospital and university trustees, but Weber seemed too firmly entrenched to be moved. Eventually the dean tried to placate Allen by offering him the professorship in gynecology—a post Allen turned down—but he would not budge on the question of adding to Allen's responsibilities in the teaching of surgical courses.

Meanwhile, a remnant of the Medical Department of the University of Wooster had continued to function on a reduced scale even after the 1881 merger with Western Reserve, and the Wooster faculty looked on with amusement at the Weber-Allen skirmishes. The dean of the Wooster school at the time was Frank J. Weed, himself a former student of Weber's and a graduate of the original Charity Hospital Medical College. After serving as an assistant in Weber's large and lucrative private practice, Weed had gone on to accumulate a number of casualty surgery contracts with local industries. He had also built a private practice of his own among some of the city's wealthier families, to whom he had been introduced while working for his mentor.

In addition to his qualities as an able physician, Weed was a charming and amusing character who inspired the same sort of patient loyalty that Weber always enjoyed. (Years later, one of Weed's colleagues would swear that he once heard a patient say, "Dr. Weed, I'd rather die under your care than live under that of another physician.") He was also possessed of a most perspicacious eye when it came to the politics of the local medical community, as evidenced by the contents of a letter he wrote to one of his own office associates who was traveling abroad in January 1889, at the height of the hostilities between what had come to be known as the Weber and Allen "factions" on the Western Reserve faculty.

Weed mentioned in his letter that he had proposed a fee of $1,000 for the annual casualty contract of the Cleveland-based Nickel Plate Railroad. "[But] I think I'll reduce my bid to $800, for I suspect Allen is laying for it," he added, noting that Allen and Judge Samuel Williamson, a hospital and university trustee and for years the Nickel Plate's chief legal counsel, were quite "chummy." Turning to the situation at Western Reserve, Weed remarked that "the fight goes on—Gustav holds the reins as tightly as ever and will probably keep on doing so ad infinitum or until his death." As for Allen, all indications were that he was to be "pocketed or shelved. He keeps wiggling, however, and like Paddy's flea bobs up serenely here and there, now and then, and scores a point unexpectedly when Weber's off duty...." Weed then offered his own assessment of Allen, whom he found to be "a good fellow, when it pays," and, even more bluntly, a "cunning, scheming wire-puller." "Just remember what I am telling you," he concluded, "and see if I don't prove right in the end."

As if to substantiate the thesis of Weed's letter, within a few weeks university president Haydn was back before the medical faculty in what proved to be a vain attempt to support Allen's request for additional teaching responsibilities. In March, at the regular monthly faculty meeting, Isaac Himes—one of Allen's staunchest backers—presented a formal motion to at last take up what was by then Allen's year-old petition. The motion was tabled by Weber and his faction, and that action was followed immediately by a Weber-inspired proposal to abolish Allen's position entirely. Although this motion too was tabled, the act itself was an unmistakable indication to Allen that he was not wanted. Bloodied in combat, he resigned his post at the school shortly thereafter, but he did not consider himself defeated. He would spend the ensuing years building a network of allies, powerful individuals whose support he could rely on when the time came to launch a new assault against the seemingly impenetrable battlements of Dean Gustav Weber.

Three years later, in December of 1892, John Lund Woods announced that he would provide the medical school with an endowment amounting to some $125,000 in securities, a gift for which Weber claimed much of the credit. (For some time the dean had been neglecting his duties at the school and concentrating on providing personal attention to Woods, who was mortally ill and who would die the following year.) But the Woods endowment ultimately proved to be Weber's undoing, because the gift only intensified the efforts of Hiram Haydn's successor, Charles F. Thwing, to regain control of the university's medical department. As Thwing later explained, the advent of the endowment strengthened the belief of many that "if the trustees did not take charge of the medical department and make a better school, the community would hold them morally guilty of a breach of trust." Accordingly, Thwing enlisted the support of Western Reserve University and Cleveland City Hospital trustees for a plan that was calculated to dislodge Weber from his palatinate. And the willing instrument of his strategy was Dudley P. Allen.

At the time, Allen had cemented friendly relations not only with Thwing and many of the trustees of both the hospital and the university, but even with a few members of the Weber faction on the faculty. And by 1893, a handful of Weber loyalists had been convinced to drop their allegiance to the dean. At a faculty meeting that summer, therefore, when Allen was nominated for the chair of surgery and his friend Benjamin Millikin proposed as professor of ophthalmology, both men were voted onto the faculty. With his faction now in the minority for the first time in a decade, Weber was confused and angered. As he had so often in the past, he attempted to regain control by resorting to the old tactic of tendering his resignation. This time, however, the resignation was accepted.

Many of Weber's partisans on the faculty subsequently resigned as well. Most were welcomed back to their erstwhile home, the Medical Department of the University of Wooster, but Weber himself was only offered the empty title of emeritus professor of clinical surgery. Spurned even by the school that he had created more than a quarter-century before, Weber was a bitter and humiliated man. He retained a portion of his private surgical practice until 1897, at which time he accepted an appointment as United States Consul at Nuremberg, Germany. Four years later, after his return to Cleveland, he suffered a debilitating stroke that left him partially paralyzed, and he never again practiced medicine.

The turmoil in the Western Reserve medical school and the fall of the seemingly invincible Gustav Weber were all covered gleefully and in great detail by the Cleveland newspapers, which ballyhooed the commotion for weeks. (The headline of one article at the time went so far as to proclaim "It's War.") Indeed, immediately after the coup that had toppled him from power, Weber himself was approached by a reporter, who asked the former dean for his own explanation of the chain of events. Surprisingly, Weber had nothing bad to say about his old nemesis, Haydn, or about the then-current university president, Thwing. Instead, he laid the blame for his downfall squarely on the shoulders of one man. "There has been for years," he said, "a steady pull on behalf of Dr. Allen by [his] influential friends and relatives."

To the uninitiated, Weber's remark might have sounded like nothing more than a petty attempt to disparage a victorious enemy. Yet the dean had indeed been outflanked by Allen, who had used the years after his own resignation from the faculty to build and strengthen his network of supporters. Frank Weed may have overstated the case when he called Allen a "cunning, scheming wire-puller," but there was no doubt that Allen's relationships with university president Thwing and various trustees had been of inestimable help in getting him reinstated to the faculty.

Allen did indeed have "influential friends and relatives" in Cleveland, among whom were such university trustees as Henry Kirke Cushing and Samuel Williamson. But perhaps the most influential of all his acquaintances was Louis Severance, treasurer of Rockefeller's Standard Oil trust and vice president of the Standard Oil Company of Ohio. Severance was the grandson of David Long, who in 1810 had been the first physician to practice in Cleveland. His mother, Mary H. Severance, had been involved with the Cleveland City Hospital virtually from its founding, and she served as an active board member and a substantial supporter for decades.

Allen's ties to the Severance family were longstanding. In 1860, his sister Emily had married Louis Severance's brother, Solon. The couple's daughter Julia eventually married Allen's friend Benjamin Millikin. And in 1892, Allen himself had married Louis Severance's daughter Elisabeth.

The obvious conclusion to be drawn from the various Severance-Allen-Millikin unions was that Allen was not only well known in Cleveland's tightknit world of wealth and influence, he was actually an integral part of that world. (The web of intermarriages also produced a genealogical tangle of nightmarish proportions: Allen's sister, for example, was also his aunt; his brother-in-law was also his uncle; and his own wife was also his second cousin.)

Allen's reliance on insiders in his struggle with Gustav Weber did not mean, however, that his professional abilities were in any way less than adequate. He was a practicing surgeon of high repute both locally and nationally, and he brought new ideas and techniques to both the clinical and educational sides of his specialty. Unlike Weber, who as a professor had relied primarily on bedside instruction and who undervalued laboratory investigation, Allen was a firm believer in benchwork, and he was instrumental in furthering the hospital's own Department of Pathology. In his own way he added substantially to the growing status of surgeons generally, who at the time were in the process of becoming the superstars of medicine.

Allen had coveted the medical school's chair of surgery for a number of reasons, not least of which were his interests in promoting pathological studies and antiseptic surgical techniques. (Of course, as professor of surgery he also gained the appointment of chief visiting surgeon at Cleveland City Hospital, which provided him with beds for his private patients and a staff of assistants to help care for them.) As he accepted his new responsibilities, he must have been determined to avoid the kinds of Weberian excesses under which he had chafed for so long.

Yet soon after his appointment as the hospital's chief surgeon, Allen would himself begin to grow more and more conservative, and before long he exhibited much the same inflexibility as his predecessor. As even one of his friends later conceded, Allen became a "severe taskmaster," capable of being "sharp and even snappy in his orders, and [making] his assistants jump as if on springs." And while still considered a "great instructor," he often resorted to "[breaking] down an opponent through an exercise of power when he was unable to convince or divert him."

Despite the obvious differences between him and many of his older, less open-minded colleagues at the start of his tenure, Allen was still something of an anachronism. He was essentially a nineteenth-century man who had been handed the job of leading the hospital's surgical service into the twentieth century. But within the divide between those two eras—a time of new discoveries and rapidly accelerating progress in medicine—Allen would lose much of the eagerness for change that had marked his earlier career. He would become, as one observer put it, the "great conventional surgeon."

Eventually, however, the staid and proper Allen would find himself coming face to face with the very embodiment of modernity, a brash young surgeon cut from nearly the same cloth as that earlier buccaneer, the archetypal wildman, Horace Ackley. For Allen it was to be a confrontation with disastrous consequences, because his long and distinguished career would end amid rancor, controversy, and humiliation.

§

In 1887, the same year that the new medical school building was opened, the City of Cleveland finally decided to build a public hospital, a larger and better equipped facility than the aging, overburdened City Infirmary at Scranton and Valentine Streets, which had been operating on the West Side since 1855. The new one-hundred-and-seventy-five-bed hospital was to be erected adjacent to the infirmary, which it was meant to augment rather than replace, and its completion would nearly double the number of hospital beds available in the city. The planned facility would, however, need a name, and after diligent consideration of all the possible appellations that could be bestowed upon Cleveland's new municipally owned health-care institution, city council settled on the one choice that was guaranteed to cause trouble. It would be called "City Hospital."

To the trustees of the privately supported Cleveland City Hospital, of course, the advent of a publicly funded "City Hospital" could only serve to cause further confusion about the identity and true nature of their operation. Unwilling to fight the city over the use of the name, however, they chose instead to redesignate their own institution, and the most obvious choice was a name that reflected its location on the shore of Lake Erie. In 1888, therefore, the former Protestant Hospital-former Wilson Street Hospital-former Cleveland City Hospital—which at the time was housed in the former United States Marine Hospital—officially adopted the name by which it would be known for the ensuing century: Lakeside.

Whether or not discarding its old name (and all the connotations of public funding attendant to it) was a contributing factor, donations to the capital-funds drive of the newly denominated Lakeside Hospital began to increase. By this time the hospital was gaining stature as a worthy local charitable endeavor—at least within the powerful and moneyed Protestant community—and it had already earned a favorable reputation among the people it served, the poor and indigent Clevelanders who daily filled its wards. If it was no longer the "City Hospital," Lakeside was still generally perceived as the "city's hospital"—the haven to which ailing destitute citizens could turn for care when they needed it the most.

At the same time, both the national and local economies were booming, and in those halcyon pre-income tax days during which monumental personal fortunes could be amassed, added to, and passed on to succeeding generations without dilution, the city's leading families began to take a more active interest in contributing a portion of their wealth to the maintenance of the hospital. The Board of Managers might continue to stage fund-raising events as they had in leaner times, but now those events were proving wildly successful and reaping vast sums. One summer's outdoor carnival, for example, netted almost $9,000, nearly one-fifth of the hospital's entire income for the year. But if accumulating donations had become less of a problem, one abiding concern simply would not go away: an unacceptably high percentage of operating funds was still being used for repairs of the building itself.

Until such time as they could afford a home of their own and at last walk away from the Marine Hospital, the trustees had to make do with the patched-up, doddering old warhorse of a building. Even as they began to contemplate a new Lakeside, a facility that might be large and flexible enough to house the hospital efficiently for decades, the trustees were still forced to contend with the galling realities of their current home. Not only were corroded plumbing, cracked plaster, crumbling foundations, and the like a continuing drain on the hospital's finances, but new additions—dormitory-like living quarters for nurses, carved out of otherwise dead space in the building's attic; and, in 1889, a fourteen-bed wing, to replace the hospital's tiny children's ward—had to be built. Each repair or modification constituted a substantial improvement for the hospital, but behind the façade of new additions and fresh coats of paint there remained a jury-rigged, forty-year-old liability.

It was time, the trustees concluded, to dust off an asset they had been holding for more than a dozen years, since the days when the hospital had first considered erecting a building of its own to replace the cramped house on Wilson Street. When Leonard Case had donated a tract of lakeshore property as a site on which to construct a new facility, the hospital had been without sufficient funds to carry out such a project. Presented then with the opportunity to lease the Marine Hospital for a nominal fee, the trustees had opted for the more conservative move. (The trustees were also of the opinion that the Case property, near what would later be East 55th Street, about two miles to the east of their then-current location, was too far from the city's center to be a practical site for a hospital.)

But the Case property was theirs to keep or dispose of as they saw fit, and by 1889, with the need for a new hospital building so acute, the trustees felt the time was right to sell the land. With $6,600 realized from the sale, and bolstered by the apparent successes of their ongoing fund-raising efforts, the trustees felt sufficiently confident to take the first major step on the road toward building a hospital of their own. They soon put a down payment on a $66,000, five-acre site east of and contiguous to the Marine Hospital grounds, between East 12th and East 14th Streets.

With a location secured, the trustees turned their attention in ensuing months to determining precisely the sort of hospital building they would actually construct. The concept they eventually agreed upon was nothing if not straightforward: they would, quite simply, create the largest, most modern, and best-equipped facility in the Midwest, an institution that represented the state of the art in health-care delivery. Motivated in part by the same charitable instincts that had driven the hospital's founders, but also by what could only be described as a sense of civic pride (with both the high-minded *and* the pejorative connotations the term implies), the trustees set out to design a major metropolitan hospital to serve the major metropolis that Cleveland had become.

Among the ten largest—and, by all measures, wealthiest—cities in the country by then, Cleveland in 1890 was awash in money, a place in which the most prosperous families thought nothing of spending the modern equivalent of several million dollars to build a Tuscan villa, Tudor castle, or Romanesque manse along Euclid Avenue, the residential street known popularly as "Millionaires' Row." If such people were to build a hospital whose primary purpose was to provide aid and comfort to those in less fortunate circumstances than their own, it was only logical that they would want to build something of heroic proportions, a living monument to the spirit of true Christian charity and, perhaps, something of a monument to themselves as well. Fueled by Calvinist impulses, a *fin de siècle* faith in modernity, and the taste for grand gestures that is so often a component of noblesse oblige, they contemplated the creation of a magnificent institution that would outlive them, their children, and even their children's children. It was all certainly a far cry from the desperate wheeze ("Will not someone come to our aid...?") with which the hospital's annual report had concluded just three years before.

To even conceive of so large and elaborate a hospital as the trustees dreamed of erecting would seem to have required an extraordinary leap of imagination on their part, given the fact that the previous structures that had housed Lakeside were nothing more than a humble old private residence and a crumbling stone building of modest proportions. But it was a notion entirely consistent with a subtle transition the trustees had been undergoing for some time. Even before 1890, meetings of the board and its various committees had begun to be held not in the parlors of local churches, as in previous years, but in the business offices of individual board members or the comfortable rooms of Cleveland's Union Club, the in-town retreat of the city's establishment. A seemingly unimportant change of venue, it was nonetheless indicative of the trustees' heightened understanding of the realities of the times. Hospitals everywhere were maturing, growing out of the weak, blundering infancies of such nightmarish facilities as Cleveland's original municipal hospital of the 1830s. Now formidable adolescents, many had become large and complex institutions that, while providing much-needed social services to the populations they served, had also to be considered at least in part as quasi-commercial enterprises. And they would have to be run as such: at hospitals around the country, business-management skills were fast becoming as important as the practice of the healing arts, because failure at the former could ultimately lead to disaster for the latter.

If the trustees harbored grandiose dreams of a new Lakeside, however, they were also sober enough to realize that they were still amateurs when it came to hospital design and management, two fields of endeavor which were becoming professions as suddenly and as rapidly as would computer engineering nearly a century later. What they needed above all else was information. How were the country's other large urban hospitals designed and laid out? What methods of operation and management did they employ? Were they flexible enough to adapt to changes in the environments in which they functioned?

A series of board meetings was held early in 1890 to determine a course of action, and in late spring, a committee of three trustees was appointed to conduct a thorough study of the state of the art in hospital construction and operation. Shortly thereafter, the aptly named "Committee on Hospitals" set out on an expedition of sorts, a voyage of discovery to the great hospitals of the East. And like John Lang Cassels, who had returned from the Lake Superior country so many years before with news of vast, untapped reserves of iron ore—news that would have a profound effect on the fortunes of his community—the committee members brought back reports detailing the latest advances in hospital design, construction, and operation, reports which would profoundly affect the new Lakeside and, through it, the city as a whole.

Beyond their service on the "Committee on Hospitals," the three trustees who traveled the country seeking out vast, untapped reserves of expertise had already contributed much to the hospital in the way of time, money, and effort, and each would continue to do so in coming years. Ralph W. Hickox, an officer and director of numerous railroads and other corporations, had been a hospital supporter and trustee for years, as had Lee McBride, a prosperous dry goods wholesaler. The third member of the committee had been a trustee for only six years at the time of the Great Pilgrimage to the East, but his tenure would eventually run well into the next century, some forty-eight consecutive years, the last thirty-two of them as board president.

Samuel Mather was in the business of shipping and iron ore—one of the many "sons" of the patriarch of Cleveland iron, John Cassels—and by 1890 he was well on his way to amassing the largest personal fortune in the state of Ohio. He was also busy determining how best to give much of it away. A descendant of the Mathers of New England, with familial ties to the pioneers of northern Ohio, Sam Mather embodied the popular conception of traditional American benevolence. In an era when grandiosity was the byword of the country's wealthiest families, Mather chose instead to be a self-effacing philanthropist. At the same time, however, he maintained the old Calvinist conviction that there was a very real gulf between the elect and the preterition—the leaders and the followers—and he firmly believed himself predestined to be numbered among the former. Indeed, Mather once told an associate that colleges "ought not to be open for the sons of mechanics or of laborers." A university education, he believed, was meant to "train the sons of leading families to take their places as leaders in the community of those who are themselves incapable of leadership."

The oldest son of the city's original iron-ore magnate, S. Livingston Mather (who had founded the Cleveland Iron Mining Company shortly after hearing Cassels' description of the bonanza of ore in Upper Michigan), Sam Mather was anything but a robber baron of the Morgan-Fisk-Gould mold; nor was he particularly conscious of the public relations value of philanthropy, as was another fairly well-to-do Clevelander by the name of Rockefeller. Mather dispensed his benefactions across the city, but he chose to do so with simple, quiet grace. Although in later years he would be dubbed by local newspapers the "First Citizen of Cleveland," he generally allowed himself to be put in the spotlight only when he thought his stature in the community might aid the cause in which he was interested. And his approach to giving did not constitute false modesty. On one occasion, his children first heard of a multimillion dollar donation he had made to Western Reserve University when they saw news of the gift headlined in their morning papers. Mather himself had not deemed the contribution sufficiently noteworthy even to mention it to his own family.

Sam Mather's abiding interest in Lakeside Hospital, and in medicine generally, stemmed in part from his genuine and deeply held religious beliefs. A lifelong member of the Episcopal church and for many years senior warden of Cleveland's Trinity Cathedral, he actively attempted to put into practice the moral precepts of his faith by investing a portion of his great wealth in the betterment of his community. Of course, Mather was also a member of the city's industrial establishment and a very pragmatic manager. He knew full well that Cleveland's inexorable march forward would be slowed if not halted entirely should working men and women experiencing ill health or temporary disability not be helped back to their jobs through the good offices of effective medical treatment.

The greatest measure of his devotion to the hospital, however, probably arose from his own experience. His mother had died suddenly of tuberculosis when he was only two years old (just two months after the birth of his sister, Katharine), so he knew from an early age how the inadequacies of medical care could affect a family. And in the summer of 1869, at the age of eighteen, his own health had been shattered when he was severely injured in an explosion at one of his father's iron mines, where he was working as a timekeeper and payroll clerk. With skull and spine fractures and neurological damage impairing the use of his left arm, he spent two years as an invalid and was forced to postpone and ultimately cancel entirely his plans to attend Harvard College. By 1872, however, he had recovered sufficiently to set out on a trip across Europe, an eighteen-month Grand Tour-*cum*-recuperative voyage. A diary he kept during the trip began with the poignant reminder to himself, "Health chief consideration...do not overdo."

When he returned to Cleveland, Mather entered his father's business, and in 1881 he married Flora Stone, daughter of Amasa Stone, the same man who had been the voice of caution at the organizational meetings of the founders of the Wilson Street Hospital. In 1883 he left Cleveland Iron Mining and went into partnership with James Pickands and Jay C. Morse, forming Pickands, Mather & Company, a small ore and shipping concern that quickly developed into a giant of the iron industry, with one of the largest fleets on the Great Lakes.

Rich as a Florentine duke, with a rather aloof, almost regal bearing and a slight lisp that some people misinterpreted as an affected British accent, Mather was in fact more of a private and, to a degree, diffident personality. He did not, for example, like talking with newspaper reporters, and he was never particularly adept at public speaking. Widely traveled and well read, he nonetheless felt keenly his lack of formal higher education, and one of the great regrets of his life was that, upon his final recovery from the injuries he sustained as a young man, he had deemed himself too old to enter the freshman class at Harvard.

For Mather, as for many prosperous Clevelanders of the city's Protestant elite, Harvard was but one of the jewels in the diadem of the East, the venerated homeland of their forebears. Aside from New York, which was for the most part dismissed as a foul and teeming sewer fit for commercial transactions and little else, the cities of the East—New Haven, Philadelphia, and especially Boston and Cambridge—were exemplars to which patrician Clevelanders always seemed to turn for inspiration and approval, for standards to follow in everything from fashion, art, and architecture to education, commerce, and, of course, medicine. It was only natural, then, that Lakeside's "Committee on Hospitals," when it finally set forth on its study trip in the summer of 1890, would journey first to Boston, to examine Boston City Hospital and the famed Massachusetts General.

One of the nation's oldest hospitals, Massachusetts General should by rights have impressed the visiting Clevelanders, but they were left curiously unmoved by their tour of inspection and barely mentioned the institution when they returned home and reported to their fellow trustees. The reason, quite simply, was that Massachusetts General had been one of the country's original "block plan" hospitals, which were ponderous multistory affairs that were set down in city centers like strange and forbidding monoliths. And by 1890, the block plan was a system of hospital construction that had been out of favor for some time.

Despite the by-then widespread acceptance of Pasteur's germ theory and the slow but growing adoption of antiseptic techniques devised by such pioneers as Lister, many doctors were still convinced that "stagnant" air and unidentifiable "noxious effluvia" were at least partially responsible for the spread of infection and disease within hospitals. "Hospitalism," as the condition was known, was blamed for everything from blood poisoning and erysipelas (a lethal skin infection also known as St. Anthony's Fire) to postoperative abscesses and what was called "hospital gangrene." Even many doctors who fully accepted the notion that specific

microorganisms were the causal agents of specific diseases still held on
to the age-old belief that additional, as-yet unidentified elements in air
itself might also be involved. The very name of the disease malaria, for
example, had originated in the fifteenth century as a combination of the
Italian words for "bad air."

When it came to building hospitals, therefore, the consensus held that
a great mass of a building in which wards and patient beds were of necessity in close proximity and in which air flow was restricted was itself
a danger to the health of its inmates. (Another, much subtler element of
the argument against block-plan hospitals may also have arisen from
their very appearance. To the individuals of wealth and refinement who
funded and oversaw the operations of big-city hospitals in the United
States, the cheek-by-jowl beds of the crowded charity wards—and the
wards themselves, stacked one upon the other—in a block-plan hospital
must have conjured up unpleasant images of that most distasteful aspect
of modern urban life, the slum tenement.) As one contemporary treatise
on hospital construction noted, "It is to be hoped that it will not be many
years before the use of the block hospital is abandoned."

The optimal method of construction for the truly modern hospital was,
it was believed, the "pavilion plan." Pavilion hospitals consisted of a
number of small, well-spaced buildings no more than two stories high,
in which patients could be separated from each other not only by ward
or by floor but by geography. In pavilion hospitals, windows and ventilation shafts were ubiquitous. Elaborate atmospheric-movement systems
were designed to ensure that bad, "vitiated" air could be vented away
from the patients while a predetermined quantity of clean and healthful
outside air—four thousand cubic feet per hour for surgical patients; half
that amount for medical cases—could be drawn indoors. Each building
was, in effect, segregated from its neighbors, connected only by a lengthy
open or enclosed walkway or, in some cases, an underground tunnel.

The pavilion plan originated in France in the middle of the eighteenth
century, and although the concept was widely praised, few hospitals
could amass sufficient land on which to erect more than a single, necessarily multistory building. Urban hospitals in particular were constrained
by the cost and lack of availability of acreage, which is why not only the
Massachusetts General but also the Boston City Hospital were built on
the block plan. Despite the fact that Joseph Lister himself had for years
insisted that it was "immaterial how many stories of wards there may be
in a hospital, provided that the details of the antiseptic method are accu-

rately carried out in all of them," the block plan was still considered dangerously out of date. Thus, the visiting committee from Cleveland, after touring both of Boston's hospitals, deemed neither a fitting candidate for emulation.

In Philadelphia, neither Pennsylvania Hospital nor Presbyterian Hospital, both block-plan buildings, proved particularly edifying, the committee members noting later that they "did not find anything in either" that they wished to recommend for the design of their own institution. And while New York's brand-new Presbyterian Hospital—recently completed at a cost of nearly $1 million—was, in the opinion of the committee, the "best of the block system [hospitals] in America," it still constituted merely the premier example of what the committee considered an outmoded technology. It was in the unlikely setting of Baltimore that the members of the Committee on Hospitals found their paradigm, the institution that most impressed them and after which they would most closely model their own.

At his death in 1873, a wealthy Baltimore Quaker merchant and financier named Johns Hopkins had left a bequest totaling some $7 million for the establishment of a university and hospital in his home city. Just three years later Johns Hopkins University opened its doors, and in 1889 the university's affiliated hospital—designed and built on the pavilion system—was completed. Unique for its time, the Johns Hopkins Hospital was the product of intense planning, was amply endowed and, most important, was specifically designated as an element of the university, the clinical component of a "campus" that would include a graduate school of medicine, to be built next to the hospital by 1893. The faculty of the medical school would be placed in charge of the hospital, not only overseeing patient care and instructing medical students—all of whom would need an undergraduate degree for admission to the school, an unheard-of requirement at a time when private proprietary medical schools were still turning out "doctors" who could barely read or write—but also utilizing the school's elaborate research facilities to pursue new understanding of the causes of and treatments for disease. And medical students, instead of simply listening to endless lectures and watching demonstrations of technique—the conventional wisdom of centuries—would receive hands-on experience in their last year, being given responsibility for a number of patients and expected to perform, albeit under supervision, a gradually increasing workload of procedures.

For the visitors from Cleveland who toured the new facility and inspected plans for the coming medical school, Johns Hopkins appeared to be nothing less than perfection, an ideal given form in a way they could not hitherto have imagined. They were wildly impressed—so much so, in fact, that upon their return to Cleveland they reported to the full board of trustees by describing Johns Hopkins as "a model institution." Yet the great revelation of Johns Hopkins—the creation of the country's first true academic medical center, a wholly contained "campus" dedicated to what was just beginning to be accorded the status of medicine's new holy trinity (patient care, laboratory research, and medical education)—seemed at first glance to have escaped the three trustees from Cleveland. Because of all the innovations and pioneering approaches evident at Johns Hopkins—particularly the concept embodied in the aggregation of university, medical school, and affiliated hospital, the sum of whose parts would, it was believed, exceed the whole—the ones that struck them most forcefully and that they reported on most enthusiastically were "the most advanced practical ideas on heating, ventilation, the supply of pure air, sunlight and many other but less important features...." In short, the lineaments of the pavilion plan.

They could not, of course, even attempt to duplicate Johns Hopkins exactly; Western Reserve's new medical school at East 9th and St. Clair, for example, while only a few blocks from the site of the proposed new hospital, was just three years old, and it would have been sheer madness to abandon the structure and then attempt to build a new one contiguous to Lakeside. But the Lakeside trustees would copy Johns Hopkins shamelessly. They would indeed build their new hospital on the pavilion plan, erecting by the turn of the century a veritable village of brick and stone structures along Cleveland's lakefront. And they would spend some $600,000 (roughly $38 million in modern dollars) to create an institution befitting the stature of their city.

Yet within just a few years of the opening of what was so proudly called the "New Lakeside," the hospital would begin to be viewed in a different light. Some of the more perspicacious members of the Lakeside board looked at their great new edifice—the most modern and best-equipped medical facility in the Midwest—and realized that after all their efforts they had really only created a very large and very expensive temporary home.

CHAPTER THREE

Thoroughly Scientific

Following the recommendation of the McBride-Hickox-Mather committee, there was virtual consensus among the hospital's trustees as early as the fall of 1890 in favor of the pavilion style of construction for the new Lakeside. Reporting its findings after visiting both block-plan and pavilion hospitals in the East, the committee had been effusive in its praise of Baltimore's Johns Hopkins, the archetypal pavilion-plan institution, with its seventeen two- and three-story buildings spread out over some fourteen acres. Indeed, even if a few board members had demurred at the idea, their objections might easily have been lost amid the general enthusiasm.

Despite its overwhelming acceptance of the pavilion concept, however, in ensuing months the board continued to send its three-member Committee on Hospitals to such cities as Chicago, Detroit, Washington, St. Louis, and Providence, to glean further information on what were referred to as "the latest scientific conclusions" on hospital construction, operation, equipment, and management. New data was assiduously collected on these trips, and the potential value of every detail, from a particular steam-heating system to a surgical-suite floor covering, was weighed carefully. It was an approach that reflected the old Calvinist tenet that the true Christian brought to the conduct of secular business a "high seriousness as in itself a kind of religion."

Still another cornerstone of Calvinist faith—the tithe—also played upon the minds of the trustees during their deliberations over the new Lakeside. Each of them knew that collectively they would bear the brunt of the cost of erecting Cleveland's new hospital. And although some of the trustees had reputations as being rather careful with a dollar in the execution of their own business dealings, all were nonetheless determined to acquire only the best for the new Lakeside.

They were fully prepared to make substantial contributions to the project for a number of reasons, not the least of which were their unquestioning faith in the nineteenth-century equivalent of high technology and their unending fascination with the very notion of modernity itself. (Such phrases as "latest scientific conclusions," "most modern and carefully thought out system," "scientific medical men," "thoroughly modern treatment," "best and most modern surgical instruments," and "the very latest improved scientific apparatus" appeared again and again in trustee-generated written descriptions of the proposed new facility.) And they saw the new hospital not as just another charitable endeavor but as further proof that Cleveland—"their" community, in more ways than one—was ready to take its place in the pantheon of great American cities, cities in which, to use Sam Mather's phrase, "civilization has attained its highest growth."

But with the lease on the U.S. Marine Hospital slated to expire at the end of September 1895, the hospital's fund-raisers had to work with all deliberate speed through the first years of the decade to accumulate adequate capital to begin construction of the new institution. Even beyond the Lakeside "family"—trustees, members of the board of managers, and longtime supporters, all of whom were expected to make at least three-figure (but preferably four- and five-figure) contributions to the fund-raising effort—Cleveland's emerging middle class was also urged to participate in the drive to build the new hospital. Soon, smaller pledges did in fact begin to come in from a variety of sources, in amounts ranging from $5 to $500.

By 1893, when Lee McBride and his co-committee member Ralph Hickox were elected president and vice president, respectively, of the Lakeside board, the trustees were at last prepared to commission an architect. George H. Smith, who had already created Euclid Avenue mansions for some of the city's elite and who had collaborated on the design of the Arcade, an innovative enclosed downtown retail gallery and office building, produced plans for a classic pavilion-style hospital. There were to be twelve separate structures, with only the central administration building and the nurses' living quarters rising higher than two stories. The entire complex would spread out across the full width of a four-hundred-foot frontage along Lake Street, between East 12th and East 14th Streets, and would run north nearly the same distance, from the street to the railroad right-of-way that skirted Lake Erie's southern shore. In all, the hospital would cover an area of more than one hundred and fifty thousand square feet, or some three and a half acres.

With their architect's drawings in hand, and with their steadily growing war chest of pledges, the trustees felt certain they could begin excavation immediately. Yet before they had a chance to turn the first shovelful of dirt, the ground itself opened up beneath their feet.

Exactly twenty years before, the nationwide bank panic of 1873 and the lingering effects of a subsequent depression had been contributing factors in the hospital's decision to forego investing in a new building of its own, a decision that had resulted in the twenty-year lease on the old Marine Hospital. Now, in 1893, another, more terrible panic again derailed the hospital's plans. For the next six years a depression of unparalleled depth ravaged the country, with the effect on individual segments of the national economy ranging from hugely destructive to utterly devastating. (By 1896 more than one hundred and fifty railroads, eight hundred banks, and sixteen thousand other businesses would collapse. And as unemployment in the areas of manufacturing and transportation rose by more than four hundred percent, the value of stocks, bonds, and other capital holdings plummeted to new lows.)

Those with cash hoarded it as a precaution against further shocks to the financial system, causing money itself to become a scarce commodity. The squeeze was felt by virtually the entire country, not least the wealthier citizens of Cleveland, who suddenly found themselves unable or unwilling to fulfill their donation pledges to the Lakeside building campaign. Victims of a painfully ironic set of circumstances, the trustees had for the second time in the hospital's short history unwittingly chosen precisely the wrong moment to set out on a course of expansion. And with few if any contributions coming in immediately after the 1893 crash, groundbreaking for the new Lakeside had to be postponed indefinitely.

Stunned by the suddenness and severity of the national economic debacle, the trustees nevertheless continued to refine their plans for the new Lakeside, waiting for the day when a semblance of stability would return to the country's economy and they could again feel confident that contributions pledged to the project would indeed be fulfilled. Meanwhile, the work of caring for the sick at the old Lakeside continued apace, and further moves to enlarge and strengthen the medical staff were still being made.

In addition to the appointment of Dudley P. Allen as chief visiting surgeon and Edward Cushing as head of the pediatric service, in 1894 the trustees boldly raided Johns Hopkins to snare an outstanding young practitioner named Hunter Robb to head the gynecology department. And in obtaining the services of Robb, Lakeside also captured another prize: his wife, Isabel Adams Hampton Robb, who was both principal of the new Johns Hopkins Nurses Training School and superintendent of nursing within the Hopkins hospital. A disciple of Florence Nightingale, the British nurse usually credited with fostering the notion and reality of professional nursing, Isabel Robb would bring to Lakeside a degree of expertise and experience unparalleled in the institution's history, and her hand would help guide the hospital's proposed school of nursing in its formative years.

The first true schools of nursing had been founded in the United States little more than two decades before Robb's arrival in Cleveland, so it was not surprising that few of the Lakeside nurses of earlier eras had much formal training in their craft. What little instruction they received usually came in the form of on-the-job training from the hospital's longtime matron, Eliza Mitchell, whose responsibilities included not only patient care but also hiring, firing, and overseeing the work of the members of the service staff. Medical education for nurses of the time was generally minimal, and historically they were treated more as drudges and lackeys than as professionals. They were, in Isabel Robb's description, mere "automatons," expected simply to follow the orders of doctors and the matron and not to ask questions.

Usually young, seldom well educated, always single (it was not until World War II that married nurses would be allowed to practice in hospitals), the typical student-nurse of the mid-nineteenth century worked a daily shift of from twelve to fifteen hours, for which she received room and board within the hospital and a small stipend for personal expenses. After a full day or night's work she would ostensibly spend her few free hours in study, but more often than not the "educational" component of her student life suffered, a victim of either her own fatigue or the hospital's lack of effort.

Around the country, hospital trustees and administrators publicly expressed pious regard for the "womanly ministrations" and "gentle, caring touch" of nurses, but in fact they were routinely worked to the point of exhaustion. Indeed, most of the earliest nursing schools were in-house institutions founded by hospitals specifically to ensure an uninterrupted flow of cheap labor; two years of "training" was offered to students in exchange for meals, a bed, and the opportunity to spend the better part of every day on their feet, not just following doctors' orders but also sweeping and dusting wards, scrubbing floors, laundering bandages for reuse, preparing and serving meals, and carrying patients between floors. Some hospitals even forced student nurses to provide their own uniforms.

At Lakeside, the practice of keeping only about a half dozen nurses on duty at any given time had produced over the years an increasingly ponderous workload for each individual, resulting in widespread dissatisfaction among the nursing corps as a whole. In fact, the first mention of the possibility of creating an in-house nursing school at the hospital, in 1882, came about as a direct result of the trustees' discovery that a number of young nurses who had trained under Eliza Mitchell were being hired away by other hospitals as paid attendants—at the time, "graduate" nurses usually commanded a salary of about $15 a month—or were entering private-duty nursing, potentially a somewhat more lucrative field. In the annual report for 1882, therefore, the "establishment of a training school for nurses" suddenly became "one of the advances which should now engage our attention."

For years Florence Nightingale and her acolytes had been advocating standardized training of nurses, with more instruction in the basic sciences and the specifics of medicine, as well as a clearly delineated chain of command for the nursing corps within hospitals. Only a handful of American institutions adopted her principles, but one of the few—New York's Bellevue Hospital Training School for Nurses—was Isabel Robb's alma mater. Robb went on to become head nurse at the Women's Hospital of New York City and later superintendent of the Illinois Training School for Nurses in Chicago, from which she was recruited by Johns Hopkins in 1889.

In Baltimore she helped to create the nursing school's curriculum, taught classes from textbooks she had written, and oversaw the daily operations of the hospital's nursing corps. She also laid the groundwork for fundamental reforms that would be instituted at Johns Hopkins the year after her departure: the establishment of a three-year course of study in nursing, rather than the generally accepted two-year course, and adoption of an eight-hour work shift for student nurses.

When Robb and her husband arrived in Cleveland not long after their marriage (the ceremony had taken place in London, with Isabel carrying a floral bouquet sent by Florence Nightingale herself), she was immediately named a member of the Lakeside Board of Managers and quickly became chairwoman of its Training School Committee. She soon began providing a "gratuitous course of lectures" to the hospital's nurses, and she offered her assistance in the planning of the curriculum of the training school, which was scheduled to open concurrently with the new hospital. At the time, however, there was still serious doubt over whether there would actually *be* a new hospital.

By the spring of 1895, with the expiration of their lease on the Marine Hospital building looming just six months away, the trustees knew that, the ongoing depression notwithstanding, work on the new hospital would have to begin soon. With a stack of pledges but far less cash in hand than they actually needed, they took the calculated risk of ordering the work to begin, and ground was at last broken on Cleveland's huge new medical complex. As excavation of the site progressed, the Board of Managers set to work on yet another fund-raising scheme, one devised to alleviate the cash-flow crisis by teasing immediate donations from the hospital's supporters in a relatively painless way.

The Lakeside Magazine was a hundred-page, single-issue publication that featured a modest assortment of donated poems, short stories, essays, and rotogravure art reproductions as an excuse to justify the scores of paid advertisements that were the real point of the exercise. The magazine was something less than an aesthetic triumph, but it served its true purpose by bringing in much-needed dollars at a crucial time. It also provided Clevelanders with their first glimpse of the impending hospital, a figurative tour through the interior of the new Lakeside as delineated in a lengthy article that appeared over the byline of that noted wordsmith, Samuel Mather.

Illustrated with a ground plan of the entire complex and architect Smith's own line rendering of the new Lakeside *in situ*, the Mather article concentrated less on a physical description of the facilities planned for the hospital than on a methodical explanation of the reasoning behind the decisions the trustees had made. And it was the latter element that most clearly revealed just how passionately the trustees had embraced pavilion-plan orthodoxy.*

---

*The Mather essay revealed not only the Lakeside trustees' reverence for pavilion-plan thinking but also what may have been a small flaw in the character of its author. Many of the phrases Mather chose to use in his article—even entire sentences, for that matter—had been lifted intact or in slightly altered form from a published address written six years before by John Shaw Billings, the planner of and guiding genius behind the construction of the Johns Hopkins Hospital.

In his article, Mather described a complex of twelve discrete structures arrayed along the waterfront to take advantage of the "fresh lake breezes and outlook" afforded by the site. Among the "cardinal principles" which governed the development of the new Lakeside, Mather placed first in importance the "most modern and carefully thought out system of heating and ventilation"—the very essence of pavilion-plan thinking. He went on to describe the system, mentioning chimneys one hundred feet high through which the "purer atmosphere of that altitude" would be drawn by powerful electric fans. The fans would in turn force the air through an elaborate system of ductwork, over coils of steam pipes and ultimately through registers set near floor level at the head of every ward bed.

"Impure air" that accumulated in the wards would sink to the floor and be drawn off through additional registers by "powerful suction," then be vented through tall shafts "to a very considerable height before being released." Heating was to be regulated by means of "patented electrical devices"—the scientific wonder known as the thermostat—and to further guard against the spread of contagion within the hospital, all "furniture, doors and window frames" would be made "without moldings or other irregular outlines in which germs might possibly lodge."

The second "great principle" governing the design of the new Lakeside was a provision for "public clinics," areas in which ward patients could be operated on by teaching surgeons before an audience of students from the medical school of Western Reserve University, just a few blocks away. Accordingly, a pavilion that incorporated a surgical amphitheater, recovery room, and ample areas for equipment and personnel was provided. Another pavilion, to house the dispensary (or outpatient department), would be located immediately to the south of the surgical amphitheater, while to its north would be an autopsy building, the laundry and boilers of the power plant, and a single large kitchen to serve the entire complex.

Fronting on Lake Street—"in the center, where it belongs," in Mather's revealing turn of phrase—would be the administration building, housing the hospital's general offices and the living quarters of the superintendent and the resident medical staff. On either side of the administration building would be pavilions for the common wards: to the west the male wards, to the east the female. Farther east of the women's pavilion were the children's wards, behind which was to be a three-story dormitory given over to residential quarters and classrooms for the nurses who would be enrolled in the new Lakeside nurses' training school. All of the structures were free-standing, but each was connected to the others by means of a ground-level covered corridor and a subterranean service tunnel.

While neither as large a complex of buildings nor as grandiose an architectural statement as Johns Hopkins' eclectic amalgam of Victorian-era styles, the new Lakeside would nonetheless constitute one of the most impressive set of structures in Cleveland. Even the simple pen-and-ink sketch that appeared in *The Lakeside Magazine* revealed how stately and imposing the new hospital would be. Indeed, with its baronial Tudor façades surrounded by manicured lawns, the whole bordered on the north by the picturesque panorama of Lake Erie, the new Lakeside resembled less a health-care institution than a holiday retreat of Old World nobility. But there were, in fact, more than the obvious reasons for the trustees to want their new hospital to be not just "modern" and "thoroughly scientific" but attractive and inviting as well—as far from the old image of Lakeside's previous homes as they could manage.

Of all the changes, improvements, and modernizations embodied in the new Lakeside, by far the most radical departure from the standard set by the Wilson Street and Marine Hospital buildings was the provision for an entire pavilion designed solely for the use of paying patients. With fifty-two private rooms—no long, dormitory-style open floors as on the common wards—the private pavilion would be the exclusive preserve of those patients who could not only afford to pay for their care but who could afford a daily rate far greater than that to be charged the paying ward patients—from two to seven times as great, depending on the room's location. They would have a separate operating room for their exclusive use, and they would be treated not by the younger house officers but by either the senior staff physicians and surgeons or by their own private doctors (at least, those deemed by the hospital to be "reputable"), who would be granted admission privileges to Lakeside.

On the very first page of his article in *The Lakeside Magazine*, in an abbreviated synopsis of the historical importance of hospitals, Sam Mather made a point of mentioning that an "appreciation of the advantages of hospitals is coming in our day to the rich and well-to-do, who are learning that they can receive better treatment and care in the modern hospital than [in] their own homes." This sentence was, as far as it went, entirely accurate, not just for Cleveland but nationally as well. The perception of hospitals as merely the havens of last resort for the poor and indigent had long since begun to change, and by 1895 hospitals were well on their way to becoming indispensable resources for all the citizens of a given community. They were at last being recognized as the most practical and efficient places in which to procure what were by then the rapidly expanding capabilities of medical science.

But implicit in Mather's statement was another profound difference in the way hospitals were coming to be perceived: a change in the point of view of hospital trustees and administrators themselves, a new awareness that was underscored in Lakeside's annual report that same year. In his yearly message to the hospital's supporters, board president Lee McBride offered his own description of the impending new Lakeside, along with the rather ominous news that at least $100,000 in donations was still needed to complete the project. (McBride then resorted to the tried and trusted method of shaming contributions from the faithful by asking, "What more God-given and glorious privilege than to minister to the wants of those who, for lack of means, cannot help themselves?") Yet within the same message, McBride took pains to mention the forthcoming hospital's newest feature, the private pay pavilion, and he spared no words in lauding it to the skies. "To this ward," he concluded, "we wish to call the special attention of the physicians and surgeons of this city, as well as of adjacent cities and country. The fact that the rooms in this ward are open to other than the medical and surgical visiting staff of the hospital, with special operating room and house staff for their use, must prove a source of great benefit not only to the physicians and surgeons availing themselves of its use, but to the patients who are so fortunate as to be sent by them to the new Lakeside."

In effect, Mather in his essay and more particularly McBride in his annual report were issuing nothing less than an open invitation for more paying private patients. The very fact that the Lakeside trustees included in their plans for the new hospital a separate pavilion exclusively for private patients meant that they were clearly hoping to increase the number of such patients, an eventuality that would, of course, increase the hospital's annual income and thereby lessen to some extent its dependence on contributions from outside. Fully twenty percent of the new hospital's proposed two hundred and fifty beds were to be in the private pavilion, with many more ward beds expected to be used by partial-pay patients who might not be able to afford private rooms. If even a third of the total number of ward patients at any one time were admitted on a paying basis (a conservative estimate based on the experience of previous years), then the trustees could expect roughly half of the hospital's total number of patients in any given year to be generating revenue of one level or another.

The private pavilion was, therefore, in part an attempt to procure not only a greater percentage of paying patients than ever before but also a greater amount of real income from them, an initial step toward weaning the hospital off the life-sustaining flow of donated dollars which in previous years had always managed to cover the institution's annual operating costs. For the first time the trustees were admitting that Lakeside could no longer afford to be so overwhelmingly an eleemosynary undertaking, that it would have to begin learning how to pay its own way through the expedient of admitting more patients from among the "rich and well-to-do." They were also openly recognizing that the growing carriage trade for medical services—not only within Cleveland but from its neighboring counties as well—was a potential bonanza, and they were expressing their determination to attract at least a portion of it to the new hospital.

The simple fact of the private pavilion did not mean, however, that Lakeside would neglect its historic mission of providing care to the poor and indigent. Nor did it mean that the trustees could ignore the ongoing need for continued fund-raising efforts. Even if they had sufficient capital to erect *two* private pavilions—as had been done at Johns Hopkins—the increase in the number of paying patients still could not possibly have made the hospital a self-sustaining entity. Donations would, therefore, continue to be sought, if anything even more aggressively. As Mather wrote in the last paragraph of his article in *The Lakeside Magazine*, "It is confidently believed that the citizens of Cleveland will take a proper pride in the new Lakeside Hospital, which it is hoped will be a model one of its kind, and will become famous, not only for the good that is done within its walls and the self-sacrificing labors of those who work within it, but also for the public-spirited generosity of the citizens of Cleveland shown by liberal contributions toward its erection and maintenance."

Shortly thereafter, a single-paragraph announcement in the December 1895 issue of the *Western Reserve Medical Journal* revealed yet another example of how powerfully Lakeside's trustees had been influenced by the innovators at Johns Hopkins. Following the lead of the Baltimore institutions, the members of the Lakeside board entered into an agreement with the trustees of Western Reserve University and the faculty of the university's medical department. The agreement gave the medical faculty sole responsibility for naming the hospital's visiting staff from among its own members, and provided for the medical school's long-standing dispensary, or outpatient clinic, to operate out of the hospital's own new dispensary quarters. Most importantly, the agreement imbued in the medical faculty "in every way full control of the clinical material [that is, the charity patients] of the hospital and dispensary."

The agreement, shepherded along principally by chief visiting surgeon Dudley P. Allen, formalized the existing ties between the university and the hospital and bound them together inextricably, making full professors in the medical school also chiefs of their corresponding clinical services in the hospital. And even before the formal agreement between the hospital and the school, Western Reserve had adopted two other Johns Hopkins-inspired initiatives: a four-year rather than three-year requirement to achieve the M.D. degree; and an extension of the academic year from six to eight months.

At Johns Hopkins, the hospital and medical school had been planned from the start as two elements of a greater whole. For Lakeside and Western Reserve, however, a formal affiliation constituted a remarkable break with convention and a bold leap into the uncharted waters of co-operation between a private university and a separate private hospital. Of the handful of medical schools in the country that enjoyed similar relationships with local hospitals, almost all were part of state universities; the others had either formulated working agreements with public hospitals or had simply started their own dispensaries and clinics.*

Of course, the ties that bound Western Reserve and Lakeside were facilitated, at least in part, by the simplest and most obvious of circumstances: fully two-thirds of the hospital's trustees were also members of the university's board. In secular terms, the two institutions shared what amounted to an interlocking directorate, and a consensus on extending cooperative efforts would not, therefore, have been particularly difficult to achieve. But the signing of the agreement was a watershed event nonetheless, and in little more than a decade the close cooperation of the two entities would earn national recognition as a model for other institutions to emulate.

The formal union of Lakeside and the medical school came at a par-

---

*As late as 1910, Lakeside was still one of only two private hospitals in the country to have such a cooperative arrangement with a private university, the other being the Barnes Hospital and Washington University, in St. Louis.

ticularly appropriate time, coinciding as it did with another, greater watershed—an era when the promise of medical science itself was finally beginning to be fulfilled. In the waning years of the nineteenth century, discoveries and new procedures were being introduced almost on a daily basis, principally from the laboratories of Europe, where researchers were, for example, able to isolate the microorganisms that were the specific causal agents of a host of diseases, from anthrax, leprosy, and tuberculosis to cholera, diphtheria, meningitis, and even plague. And with the discovery of the causes of these diseases came the hope that treatments, cures, and even immunizing serums might soon follow.

In 1895, Wilhelm Roentgen demonstrated what overnight became one of medicine's most valuable diagnostic tools, the X-ray. (Three months later, Dayton C. Miller, of Cleveland's Case School of Applied Science, made one of the first X-ray exposures in the United States.) On the domestic front, William Halsted, chief surgeon at Johns Hopkins, had begun to wear sterile rubber gloves in the operating room. The use of gloves (which were made for Halsted by the Goodyear Tire and Rubber Company of Akron) was yet another step in the journey up from the chaos and filth of pre-Lister surgery to antiseptic environments and beyond, toward unconditional aseptic, or totally germ-free, conditions. At the same time, Halsted was perfecting the radical mastectomy, the first effective treatment for cancer of the breast, which in the past had proved almost universally fatal.

Also at Johns Hopkins, Cleveland native Harvey Cushing (son of the Wilson Street Hospital's Henry Kirke Cushing and younger brother of Lakeside's Edward Cushing) was pioneering the technique of monitoring blood pressure during surgery in order to avoid the all too common incidences of surgical shock—massive blood loss—which for centuries had proved lethal to otherwise healthy patients. Cushing, who in later years would come to be regarded as the father of American neurosurgery, was also beginning to map out new paths in what was at the time the virtually unexplored field of surgery on the brain.*

Of course, despite all the progress that medicine had made by that time, every turn-of-the-century patient knew that submitting himself to

---

*At the height of his career, Cushing's reputation as a brilliant practitioner in his area of specialization was so widely known that he may well have been the inspiration for an addition to the American idiom. Henceforth, a person displaying only limited mental capacity would often be dismissed with the phrase, "He's no brain surgeon."

medical treatment also meant subjecting himself to a high degree of risk. With no reliable means of controlling infection, for example, patients— especially surgical cases—continued to die at rates that even then were considered immoderately high.

Part of the problem lay in the fact that side by side with the advent of new ideas and techniques, many of the old ways continued to linger on. Progressive surgeons like Halsted, for example, were indeed wearing sterile rubber gloves in the operating room, yet no one had yet thought to take the seemingly obvious further precaution of wearing a mask to cover the nose and mouth. Risk, therefore, was still the inevitable concomitant of treatment, and it was ever-present not only for the charity cases but for the paying patients as well. Once, Harvey Cushing himself, when faced with the necessity of undergoing an emergency appendectomy, actually put off the procedure until he was assured that the surgery would be performed by no one but his chief, William Halsted. And even then, moments before the operation, Cushing sat down and wrote out a will.

§

In September of 1895, with only limited progress having been made on the construction of the new Lakeside, the trustees petitioned the federal government for an extension of their lease on the Marine Hospital. In a response either cynical by design or imbecilic by default, the government did grant an extension—of exactly six months, to April Fool's Day of 1896. The value to the contractors of the extra six months, most of them in the dead of winter, was minimal at best, and by April 1st the new buildings were still far from completion. In addition to the effects of the ongoing depression, which had delayed the start of the project for two years, construction itself had also been slowed by unforeseen problems on the site. Some of the first foundation footings to be set, for example, had been swallowed up in what amounted to quicksand on the sloping land overlooking the shore of the lake, and all of the work had to be redone.

By the deadline date of the lease extension, there simply was no hope that even one or two of the complex's new buildings would be available for use in the near future. Faced then with the imminent loss of its home,

Lakeside was forced to exercise its only remaining option. Just as it had nearly twenty years before, during the great Allopath-Homeopath war of 1867, the hospital ceased all activity and closed its doors. Those patients who could not be discharged safely were, however, provided with an alternative; they were transferred to, of all places, St. Vincent's Charity Hospital, which granted Lakeside's staff physicians temporary privileges until their new facilities could be finished. Despite the enmity that had divided the two institutions at the time of their founding, the cooperative stance adopted by St. Vincent's during the second Lakeside closing was actually not surprising. As early as 1878—even while the volatile Gustav Weber was still suzerain of St. Vincent's—relations between the Catholic hospital and the Protestant community had already warmed appreciably. Indeed, that year St. Vincent's granted limited clinical-teaching privileges to the faculty of the then-Medical Department of Western Reserve.

While work on the buildings continued, numerous details still had to be attended to in preparation for the eventual opening of the new Lakeside. Among the first requirements was the hiring of supervisory personnel, and by September of 1897 James S. Knowles had been named superintendent of the hospital. Knowles was a rotund and easygoing man with more than a dozen years of experience as a hospital administrator in New York and as an inspector with the New York City Department of Charities. He immediately set to work creating a management structure and administrative guidelines for the new Lakeside, in addition to ordering equipment and supplies and overseeing the final stages of construction of the buildings themselves.

Just a month after Knowles' hiring, M. Helena McMillan was named the first principal of the Lakeside Training School for Nurses. A graduate of McGill University in Montreal and the Cook County (Illinois) Training School for Nurses, McMillan had been principal of a training school in Kingston, Ontario. Together, she and Knowles collaborated on the creation of the Lakeside school's structure, and in November they presented their plan to the trustees for their approval.

Incorporating many of the suggestions of Isabel Robb, much of the new training school's organization and curriculum reflected Robb's own background in Nightingale-style education. As recommended to the trustees by Knowles and McMillan, the Lakeside school would, for example, offer a three-year course of study rather than the old standard of two years, and a substantial portion of the instruction was to be presented by the hospital's own doctors and surgeons.

The first year of schooling would include weekly lectures by the hospital's medical staff on elementary anatomy and physiology, materia medica (drugs and their application), bacteriology, and hygiene. These courses were to be augmented by classroom study of nursing texts devoted to practical nursing for surgical, medical, and gynecological patients, as well as additional instruction in "practical and theoretical cooking." Second-year students would learn obstetrical nursing, care of newborns and children, operating-room procedure, care of the "nervous and insane," advanced medical subjects, and "practical and theoretical cooking."

Each third-year student would begin to work as a head nurse on the wards and as a special nurse to the private patients. There was no classwork to speak of for third-year nurses, but they were expected to attend medical-staff lectures on "eye, ear, throat, skin, electricity and massage," and they were to be given special instruction in "management of wards," "management of small hospitals," and even "training school administration." Further cooking lessons were not, however, deemed necessary.

Applicants would be limited to women between the ages of twenty-two and thirty-three "with no exceptions," because it was generally agreed that "girls under twenty-two...are seldom strong enough and sufficiently developed to stand the work," and women over thirty-three "seldom make successful nurses." Student nurses would receive no compensation other than room, board, uniforms, and books, but "as an incentive to good work," prizes of $50 each would be awarded to the two best students in every class.

Together, Knowles and McMillan estimated the nursing requirements of the new hospital's eight wards, two operating rooms, and dispensary to be one day supervisor (McMillan herself), one night supervisor, ten head nurses, thirteen day (graduate) nurses, seven night (graduate) nurses, eight to ten student nurses, and four orderlies. But since the school could not produce head nurses before it had been in existence for at least three years (four years for graduate nurses), and since the school itself would open concurrently with the new Lakeside, the hospital would be forced to hire paid graduates to make up fully three quarters of its nursing corps for at least its first three years of operation.

The estimated cost of these extra nurses, according to McMillan, would be $40 per month for a night supervisor, $30 per month for each head nurse, and $20 per month for each graduate nurse (the latter to provide their own uniforms). The trustees directed McMillan to write to various graduate nurses in the city with an offer of temporary employment in the new hospital at the rate of $20 per month, with the understanding that they would eventually be replaced by training school students as the latter progressed.

Shortly thereafter, McMillan was obliged to inform the trustees that, while she had indeed written to a number of nurses in the city, "some of these letters have remained unanswered [while] others have expressed indignation at the [salary] offer." The trustees reluctantly agreed to up their offer to $25 per month, and they informed McMillan that she could promise as much as $30 if necessary. Under no circumstances, however, was she to exceed the latter figure.

The board's initial reluctance to offer more than $240 per year—a pittance, even in 1897—for the services of a trained graduate nurse would appear to be nothing more than the worst sort of shortsighted parsimony. In truth, though, the Lakeside trustees were at last coming to the realization that the cost of operating their elaborate new facility would be enormous, and they would have to take advantage of every opportunity to effect savings of even the smallest amounts. The new Lakeside, so much larger and demanding of so many more services and service personnel than the hospital's previous homes, would consume dollars the way a roaring fire burned fuel.

The existing service payroll, for example—which included the salaries of Knowles ($2,250 per year) and McMillan ($1,000), as well as those of a chief engineer ($1,200), one assistant engineer ($600), one steward ($600), one housekeeper ($600), one carpenter ($540), one gardener ($540), one laundryman ($480), one apothecary ($480), one fireman ($480), one clerk ($480), one night watchman ($420), and one porter ($360)—already totaled out at slightly more than $10,000 per year, roughly ten percent of the projected annual operating budget of the new hospital. And even more personnel—cooks, orderlies, porters, doorkeepers, charwomen and laundresses, clerks, bookkeepers, and the like, a payroll of about one hundred people in all—would eventually have to be added.

Contrary to their attitude toward increasing the pay of nurses, however, the trustees did not so much as quibble when Superintendent Knowles raised the possibility of increasing the number of visiting physicians on staff, a move that would ultimately entail considerably more expense. Knowles had, however, a perfectly good rationale for suggesting the addition of another visiting surgeon and an additional visiting gynecologist, and he summarized his reasoning in a lengthy memo to the board in November 1897.

"Medical men, perhaps more than any other profession, are subjected to the likes and dislikes of the laymen," wrote Knowles, who had a keen understanding of public perceptions but something of a problem with written English. "The more widely known one becomes, the more enemies he has.... Many [prospective] patients would go elsewhere for treatment, simply because of some fancied grievance or prejudice against the one available operator here...." By adding, however, "at least one prominent name to each of the [surgical and gynecological] staffs," he continued, "[we] will certainly increase the attraction for patients to enter the hospital. Furthermore, these appointments, if made from the ranks of men prominent in their particular line of work, would naturally be an influence in securing a greater private-room attendance, and, as a result, more revenue and popularity for the hospital."

In his own convoluted way, Knowles had delineated a theory that would eventually be put into practice not only by hospital administrators but, in later years, by shopping mall developers and movie producers as well. Creating a confederation of two or more luminaries—be they in medicine, retailing, or entertainment—should increase exponentially the number of customers who might not otherwise be willing to pay for the goods or services offered by an individual component of the confederation.

On paper, at least, the theory of the drawing power of star quality was a viable one, and in practice it would work quite well in various applications. Even at Lakeside, for example, its implementation some two years later would, for a while, yield substantial dividends. But the theory failed to take into account one very real possibility: the luminaries themselves might grow to loathe one another—so much so, in fact, that their mutual discontent could threaten the stability of the institution that had brought them together in the first place.

At the time of the Knowles memo, however, the Lakeside board had more immediate questions to address than the addition of a new doctor or two. Their hospital, the great stone and brick complex on the lakefront, was at last nearing completion, and the trustees and Board of Managers were busy attending to last-minute details and arrangements for the dedication of the new institution. By the beginning of the new year the final coats of paint were being applied, and at two o'clock on the rainy Wednesday afternoon of January 12, 1898, a select group of nearly six hundred supporters and guests crowded into the cavernous waiting room of the hospital's dispensary building to see the new Lakeside for the first time.

The hospital's old ally, the Cleveland *Leader*, had already devoted almost an entire page to a description of the new hospital facilities on the Sunday preceding the inaugural festivities, and with typical *Leader* hyperbole the newspaper had lauded the new Lakeside as "the best exemplification of an ideal hospital in the light of the science of the present day." But to the guests who toured the vast complex at its dedication—particularly those who recalled the early days at the little house on Wilson Street —the *Leader*'s characterization of the new hospital might not have seemed particularly overblown.

The three-story central administration building alone was so large that it could accommodate the hospital's general offices, the apothecary's room, a small kitchen and dining room, living apartments for the superintendent and the dozen house officers (the senior and junior residents), a reception room, and even a sunroom. Running east and west at the rear of the administration building was the four-hundred-foot-long, ten-foot-wide main corridor, which connected almost all of the buildings of the complex. To the east was one of the hospital's twin two-story common ward pavilions and, beyond that, the children's ward, another separate pavilion.

The wards themselves were sixty feet long and thirty-two feet wide, with fourteen-foot ceilings and large windows along their eastern and western walls, to afford ample sunlight at all times of day. Described by the *Leader* as "exceedingly cheerful," the interiors of the wards featured polished hardwood floors, white iron bedsteads (or cribs in the children's wards), glass-topped white iron bedside "antiseptic tables," and walls and ceilings painted a dark yellow, with matching window blinds. As the *Leader* noted, "Long experience and many experiments with colors have proved conclusively that ocher is the most desirable color for the sickroom."

At the south end of each floor a solarium with large bay windows, couches, easy chairs, and "soft rugs" provided a pleasant open sitting area for recuperating patients. Bathrooms on either side of the sunroom featured walls of white marble and porcelain bathtubs "imported from Europe." And each ward pavilion had a laundry chute running from the top floor to the basement, a feature that obviated the necessity of carrying soiled linen through the wards and halls. Ever inclined to boosterism, the

Leader claimed that "no other hospital in the world" could boast of a similar innovation.

To the north of the children's ward was the three-story nurses' home, whose basement held lecture and dining rooms while the first floor housed living apartments for the school prinicpal and the matron as well as a large reception room. The two upper floors were reserved solely for living quarters for the hospital's twenty nurses, each floor having a common sitting room as well. Just west of the nurses' home was the private pavilion, two stories high like the ward pavilions but divided into fifty-two individual patient rooms, with sunrooms on the north end of the building—the end with the best view of the lake.

To the west of the administration building was the second adult common ward pavilion. Farther west, at the southwest corner of the hospital's property, was the huge dispensary building, another three-story affair that boasted a number of small examination rooms surrounding a twenty-four-hundred-square-foot, fifty-foot-high waiting room large enough to accommodate three hundred and fifty people at one time. The third floor of the building was given over to lecture rooms for medical students and younger house officers.

Immediately to the north of the dispensary was the surgical amphitheater, also used for instruction of students and house officers. The main operating theater—all white, except for the glass skylights and the brass railing that separated the tiered seats from the operating stage—was surrounded by four private operating rooms. The basement housed an X-ray room and the hospital's emergency admitting ward, which was to be staffed day and night.

Due north of the amphitheater were the laboratories of the pathology building and the autopsy and morgue facilities. At the northwestern corner of the property was the powerhouse and laundry building, with its four steam boilers, two electric dynamos, and ice-making facilities on the first floor, and, on the second, a laundry capable of processing up to fourteen thousand pieces per week. The powerhouse basement was constructed to extend under the adjacent tracks of the Lake Shore & Michigan Southern Railroad, so that entire cars of coal could be unloaded directly into the furnace room.

Next to the service building was the three-story kitchen building, whose uppermost floor served as housing for the hospital's live-in domestic staff. The second floor was the great kitchen itself, with its huge stoves and ovens and the dumbwaiters that would take prepared meals to a basement corridor for transport in rolling heated carts to the other buildings of the complex.

All of the hospital's dozen buildings were illuminated with electric lighting, and all of the drinking water to be used would first be filtered and then boiled in the complex's own equipment. Floors and walls were constructed of fireproof materials, so that, in board president McBride's words, "the danger of a holocaust is entirely obliterated." McBride also described the hospital's sewer system as being "as near perfect as can be made" because it emptied directly into the lake "without any connection whatever with the city sewers."

An elaborate internal telephone system, complete with switchboard, provided communication between the buildings. Normal capacity of the hospital would be approximately two hundred and fifty beds, but there was easily sufficient space to accommodate three hundred in an emergency situation, such as an epidemic. There was also ample room to build additional wards if they were needed; in addition to a separate but contiguous lot to the east of the complex, which the trustees had purchased with the hope that a maternity hospital could eventually be built there, the open lawns surrounding the existing buildings were so ample that in the summer, awning tents and settees could be set up for those patients who were sufficiently recovered to avail themselves of the sunshine and lake breezes.

No patient, it was promised, would ever be turned away; admission would be open "irrespective of race, creed or color." Indigents, of course, would pay nothing for their care, while paying patients on the open wards would be charged $1 per day, and private patients would pay between $12 and $50 per week, the higher prices being charged for those rooms in the private pavilion with the best views. Every patient from outside the city would be charged full price for all services.

Although the hospital did not own an ambulance and had no intention of buying one, Superintendent Knowles had already procured a service to transport emergency cases to Lakeside. Following standard business practice of the time, Knowles contracted with a firm called Hogan and Sharer, one of the "several undertakers [who] have applied to me for the privilege of running their ambulance in connection with this hospital." Knowles also initiated a new practice with the ambulance service, sending along on every call "a Lakeside surgeon, properly equipped to meet any ordinary emergency that is likely to arise." (The superintendent had sold his idea to the trustees by saying that he believed "if this method is established…it will do a great deal towards popularizing [Lakeside] with the people….")

The entire complex—buildings, equipment, and land, including the additional lot next door—constituted a $600,000 investment (some $38 million in equivalent modern dollars), with roughly $400,000 of the total already raised in donations. Superintendent Knowles estimated the hospital's annual operating budget at about $95,000, with annual revenues of $25,000 from paying patients and $10,000 from endowment earnings— figures that left a substantial difference to be made up each year by contributors.

The specter of unpaid construction bills and inevitable annual operating deficits did not, however, dampen the enthusiasm of the guests at the new Lakeside's dedication, even when the subject came up in an address by one member of the board of trustees during the hour-long ceremony that preceded the open-house tours of the complex. The other speakers that day—visiting staff chairman Hunter H. Powell; the Board of Managers' Isabel Robb; Western Reserve University president Charles F. Thwing; Worcester R. Warner, president of the Cleveland Chamber of Commerce and partner in the machine-tool manufacturer Warner and Swasey; and C. Irving Fisher, superintendent of New York's Presbyterian Hospital—all addressed topics that reflected the high ideals and accomplishments of medicine in general and hospitals in particular. But it was Lee McBride, president of the Lakeside board, who would add a more somber note to the festivities.

Charged with relating the by-then standardized historical sketch of the hospital and its many previous incarnations, McBride made a slight detour toward the end of his speech, turning off onto a path well worn in many a previous annual report. "When we open the doors of new Lakeside, we shall not do it without some apprehension for the future," he intoned. "We shall have to face that American entanglement—debt. We ask you, and all citizens of Cleveland, to open your hearts and your purses, that new Lakeside may be freed from this burden."

It was also, in all likelihood, McBride himself who later buttonholed a reporter to dictate what turned out to be the most appropriate ending for the *Leader*'s coverage of the dedication ceremony. "'Make prominent this idea [in your article],'" the unnamed member of the board was quoted as saying. "'The opening of the hospital offers opportunity for the giving of useful donations, endowments and bequests.'"

§

Five days after the dedication ceremony, both the new Lakeside and the new Lakeside Nurses' Training School officially opened their doors. For nearly two years Lakeside Hospital had simply ceased to exist, and the return of the three-decade-old institution—housed, now, in its grand new buildings on the lakefront—was cause not only for celebration on the part of the people who had made it all possible, but also for thanks from those who most needed the services the hospital could provide. Clevelanders believed they had one of the finest health-care facilities in the country, a hospital that had weathered untold storms and survived to take a permanent place in the very heart of the city, its future assured.

Or so it must have seemed. Although no one realized it at the time, however, a number of factors had already begun to undermine the future of the new Lakeside, not the least of which was the very location of the hospital itself. The railroad along the lakefront—proximity to which had been considered an asset because it minimized the time and expense involved in receiving shipments of coal and other supplies—would soon be perceived as a distinct liability, as increasing rail traffic produced increasing amounts of smoke, dirt, noise, and vibration. Teaching clinicians might tell their students that putting a stethoscope to a patient's chest just as a westbound freight roared past was a valuable experience because it forced the student to concentrate fully on the task at hand, but before long no one could deny the overall deleterious effect of being so close to the railroad right-of-way.

Perhaps the most devastating factor for the new Lakeside, however, had its origins in an event that occurred fully four years before the opening of the lakefront complex. In 1894, the same year that Lakeside recruited Hunter Robb from Johns Hopkins, another Baltimore alumnus, William Travis Howard, was enticed to Cleveland to establish the position of visiting pathologist at Lakeside, a position which had not theretofore existed. The hiring of Howard—for that matter, the inclusion of a well-equipped pathology laboratory among the new hospital's buildings —was a reflection of the growing importance of scientific research in the pursuit of a clearer understanding of disease. And it was this new understanding, achieved over a period of years, that would ultimately seal the fate of the new Lakeside.

If the germ theory and the concepts of antisepsis and asepsis were on the scene long before the advent of the new Lakeside, they were, nonetheless, not wholly accepted immediately. None of the ideas that marked turn-of-the-century medicine's watershed era of change emerged full-blown, and none was quickly accorded the status of conventional wisdom. John Shaw Billings, revered as the designer of Johns Hopkins, had, for example, accepted early on the premise that minute bits of organic matter—at the time, agents of unknown origin and mode of propagation—were probably responsible for disease. But Billings also believed that impure "emanations" from such sources as the ground itself would cause disease when disseminated through the air. He could not renounce the old notion that "purified" air would in some way lessen the incidence or spread of disease in hospitals. Indeed, Billings was such a clean-air fanatic that he did not include elevators in the Johns Hopkins buildings, believing their shafts to be nothing more than natural conduits for miasmatic "bad" air. As a result, for years Johns Hopkins patients on stretchers were carried between floors by hand.

But as the watershed era of change wore on, all of medicine finally came to accept and embrace the concept of asepsis—which, by definition, made Cleveland's newest hospital an outmoded institution. The new Lakeside may well have been a grand and beautiful creation—the pride of its community—but it was a monument to yesterday's notion of modernity, and it was obsolete even before it opened its doors. The work of such investigators as the German Robert Koch, who isolated individual organisms and identified them as specific causes of disease, would prove that air in and of itself was not a growth medium for mysterious unknowable agents.

The real agents of disease could be seen, labeled, and targeted for destruction with specific remedies, and hospitals themselves could, just as Lister had always insisted, be made as close to germ-free as possible. And if the wards, beds, bandages, surgical instruments—everything, including the doctors' hands—with which the patient came in contact during his hospital stay were to be kept free of contamination, then the precautions taken to assure the removal of the unseen and unknowable agents of disease thought to exist in so-called "bad" air were a complete and utter waste. The elaborate atmospheric-cleansing mechanisms of hospitals like Johns Hopkins and Lakeside—all the chimneys, ducts, screens, shafts, filters, coils, fans, and vents that were designed, built, and installed at such great expense—would, in the event, be virtually pointless. And if all the variegated paraphernalia of the pavilion plan's pure-air crusaders had no real value, then a pavilion-plan hospital was less a marvel of the modern age than an untenable cluster of a great number of small, inefficient structures spread out across a few acres and connected by long walkways that made movement between buildings a tiring and time-consuming business and militated against efficiency at the very time when it was most needed, as urban populations (and, by extension, *hospital* populations) began to increase dramatically.

For the new Lakeside in its first year, however, a nearby railroad and even the possibility that it was housed in an outdated, ridiculously expensive physical plant were not questions of immediate import. By 1899, when Samuel Mather was elected president of the Lakeside board of trustees, the hospital's annual report was the cause of alarm, because it revealed painfully disappointing numbers for the first twelve months of operation.

True, some members of the burgeoning middle class were beginning to come to the hospital for paid health care, as evidenced by a patient roster that listed merchants and bank clerks along with blacksmiths, coopers, slate roofers, a cigar maker, and even an elevator boy. But of all the categories of labor represented by the patients at Lakeside, by far the largest was "No Occupation"—an indication that the carriage trade, the moneyed captains of industry and their families who were the hospital's most constant supporters, were still reluctant to enter Lakeside as anything but interested visitors.

The hospital's most pressing problem was revenue, and the only way to generate more was to attract more private patients. Just as Superintendent Knowles had advised even before the hospital opened, more high-profile doctors had to be added to the visiting staff if Lakeside were to make any progress in drawing the "rich and well-to-do." But if the trustees acknowledged Knowles's theory—that new recruits should be men prominent in their "line of work" to attract more potential admissions—they were also mindful of their responsiblity to the hospital's historic mission and to the institution's role in the greater venue of medicine itself. The Lakeside board therefore determined to seek candidates for the visiting staff from among the brightest of the bright young men of the era.

One such man was to be found, not surprisingly, at the Johns Hopkins Hospital. Just thirty years old at the time, Harvey Cushing combined a penetrating intellect and a superhuman capacity for work with a deft and delicate touch in the operating room, and he was clearly destined for greatness. A graduate of Yale and the Harvard Medical School, his professional reputation—even then, early in his career—was already beginning to pique the interest of a number of institutions, each searching for a luminary of precisely those qualities that Lakeside sought. But Cushing was just completing his third year as resident surgeon under his mentor, Halsted, and although the offer to return to Cleveland was tempting—he would have particularly enjoyed being closer to his family and practicing medicine alongside his brother Edward—he decided that the prestige of and resources available to him at Johns Hopkins would more readily enable him to achieve his goals.

With Cushing's refusal, the Lakeside trustees and Western Reserve faculty were forced to continue their search for a new associate visiting surgeon. If they could not get Cushing, they reasoned, they would look for someone like Cushing, a young doctor who was not only a skillful practitioner but also a competent teacher and dedicated researcher, a man without fear of the new, with a willingness to find inventive solutions to old problems, with the ability to keep abreast of and contribute to the great stream of breakthroughs that ran so rapidly through medicine's era of change.

After searching for nearly a year, they ultimately found the man they sought in their own backyard. He was a peripatetic surgeon who was already straining the facilities of six different Cleveland area hospitals and who, in his spare time, conducted experimental research on a raft of timely problems. He was, to be sure, a second choice, but a second choice with whom the trustees were perfectly comfortable. In the autumn of 1900, therefore, the post of associate visiting surgeon at Lakeside Hospital was officially offered to and accepted by a thirty-six-year-old former farmboy by the name of George Washington Crile.

CHAPTER FOUR

War of the Ages

Lakeside Hospital's annual report for the year ending December 31, 1898 —the first report reflecting operations in the newly opened multistructure facility on the lakefront—presented a study in contrasts and mixed emotions. With pardonable pride the trustees included such phrases as "magnificent institution," "beyond comparison," and "second to none" to describe the new Lakeside. But the report also mentioned the clear need for a separate maternity building and an isolation ward, neither of which would be attainable in the near future without new and decidedly large gifts from the community. And the report went on to describe the new hospital's preceding twelve months as "a year of perplexities," foremost among which was a "mortgage indebtedness of nearly $200,000...on which we pay interest at the rate of four percent per annum."

The hospital's supporters were, therefore, "earnestly requested" to help liquidate this debt by means of "generous gifts or bequests." Indeed, in what was virtually his last official act as president of the board of trustees before turning over that office to Sam Mather, Lee McBride once again wrote out a plea for funds, offering the reminder that "it remains very largely with our friends to determine how far we can extend [Lakeside's] field of usefulness—whether or not we can use every facility to its utmost limit, or be obliged to restrict our work for lack of sufficient income."

Nothing if not punctilious, the annual report included complete lists of all the donors to the new hospital's various funds. Sam and Flora Mather, for example, had contributed a total of more than $73,000 to the land acquisition, construction, and maintenance accounts. Mrs. Stephen V. Harkness, widow of the Standard Oil partner, had provided some $50,000, while Mary H. Severance and her son Louis together gave more than $41,000. Even John Lund Woods, the benefactor of the Western

Reserve School of Medicine back in 1885, was duly listed as having contributed nearly $50,000 for the new Lakeside, and at the time of the re-
port, Woods had already been dead for five years.

Of course, not all donations to the hospital were as large (the modern
equivalent of from two to three million dollars), nor were all contributions monetary in nature. There was a $20 gift from the Women's Benevo-
lent Society of the Woodland Avenue Presbyterian Church, $25 from the
law firm of Squire, Sanders & Dempsey, $150 from the White Sewing
Machine Company, and $300 from Mrs. Isaac Leisy, wife of one of Cleve-
land's most successful brewers. There were also a dozen "white flannel
blouse waists" from Mrs. Charles Bingham, wife of the local iron magnate, and five pairs of bedroom slippers from the Ladies' Auxiliary of
Trinity Cathedral. At holiday time, the Board of Lady Managers traditionally provided the ingredients for festive meals for the patients: Mrs.
William Chisholm, whose family fortune also derived from iron and steel,
gave two turkeys and one bunch of celery, while Mrs. Benjamin Rose,
wife of Cleveland's largest meat packer, gave one box of cranberries. Mrs.
E.W. Oglebay chipped in with three dozen oranges and three dozen bananas, and Mrs. R. Livingston Ireland (iron, steel, the American Ship-
building Company, *et al.*) provided four quarts of mincemeat and two
quarts of pickles. There were also ongoing gifts of sheets, pillow cases,
and lengths of cheesecloth, as well as towels, socks, mosquito netting,
nightshirts, sponges, combs, tablecloths, handkerchiefs, and even bottles
of wine. On Christmas Day, a visiting entertainer from Chicago named
C.C. Case donated his time and talent to sing in each of the wards.

In his report to the board, superintendent James Knowles called the
new hospital's first year of operation "creditably successful," but this was
something of an exaggeration. Revising downward their occupancy estimates even before the 1898 opening, the trustees had already abandoned
the original concept of separate male and female ward pavilions. The two
structures were redesignated as "medical" and "surgical" pavilions, with
males to be housed on the first floor of each building and females on the
second floor. And even after that downsizing, in the hospital's first years
the medical ward would still not be opened; medical patients were relegated to one floor of the children's pavilion "until the number of patients
and increased revenues of the hospital permit the opening of the medical
building."

Noting that on opening day Lakeside was not yet equipped to receive
its full complement of two hundred and fifty patients—in fact, there were

sufficient beds for just sixty percent of the hospital's planned capacity—Knowles acknowledged that less than fourteen hundred patients had received treatment in the wards and private rooms, and of these only about forty percent were paying patients. The number of patients actually in the hospital on any given day averaged out to a paltry seventy-seven, slightly more than half of even the reduced capacity. Reviewing these numbers at the time, Dr. E.P. Carter, the senior medical resident, openly expressed his disappointment with what he termed the "paucity of [clinical] material" available in the charity wards. Other Lakeside physicians wondered aloud if the hospital would *ever* fill all of its beds.

Among the patients admitted in the first year were the usual cases of tuberculosis, influenza, chronic nephritis, gastroenteritis, and pneumonia—the latter the most consistently lethal of all the diseases seen—along with nearly two dozen cases of chronic alcoholism. The surgical division recorded twenty-eight fractures, thirty-four cases of appendicitis, twelve uterine tumors, and fifteen cancers of the breast. And before long, entire wards were filled with typhoid patients, further evidence of what pathologist William T. Howard called the "stupid ignorance" of Cleveland's city government, which seemed intent on ignoring the basic necessities of "modern hygiene."

But the Lakeside doctors, particularly the surgeons, were already beginning to undertake much more demanding work with far more confidence than they could have had only a few years before. As they came closer to achieving a true aseptic environment in the operating room, they were able to perform all manner of previously impossible procedures, particularly in the abdominal cavity, theretofore a region into which surgical invasion more often than not proved a lethal gamble. Still, the mortality rate for such operations was roughly twice that of surgery on other regions of the body. Peritonitis, for example, was a major killer, as were a host of infections directly attributable to the very act of opening the body under less than perfect aseptic conditions.

Of course, Lakeside's mortality statistics were skewed somewhat toward the negative because so often patients—particularly charity cases—retained the old fear of hospitals as houses of death. As a consequence, they tended to put off seeking treatment until they were in such desperate condition that nothing could save them. Others had more valid reasons for avoiding the hospital until the last minute: in some years, for example, nearly thirty percent of the deaths in the gynecological division were of women who arrived at Lakeside with advanced infections resulting from illegal backstreet or self-induced abortions. And the children of poor and uneducated immigrants were often the innocent victims of their parents' lack of knowledge. In one case, an eight-year-old girl who died from a streptococcus infection had first been brought to the Lakeside dispensary only after experiencing a "purulent vaginal discharge" for *two years.*

Despite such factors, however, by 1899 the combined services at Lakeside were able to discharge nearly ninety percent of their patients as either materially improved or fully cured. Some of this record should have been attributed to the human body's own recuperative powers, however, because as yet surgeons still did not wear masks and Lakeside's operating rooms actually had windows—windows that, even when closed, allowed small amounts of dust to blow in directly from the unpaved street that ran parallel to the hospital's western edge.

Fortunately, chief surgeon Dudley P. Allen was a firm believer in antiseptic surgical techniques, particularly the use of sterile rubber gloves. Some of his peers, however, still dismissed gloves as valueless impediments. Even one of the Mayo brothers, founders of the famous Minnesota clinic that bore their name, was opposed to the idea. Once, when a visiting surgeon credited his success with a dangerous operation to the fact that he had worn gloves during the procedure, Mayo replied that he had achieved the same results while wearing rubber *boots.*

If patients in the new Lakeside received more able care than they would have even a few years before, they were, nevertheless, expected to follow all of the same guidelines for proper behavior that had applied in the hospital's previous homes. Indeed, house rules in the new facility were even more stringent than those in the hospital's original Wilson Street building. In addition to the old strictures against drinking, smoking, card playing, and profanity, for example, the new rules also forbade patients to "express immoral or infidel sentiments," a rather expansive prohibition open, it would seem, to broad interpretation. And in a throwback to 1865, when the fear of proselytizing Catholics had so dominated the minds of the hospital's founders, visiting clergy of all faiths were instructed to "confine their conversation to persons of their own creed or denomination, and to refrain from addressing or distributing books or pamphlets to other patients...." As in previous years, ambulatory charity patients were still expected to help out with light housekeeping chores. Not long after the opening of the new Lakeside, it also became necessary to post a rule forbidding friends of patients from entering operating rooms without the superintendent's consent. Some visitors had been wandering into surgical suites in mid-operation, to check on the progress of their loved ones.

By far the most successful element of the new hospital complex was the dispensary operated jointly by Lakeside and the Medical Department of Western Reserve University, although even this most accessible part of the hospital was operating far below capacity. Nonetheless, Cleveland's poor did come by the score for the free care offered there. In its first year of operation the dispensary recorded some eighteen thousand patient visits: children suffering from malnutrition, worms, typhoid, rickets, and whooping cough; men and women with crushed fingers and fractured limbs, sprains, wounds, typhus, heart ailments of every description, neurasthenia (the latter a new moniker for the old catchall, "debility"), and sciatica. One man came in and asked to have a fishhook removed from his hand.

The dispensary was valuable in a number of respects, not least in that it provided opportunities for medical students to see at first hand a wide variety of diseases, ailments, and injuries, and it allowed interns to gain experience in diagnosis and treatment. The community, of course, benefited most of all, because aside from a ten-cent charge for prescriptions and surgical dressings, the care provided was free. But the latter fact also meant that the dispensary would always run in the red, and although the hospital and medical school shared most of the costs of the facility—the university subsidized the facility with an annual $1,000 payment to Lakeside—the expenses drew down even further the hospital's meager resources. Indeed, the very popularity of the dispensary only served to increase Lakeside's first-year total operating deficit of some $57,000.

Just how far below capacity the hospital was operating was made amply clear in September and October of 1898, when the new Lakeside underwent its first large-scale emergency. Nearly two hundred members of the Fifth Ohio Volunteer Infantry, a unit called to service in the Spanish-American War, which had erupted in the spring of that year, were brought to the hospital for extended care. Suffering primarily from typhoid and malaria (far more soldiers were disabled by disease and accidents than by combat wounds in the war's short duration), the soldiers were placed in the one unopened charity ward building and on the as-yet unused second floor of the private pavilion. But if Lakeside had ample room for a sudden influx of new patients, there was still insufficient equipment to accommodate them all. With its anemic income from paying patients and its constantly growing expenses, the hospital simply could not afford to furnish and open wards that would not be used to their capacity. The veterans from the Fifth O.V.I. would, therefore, receive care at Lakeside, but they were forced to sleep on cots borrowed from various sources around town.

One reason for the paucity of private, full-pay patients at Lakeside was, quite simply, competition. By the turn of the century, Cleveland and its environs boasted of more than a dozen hospitals, many of them less than ten years old. Most of these institutions had religious affiliations, having been founded by the various denominations represented in the great flow of European immigrants that was swelling the area's population. Each tended to attract potential patients—especially paying patients —from its own relatively homogeneous neighborhood. The quality of care available at the new Lakeside was still not sufficient inducement to bring these people across the length of the city. Each new facility, sectarian or not, therefore represented an increasing drain on the available patient population.

By the end of 1899, after accumulating another substantial operating deficit for the year, the hospital's board tried a more systematic and businesslike approach to fund raising. Trustees and members of the board of managers were assigned lists of potential donors—usually their friends and business acquaintances—and given small, bound subscription books in which to record names and contributions. The innovation had the advantage of being more methodical than previous fund-raising efforts while still retaining the personal touch of one-on-one canvassing, and its effectiveness was soon proved.

In addition to blank pages on which to record donations, each subscription book also contained a message from board president Mather outlining the hospital's needs. According to Mather, the most urgent necessity was for "large gifts" to the endowment funds, followed in importance by sufficient donations to liquidate the operating deficits that had accumulated over the preceding two years. Finally, additional monies were needed in the form of "guaranty pledges," amounts which individuals would promise to provide on an annual basis until income from the endowment funds could meet the yearly budgets.

In truth, Mather had listed the hospital's needs in inverse order, either by design—perhaps to alleviate the fears of the hospital's supporters—or through wishful thinking. Lakeside's most urgent requirement was, in fact, a positive cash flow, and with little in the way of income from patients, the "guaranty pledges" took on added importance. Historically, endowment funds were the most difficult and time-consuming to develop, and the hospital needed monies more quickly to deal with daily expenses and the ever-growing deficits. A more business-oriented sensibility was clearly called for at the time, and although it was not apparent from Mather's written plea for contributions, new hospital policies would reveal that the trustees were indeed thinking along those lines.

To improve cash flow and minimize the possibility of uncollectable billings, for example, the new Lakeside began to demand from patients occupying private rooms an advance deposit the equivalent of two weeks' worth of room and board charges. And for the first time in its history, the hospital started to monitor the precise nature of its charity work. Too many patients, it seemed, were sneaking through the system as charity cases when in fact they had the wherewithal to pay. In May of 1900, therefore, the hospital hired a clerk whose primary responsibility was to search for possible hidden financial resources of individuals applying for care as indigents. The message to patients was clear: if they could afford to pay even a small sum toward the actual cost of their treatment they would have to do so.

Within months of its introduction, the trustees' subscription-book fundraising plan was succeeding so well that the hospital's combined two-year operating deficit was reduced to just $21,000. And in March of 1900, even that balance was retired when John D. Rockefeller—an unlikely source, since his philanthropies had usually been directed toward the city's Homeopathic hospital—made a one-time donation to cover the amount. The number of paying patients also increased during the year, so much so that the second floor of the private pavilion was at last furnished, equipped, and opened.

Free of at least one portion of its debt for the first time, the new Lakeside should then have begun to settle into a stable operating routine. Yet internal divisions among the medical staff itself would soon cause new headaches for the board. Obstetrician Hunter Powell, the hospital's chief visiting physician, was, for example, chronically unhappy with the absence of a separate maternity building on the Lakeside grounds, and he missed no opportunity to lobby for such a facility. At the time Cleveland claimed two maternity "hospitals" within its borders, but each was small, understaffed, underequipped, and underfunded. Indeed, the accommodations available locally for "confinement" cases were so inadequate that the Lakeside Nurses' Training School was forced to send its students to

the Society of the Lying-In Hospital in New York to receive their required
three months' training in maternity work. As for the new Lakeside, Powell insisted repeatedly, it could never be considered "complete" without
maternity wards.

Everyone associated with Lakeside agreed that a maternity building
was a necessary adjunct to the general hospital; additional property had,
after all, been purchased for just that reason. But nothing could be done
without donors to underwrite the project, and the trustees were more
concerned with maintaining daily operations than with mounting another
building campaign. Powell was therefore reduced to frequent grumbling
to the board about the inadequacies of the "finest hospital west of the
Alleghenies."

But the consequences of Powell's dissatisfaction were minor in comparison with the bitter feelings engendered late in 1900, when a full-scale
territorial war erupted, the first of many that would flare up repeatedly
over the years in various departments of the new hospital. In the new
century's first major internal battle, Dudley P. Allen led the surgery
department in competition against Hunter Robb and his gynecology department, each camp seeking more control over female surgical candidates admitted to Lakeside's charity wards. Unable to reconcile their differences, both sides ultimately vied for the favor of the trustees, putting
forth their own formulas for determining just where general surgery left
off and gynecological surgery began.

After protracted wrangling, a trustee-mediated compromise was
reached and specific new rules were formulated. Thenceforth, all female
general surgical cases, as well as "all abdominal cases not connected with
the female organs of reproduction," would go directly to the surgery department. All "diseases of the female external genitalia...including lacerations, [all] diseases of the cervix, malposition of uterus and all operations pertaining to adherent tubes and ovaries and suspension of the
uterus" would go to gynecology.

A further element of the compromise, one revealing clearly to what
depths of childishness the squabbling had descended, called for all cases
"in which there is a question of disease...requiring abdominal operation"
to be examined first by the gynecology department. The resulting diagnosis would then be filed in a book in the superintendent's office, where
it would be open to the "inspection" of the surgical department. If the
diagnosis were questioned by any member of the surgical department—if,
in other words, the general surgeons believed the gynecological surgeons

were making off with what should have been one of *their* patients—the entire matter would be turned over to the consideration of a three-member committee consisting of visiting pediatrician Edward Cushing, visiting opthalmologist Benjamin Millikin, and visiting dermatologist William Corlett, "whose decision with regard to such cases shall be final." And just to ensure absolute fairness and an end to the conflict, "all cases of…abdominal hysterectomy and [operations] for ovarian cysts and hernia of the abdominal wall…shall be divided between the two departments alternately."

The net result of the war between the departments of surgery and gynecology was to force the trustees to act as parental authorities, in effect doling out candy equally to two squalling siblings. And in a sense that is exactly what was happening—the candy in this case being access to surgical candidates. Because for a number of reasons it was in the interest of each service to perform as many operations as possible.

Each department chief was, of course, paid for his services by patients when operating on either private or pay-ward cases, and any successes that added to the chief's reputation as a skilled practitioner increased his prestige among both his colleagues and the public. But even though the bulk of the surgery on charity cases was supposed to be performed by each service's house staff, department chiefs still found the "clinical material" of the wards to be of particular value, both for teaching purposes in the twice-a-week clinics held for medical students in the surgical amphitheater, and as subjects upon whom they could try out new techniques. (No surgeon in his right mind would attempt an unproven procedure on a private patient, unless the situation was of such an extreme nature that no other alternative presented itself.)

Even the house staff—a resident surgeon in charge of the wards (appointed at the discretion of the department chief) and his junior resident and intern assistants, all of whom received room and board and small fixed salaries from the hospital, but for whom additional charity cases did not result in additional income—welcomed the chance to perform more surgery. The object of surgical residencies was, after all, that the neophytes should achieve competence in their craft. More work meant more opportunities to hone their skills, which might also result in favorable reputations of their own and, ultimately, paying patients.

There was, of course, a less tangible but no less real incentive for both warring departments and their chiefs. As in virtually all large organizations, power accrued to individuals who controlled resources and territorial prerogatives, and power and its exercise were alluring attractions to many of the more dominating personalities within the hospital.

The trustees were forced, therefore, to turn their attention to refereeing an interdepartmental fight rather than concentrating their energies on promoting new contributions to Lakeside's sustaining funds, at the time the very life blood of the hospital. And the contretemps between the surgeons and the gynecologists was but one of many such altercations, most of them resulting from the department chiefs' disquieting propensity to allow simple disagreements to turn into insoluble problems, with the combatants unwilling to enter into reasonable discussion to work out a compromise between themselves. Time and again an ember of resentment would smolder for long periods and then burst into flame, at which point the trustees would be forced to intervene.

As the surgery-gynecology war illustrated, chief visiting surgeon Dudley P. Allen was never loath to turn to the trustees when he perceived either a challenge to his authority or some incursion into his territory. Allen acquaintances and family members were, after all, well represented on the board, and Allen himself had gained an appreciation of the power a board could wield during the 1893 coup that had so successfully ended the reign of Gustav Weber and brought Allen back from exile and into the hospital and the medical school. As Allen would soon learn, however, the trustees' influence was a two-edged sword.

In the midst of his squabble with the Department of Gynecology, Allen was approached repeatedly by two board members, Ralph Hickox and General George Garretson, the latter a retired army officer who had become a wealthy Cleveland banker. As Allen later recalled, the two trustees expressed their desire that he "make a place" at the hospital for a local surgeon of their acquaintance. Although Superintendent Knowles was still lobbying for the addition of a "name" surgeon to the Lakeside staff even after Harvey Cushing indicated his intention of remaining at Johns Hopkins, Allen was hesitant about adding a new man. By midsummer of 1900, however, the local surgeon touted by the two trustees was himself speaking with Allen, indicating that he would appreciate any spot in the hospital no matter how unimportant, because, as Allen later described the conversation, "what he [mainly] desired was an opportunity to care for his private patients advantageously."

With two interested board members breathing down his neck, Allen must have felt constrained to proceed with discussions, but he insisted that if a position were to be made available, "it must be a wholly subsidiary one"—subsidiary, that is, to the chief visiting surgeon, Allen himself. And as a prerequisite to the offer of any position, the candidate would have to sever his ties to the other local hospitals with which he was associated. These conditions proved acceptable to the new man, however, and before long formal negotiations were held that resulted in an appointment to the Lakeside staff for George W. Crile.

The thirty-six-year-old Crile was already a well-known commodity in much of Cleveland, and had been for most of the preceding decade. Born in 1864 on a farm outside the tiny southern Ohio community of Chili, his quick and agile mind had matured so rapidly that by the age of fifteen he was already teaching in a small country school. A growing interest in medicine led him to Cleveland in 1886 to matriculate at the Wooster Medical School, the reorganized remnant of the old Medical Department of Wooster University that in 1881 had been assimilated into Western Reserve.

The new Wooster school, then under the leadership of Frank J. Weed, was housed in a dilapidated old building in the center of the city. Its two-year course of study included clinical experience in a nearby "hospital"—actually two old homes converted to accommodate a total of thirty beds. Upon his graduation, Crile interned for a year in the small hospital before joining Weed's private practice as his second assistant in 1889.

In addition to his lucrative casualty contracts with the local railroads, Weed also maintained one of the largest private practices in the city, a practice that catered to many of the more prosperous families on the west side of the river. It was through Weed that Crile was initiated into the world of the wealthy, and it was from Weed that he learned the diplomatic skills necessary to win and retain the favor of the well-to-do. Weed himself, of course, was a virtuoso of the art, having learned at the feet of a past master—his old mentor, the redoubtable Gustav Weber.

After Weed's death in 1891, Crile and his co-associate, Frank Bunts, purchased Weed's equipment from his estate and assumed the lease on their old office on the city's west side. They and their own new associate, Crile's cousin, William E. Lower, maintained both the casualty and private practices of their late chief. Crile eventually performed thousands of operations, in hospital settings, private homes, railroad yards, and the hovels of the working-class poor. Through this experience he became a deft and expeditious operator, two attributes that, while no longer absolutely mandatory as in the preanesthetic era, were nonetheless still desirable for surgeons of the day.

Crile's speed with the knife and his apparent boyish glee in tackling prodigious surgical workloads had already earned him a nickname among some of his more mature colleagues, who occasionally referred to him as "The Carver Kid." His abiding interest in discovering solutions to the myriad mysteries still extant in medicine also led him into experimental research, particularly in the area of surgical shock. In 1897 he published a paper on that subject and was awarded the prestigious Cartwright Prize for his efforts, further enhancing his reputation and fulfilling the promise of yet another of his earlier nicknames: "The Warm Proposition from Chili."

In 1898, at the outbreak of the Spanish-American War, Crile finagled a commission as a brigade surgeon in the army. After the war he returned to Cleveland and took up his practice and his research. By the turn of the century, Crile enjoyed a wide circle of acquaintance within the medical community, both at home and abroad, and his abilities were recognized by some of the world's most prominent physicians. He did have his detractors, however, most notably the members of various antivivisection societies around the country, who strenuously opposed the use of animals in medical research. The antivivisectionists targeted a number of prominent doctors and scientists with accusations of cruelty and barbaric treatment of their laboratory subjects, and Crile's prize-winning paper on shock—in which he detailed his experiments on more than one hundred dogs—left him open to some of the group's most virulent rhetoric.

In 1899, a national magazine reprinted excerpts from an article on Crile that had previously appeared in an antivivisectionist publication called "Our Fellow Creatures." Responding to Crile's shock study, the antivivisectionists relied on the simple expedient of cataloguing his own experiments to portray him as having "tortured one hundred and forty-eight dogs to prove what any intelligent person would comprehend with a moment's thought—namely, that 'clean cuts with a knife produce less shock than rough manipulations and lacerations.' So he [proceeded to] tear out nerves, to crush paws and other parts of the body, to open the abdomen and pour boiling water on the intestines, amputate the hip joint, cut the sciatic nerve, apply a gas flame to the knee joint and bowels and paws, and a long list of other atrocities worthy the ingenuity of Satan himself."

Crile's professional reputation was, if anything, enhanced by such attacks, at least among his peers. Many had themselves incurred the wrath of the antivivisectionists, and most could sympathize with Crile's predicament. Surprisingly, the adverse publicity never seemed to affect the number of patients who sought him out. Charming and gregarious, Crile was a genuinely likable fellow, and as his fame grew, Clevelanders expressed pride in their bright new star of medical science. Indeed, by the time of his appointment to Lakeside, Crile was one of the busiest surgeons in the city.

Late in the summer of 1900, the particulars of a working contract between Crile and Dudley P. Allen had already been decided. The gist of the agreement was that a new position—associate visiting surgeon—would be created for Crile. While Allen was on duty—that is, in the city and available to fill his post—Crile would not be considered a member of the staff of the hospital. He would, however, have the use of four beds in the male charity ward and two beds in the female ward, these patients to be cared for on a daily basis by the surgery department's regular assistants. He would be allowed to admit all of his private cases to Lakeside, and he would also be allowed to retain his affiliation with one other hospital—St. Alexis, on the city's southeast side—a privilege that no other member of the visiting staff enjoyed.

When Allen was not on duty, Crile would assume Allen's role as director of the surgical department, taking charge of Allen's ward patients, presenting Allen's teaching clinics to medical students, and acting in every way as a member of the visiting staff. Allen would nominate Crile to a professorship in the Medical Department of Western Reserve University, and, as the terms of their contract pointedly spelled out, Crile was to be "nominated annually by Dr. Allen to his position as associate surgeon...."

As Allen later described the contract to board president Mather, it was "a very generous agreement on my part and a very advantageous one to Dr. Crile."

On August 17th, then, Allen asked his colleagues on the medical school faculty to recommend to the trustees of both the university and the hospital that George Crile be named professor of clinical surgery in the Medical Department of Western Reserve and associate visiting surgeon at Lakeside.

§

In many ways George Crile embodied the spirit of his age, at least as the era was perceived in the United States. Simultaneous with the advent of what would be known as the "American Century" came the century's quintessential brash young man, a former farmboy who had migrated to the city and entered an exciting, rapidly progressing profession which, it seemed, he fully expected to mark with his imprint. He was the classic go-getter, a man who embraced modern thinking and sought to add his own ideas to the intellectual stew that bubbled at the time. With the try-anything attitude of the born adventurer, he seemed to personify the country's growing self-confidence. It was not surprising, then, that the trustees of Lakeside Hospital—despite their inborn conservatism and the baggage of nineteenth-century attitudes they brought with them—eventually found themselves charmed and beguiled by their new associate visiting surgeon.

Lakeside's chief visiting surgeon, however, would soon be harboring a much different opinion of his younger colleague.

In September of 1900, just a few weeks after signing his agreement with Allen and just days before the latter was due to leave on a month-long vacation, Crile appeared at a meeting of the Lakeside Hospital visiting staff. Although the terms of his appointment stipulated specifically that he was not to be considered a member of the staff while Allen was on duty, Crile not only attended the staff meeting but rose to ask that the assistants in the hospital's "outside service"—the interns and junior residents designated to assist those private surgeons with admission privileges who brought their patients to Lakeside—be placed under his sole control. Allen pointed out to the meeting that such a move would violate both the terms of his agreement with Crile and the by-laws of the hospital, because in effect it created a separate surgical service outside the control of the chief visiting surgeon. Yet despite Allen's protest, a majority of the full visiting staff voted to put control of the assistants in the hands of a committee consisting of Hunter Powell, Edward Cushing, and Crile.

By the end of the year, Crile, after making repeated requests of Allen, also received permission to bring in two assistants from his own office practice—Clyde Ford and William E. Lower—to direct the care of his patients on the wards. Although this, too, went far beyond the provisions of the written agreement between chief and associate, Allen, apparently worn down by Crile's persistence, had finally acceded to the request. But even as Crile enjoyed the fruits of his two victories, Allen was beginning to look at his young associate with marked distrust, and before long he was letting his feelings be known.

Years later, writing in his autobiography, Crile professed astonishment at what he claimed to perceive at the time as Allen's sudden shift in attitude toward him. "Scarcely had I begun the work at Lakeside when Dr. Allen looked upon me as a rival," he marveled, seemingly incredulous that Allen could have made so inexplicable and unwarranted an assumption. After all, Crile wrote, Allen was "a well-trained, able, ambitious and successful surgeon, with influential friends and relatives" (the latter phrase, coincidentally, being precisely the same wording that Gustav Weber had used to describe Allen back in 1893). And when compared with Allen, Crile added, "I, who had made my own way, was an alley cat."

That Allen might show concern over Crile's intentions was not, however, particularly surprising. By then approaching the age of fifty, Allen had long since grown accustomed to giving orders and seeing them followed. A prideful man, he expected the obedience and respect he saw as his due as chief visiting surgeon of one of the country's largest medical institutions. Possessed of a personality virtually addicted to the notion of order, he had retooled the surgery department until it functioned with clockwork precision, and it was even said of him that he knew the precise location of every scalpel, syringe, and roll of gauze in the hospital. It is more than likely that the presence of any foreign body in the smoothly running system he had created would have caused him at least some disquiet. And when the foreign body in question was an eager and dynamic younger man who was accustomed to pursuing his own agendas and who seemed to blithely ignore both the letter and the spirit of a very specific written agreement, it is difficult to believe that Allen would not have felt at least concern, if not the beginnings of alarm, as he watched the foundations of his control beginning to erode.

Crile, on the other hand, was wholly disingenuous when he described himself as a mere "alley cat" when compared with the patrician Allen. He already had longstanding relationships with some of the city's better families, thanks to the "silver doorbell" portion of the practice he had inherited from Frank Weed. And he had numerous other "influential friends and relatives" of his own, many of them on the hospital's board of trustees. He had, for example, secured his appointment as a brigade surgeon in the army through the intercession of U.S. Senator Marcus A. Hanna, who had obtained the commission as a favor to their mutual friend, General George Garretson. (The three Hanna brothers—Marcus, hospital board member Leonard, and Howard [who would become a Lakeside trustee in 1903]—were the founders of M.A. Hanna & Company, a huge coal and iron-ore shipping concern. All three were among Crile's wide circle of acquaintance.) Trustees Garretson and Ralph Hickox had already proved their friendship by approaching Dudley P. Allen on Crile's behalf. But by far the most interested party on the Lakeside board was former president Lee McBride, because in February of 1900, Mc-Bride's niece Grace had become Mrs. George W. Crile.

Even before his appointment to Lakeside, therefore, Crile had his own coterie of powerful friends and relations, in the city at large and even on the board of Western Reserve University, where his father-in-law, John H. McBride, was a trustee. And Crile did not hesitate to call on them when he thought they could be helpful.

By midsummer of 1901, Crile—in a move that set the pattern for his tenure at the hospital—was already making a request of the Lakeside board. In this instance he asked that a small room in the hospital be made airtight for use in some experiments he was planning. Superintendent Knowles informed the board that for $30 he could fit up a seldom-used room that had originally been meant for delirium tremens cases, and the board's executive committee issued its approval. The actual cost of the alterations turned out to be $183, but no one on the board expressed even slight concern at still another addition to the year's operating deficit.

Ironically, Knowles's championing of Crile was one of the superintendent's last official acts in the hospital. At the same executive committee meeting at which Crile's request for a laboratory was taken up, board president Mather revealed the results of "careful investigations" he had made pertaining to "certain charges" about the "personal habits" of Knowles, charges that had been submitted to him in writing by an unnamed source. Convinced of the "substantial truth" of the allegations, Mather felt it was "incumbent upon him to recommend that Superintendent Knowles be requested to [submit] his resignation." The executive committee, after inspecting unspecified "evidence" which Mather produced, agreed with his conclusion.

By the beginning of August, Knowles was gone. The exact nature of his "personal habits" that had so disturbed the trustees was never mentioned in the minutes of the meeting at which they were discussed. Indeed, the record of the discussion itself was handwritten by board treasurer Harry A. Garfield (oldest son of the late president) beneath the typed transcription of the minutes of the full committee meeting that had preceded the vote on the Knowles case. The trustees apparently believed the subject to be so sensitive they would not even trust a secretary to know all of the details. No mention of the true nature of Knowles's difficulties ever reached the newspapers, and even the Lakeside annual report that year merely stated that the board had been "compelled to request" the superintendent's resignation "by reason of dissatisfaction with his services."

Soon after Knowles's dismissal, Sam Mather reported on his interview with a candidate for the superintendency, Dr. Archibald J. Ranney, then the thirty-three-year-old superintendent of the Long Island Hospital in Boston. Protracted negotiations with Ranney dragged on for months, but early in December he finally accepted the job.

Just two months later, an incident with overtones similar to the Knowles case resulted in the dismissal of two young residents. The two men had left the hospital for little more than an hour one evening and repaired to a nearby tavern. Upon returning to the hospital they were met by Ranney, the new superintendent, who judged them unfit for duty and ordered them to their rooms. Neither man offered an excuse to the trustees, but each pleaded for clemency on the grounds that dismissal would destroy their careers. The trustees nevertheless voted unanimously to dismiss both men from further service. And as with the Knowles dismissal, no mention of the incident would appear in the local newspapers.

The gag order that the trustees imposed on both cases was typical of the pains they took to avoid news that did not reflect well on the hospital. They were, by and large, fearful of even the slightest negative publicity, both for its potential impact on the public's trust in the institution and for its potential effect on their ability to successfully raise funds. But the trustees were also concerned with maintaining what they perceived as the high moral tone of the hospital, an institution that was, after all, founded as a virtual extension of the church. Thus, patients were required to abide by rules of behavior so strict that they seemed less regulations than commandments, and members of the staff were held to an even higher standard.

Perhaps the most revealing incident of this sort would occur a few years later, when a senior nursing student was absent from the hospital overnight without permission and was seen "drinking wine in the Grill Room of the Hotel Euclid between 12:30 and 1 [a.m.] with two men and another woman." Although the infraction was a seemingly minor and relatively harmless first offense, the nurse involved was given neither reprimand nor warning but was, rather, summarily expelled from service. How much of that decision could be laid to the fact that a rule had indeed been broken and how much to the extremes of moral judgment that the trustees had always adopted toward the hospital is problematic, but it was entirely representative of the standards they imposed, particularly in cases involving junior members of the hospital's staff. It was typical of the trustees' point of view that they would not perceive their sentence of the ultimate penalty—dismissal, with its concomitant black mark on the subject's professional record—as unduly harsh judgment for a first offense when that offense even hinted of moral taint.

The dismissal of an otherwise qualified nurse was, however, a difficult decision at the time, if for no other reason than that the hospital population was at last beginning to rise appreciably and nurses were a precious commodity. By 1902, the average number of patients in the hospital had grown to one hundred and forty-five per day, twice that of the first full year of operation. Although never completely filled on any given day, all of the charity wards were at least now in use; the larger children's pavilion had been converted to accept male medical and surgical patients, while the children were moved to the ground floor of what had been the female pavilion. And both floors of the private pavilion were also in full operation. Pupils in the Lakeside Nurses' Training School, working under the supervision of graduate head nurses, provided the bulk of the nursing services in the hospital, and as the hospital population increased it was not a particularly good idea to lose nurses for whatever reason.

Coincidentally, a nursing-staff change was the precipitating factor for another run-in between chief visiting surgeon Dudley P. Allen and associate surgeon George Crile. In the summer of 1902, while Allen was vacationing out of the city and Crile was temporarily in charge of the hospital's surgical division, Allen's longtime head operating-room nurse resigned to take a similar position at another hospital. Superintendent Ranney hired a graduate nurse to fill the vacant position, presumably after at least some consultation with Crile.

Upon his return to Cleveland, Allen was livid when he discovered the new arrangement, and he resorted to his favored means of resolving disputes: he first took the matter to the visiting staff's monthly meeting with the board's executive committee, and then, two days later, submitted the same issue for the consideration of the full board of trustees.

Allen had previously insisted of Ranney that no head nurses be appointed without first consulting him. Now that a nurse had indeed been hired without his knowledge, Allen wanted the board to authorize the hiring of a second graduate nurse for his operating room, someone of his own choosing. The nurse already hired could, according to Allen, serve as an "alternate"; in effect, she would serve only when Allen was out of town and his duties were taken on by Crile. Board president Sam Mather, who raised the question at the board meeting only because Allen had officially requested he do so, was opposed to the surgeon's suggestion. He dismissed the idea with undisguised annoyance, saying that Allen "had not much reason to complain and should not have brought the matter up" at all. The full board eventually vetoed the proposal on the basis of cost; at a time when the hospital was still running a deficit, it was unwise to take on another nurse's salary, even when the salary was just a few hundred dollars a year—little more than the cost of outfitting Crile's laboratory in the old delerium tremens room.

Allen received more bad news in 1902 when Mary Severance, one of his staunchest supporters on the board, died. The following year saw the death of Samuel Williamson, another Allen friend, whose place on the board of trustees was filled by Howard M. Hanna, a Crile partisan. It was a particularly bad time to be losing allies on the board, because relations between Allen and Crile had by then reached a new low point. Allen felt aggrieved on two counts: not only had Crile managed to gain virtual control of the outside surgical assistants—in effect, a separate surgical service beyond what Allen called his "sphere of influence"—but he was also negligent in overseeing the work of Allen's assistants and enforcing the strict discipline of Allen's service when the older man was absent from the city.

At a luncheon meeting at the Union Club in mid-1903, Allen spelled out his discontent to three trustees: the Crile loyalist Ralph Hickox; Allen's own father-in-law, Louis Severance; and the apparently neutral board president, Sam Mather. Allen's main point at the meeting was his dissatisfaction with "the manner in which Dr. Crile [has] met what I considered his obligations to me as Chief of the Surgical Service at Lakeside Hospital."

Mather assured Allen that he would address the situation and that some remedy would be devised, a proposal that Allen accepted. In all probability Mather or another trustee did discuss Allen's problems with Crile, but apparently no one pushed the associate visiting surgeon too strenuously to at least make a show of obeisance toward his nominal superior. In the event, Crile continued to function exactly as he had since first arriving at Lakeside. For his part, Allen was forced to wait and watch as he kept a running account of what he considered the continuing outrages of George Washington Crile.

The trustees' apparent lack of desire to discipline Crile could be attributed to a number of factors, including their growing impatience with Allen's habit of turning to the board for redress of all injustices, whether real or imagined. But Crile himself was also creating his own fairly strong position. In 1902, for example, it was Crile supporter Leonard C. Hanna who had donated some $30,000 to the hospital to build and equip an isolation ward, one of the long-hoped-for elements of the Lakeside complex. Most importantly, though, the surgical service over which Crile presided was running smoothly and producing more revenue than ever before.

Although the hospital still faced annual operating deficits, the fees generated by the private ward—and particularly Crile's own paying admissions—added substantially to the more than $40,000 in patient revenue earned in 1903, a figure that actually exceeded the interest income derived that year from the hospital's $600,000-plus endowment. And scores of local physicians not affiliated with the hospital were by then admitting their patients to Lakeside's private ward, thereby producing a steady stream of revenue. Unfortunately, the year 1904—described by Mather in the annual report as "uneventful"—saw fewer patients in the hospital, smaller revenues, and therefore an even larger deficit. But in 1905, when patient revenue was combined with endowment income, the hospital for the first time not only met its expenses but actually showed a small surplus of $7,300. After four decades, Lakeside had finally managed to accumulate an endowment large enough to produce income sufficient to make a sizable dent in its annual operating deficits.

All was not euphoria, however, as the trustees faced a new problem that, although apparently minor at first, before long grew to intractability: the viability of Lakeside's very location. As early as 1902, just four years after the new hospital opened with such fanfare, the trustees had turned down an offer of $10,000 from the Gund Brewing Company for the empty lot to the east of the hospital, a parcel of land that separated Lakeside from the brewery and its stables. Being situated within a few hundred feet of the existing Gund buildings was, to the board, bad enough, but to see that facility grow to the hospital's very doors was unthinkable. In addition to the prospect of subjecting patients and staff to the effluvium of the brewing process (not to mention the odor and noise of the stables, which housed the motive agents for the wagons that transported the brewer's finished product), the trustees fretted over another and, in their eyes, more worrisome possibility. Reverting again to the role of moral guardians, they harbored the fear that a building so close to the nurses' living quarters would prove an irresistible temptation to brewery workers to peep into the windows of the dormitory.

The few residences still in the area were also cause for concern, and in 1905 the board gave Superintendent Ranney a raise sufficiently large to enable him to move himself and his family out of his living quarters in the hospital and into a home of his own. The reason given for the move was that the neighborhood of the hospital "had steadily been growing worse and more and more disagreeable for Superintendent Ranney's family, [and] that most of the houses opposite [the hospital] were now occupied by a very low order of Negroes...."

Meanwhile, in September of the same year, board president Mather reported to his fellow trustees that two wealthy Lakeside supporters had expressed—"through Dr. Crile"—their interest in making sizable donations to the hospital. Gifts offered by individuals (particularly appreciative patients) "through" a particular doctor or surgeon were fairly common at the time and a practice that was encouraged by the physicians themselves. Not only did the hospital benefit from such gifts, but the doctor-intermediaries were not averse to having their names before the trustees in conjunction with incoming contributions. Being known as the party "responsible" for a patron's donation was one way to build up a store of credits with the trustees, who might thereafter be more responsive to requests for special favors.

For Crile, the fact that he could produce two prospective donors at the same time was a clear indication that he could move with a delicacy far beyond that of which a self-described "alley cat" should have been capable. And although only one of the two gifts actually came to fruition— Emeline Bolton, widow of prominent attorney Thomas Bolton, eventually donated $1,000 for the purchase of a new and modern X-ray apparatus— it was obvious to even a casual observer that Crile's stock was rising appreciably with the hospital's board.

Dudley P. Allen, who may have been the least casual observer at Lakeside, was growing more disturbed with his nominal associate, however, and Allen's smoldering discontent flared forth at the very end of 1905.

Crile had instituted a new protocol by which the staff of the regular surgical service would, during Allen's absences from the city, be restricted to treating ward patients only, leaving all of the hospital's private cases—including Allen's private patients—to Crile and his own staff of associates. For Allen, this constituted the most presumptuous infringement on his authority to date, and he soon informed Crile that he would not be renominated to his post for the coming year.

On January 10, 1906, Allen wrote to board president Mather, outlining his ongoing problems with Crile and even including a copy of the written agreement the two men had signed six years before. Characteristically, Allen wrote with an almost palpable tight-lipped restraint, choosing words and phrases that conveyed his displeasure more with the current state of affairs in the hospital than with Crile himself. There was, he wrote, "to all intents and purposes a second surgical service" within Lakeside, and "to make further concessions [to Crile], and even to continue present conditions, seems to me incompatible with the preservation of an efficient surgical service and teaching clinic."

"The encouragement and reward of the assistants in the dispensary is very unsatisfactory," he continued. "I find it increasingly difficult to keep my assistants, both in the dispensary and in the house, satisfied and doing good work." Furthermore, Allen felt "compelled" to add that, upon returning from each of his absences from the city—during which Crile would have been in charge of the entire department—"a long time is required to get my service into proper working order."

"Dr. Crile solicited from me his position in the hospital as a favor to himself," Allen wrote, giving his version of the events of 1900. "Previous to this time my acquaintance with him had been very slight. I granted his request out of deference to the expressed wishes of two trustees of the hospital, who had said to me they hoped I would do something for him...."

Allen complained that his "sphere of influence and activity" had become more limited than Crile's, a state of affairs he found unacceptable. "It is only after deliberation extending over several years that I have decided to lay the matter before you," he concluded. "Unless existing conditions can be remedied, the present position of the surgical service seems untenable."

After reading Allen's letter, Mather passed it along to Superintendent Ranney with a request for his thoughts on the matter. Ranney responded five days later in a four-page memorandum, and if Allen had ever wondered why, after so many years of faithful service, he seemed to be so unappreciated at Lakeside that his own subordinate could feel free to undermine his authority, Ranney's memo would have supplied the answer.

Ranney described as "far-fetched" Allen's assertion that there was a second surgical service operating in the hospital. "As far as my observations go, I believe Dr. Crile is acting wholly within his authority," he wrote, adding that the hospital rules called for a committee to govern the "outside service" and that Crile was, in fact, a member of that committee. "We would [also] find it very difficult to secure good men for positions on the private ward service if it were not for Dr. Crile's private patients," he added. "The staff seems very well satisfied with the service as it is now organized."

Addressing another Allen complaint, Ranney defended the practice of limiting Allen's assistants to ward work when Allen was out of town, a plan that he said had "worked very well and to the satisfaction of both services." It was, he insisted, only Allen who had felt "grieved [sic] and provoked." As to Allen's men on the dispensary service, they were "well cared for," thought Ranney, who believed that their connection with Lakeside not only added to their reputations but also gave them "a varied experience which they could not and would not obtain in private practice in many years' time."

Allen's house staff, however, was indeed dissatisfied with the status quo, but according to Ranney it was because "Dr. Allen gives them little or no opportunity to operate on charity cases. When Dr. Allen told me that his staff showed lack of interest in his work, I suggested that if he would allow his men to do more minor surgery under his direction, they would become contented." Crile, on the other hand, commanded "respect and loyalty" from his staff, although, in Ranney's opinion, "he allows the men too many liberties, and does not give their work as close supervision as it ought to have."

Ranney then praised Allen for being "thorough and painstaking," and noted that it would be a "great loss" if he were to leave Lakeside. "I have never known anyone to show so much interest in the patients; the poorest and humblest person in the hospital receives the same consideration from his hands as the rich," he wrote. "He sees every patient daily and is able to tell you instantly their condition."

Yet immediately after this panegyric to Allen's qualities, Ranney added two devastating criticisms. "Dr. Allen," Ranney wrote candidly, "has annoyed me many times because of his selfish and pecuniary traits. He nearly always desires to get his [private] patients in at a very low rate, when they are amply able to pay five or ten dollars per week more for their room." And, most damning of all: "During the past two years I have noticed that Dr. Allen's practice has fallen off perceptibly and that Dr. Crile's practice has increased."

Lest Mather not get the point of his last remark, Ranney continued, "I would welcome any change at the hospital which would increase the number of patients.... I must say now that I feel much discouraged about the hospital affairs. I cannot understand why this hospital should not be turning away patients because we have no room for them instead of running along with our wards half occupied." Summing up, Ranney expressed his belief that "the existing condition is due partly to the organization [of the surgical service] and that too much attention is given to teaching the [medical] students...and too little attention to developing the different services."

The implication of Ranney's comments was clear. While still an asset to Lakeside, Allen was actually approaching ossification in his management of the surgical service. His declining practice—at least in part a result of his devotion to teaching—was having a detrimental effect on the hospital's balance sheet, as was his tendency to offer discounted room rates to his private patients. If harmony were to be restored and the hospital set on a course toward realizing its full potential, a change of some sort would have to be contemplated.

After reading Ranney's memo, Mather approached Allen and asked him to offer concrete suggestions for resolving his problem with Crile. Allen responded a few days later with a two-page letter in which he proposed six changes to be effected immediately. First, he would terminate his official relations with Crile, thus relieving Crile of "the conditions by which his service is subject to my annual nomination." Crile should then be appointed directly by the board as "Surgeon to the Private Room Service," with the clear understanding that he could in no way control "the staff of any other service now existing in the hospital, nor their patients."

As long as Allen was chief of the regular surgical service, Crile would be allowed no patients other than those in the private rooms, and during Allen's absences, one of his own assistants, rather than Crile, would be in charge of ward patients. Allen also insisted that Crile have neither a seat nor a vote in meetings of the visiting staff. And finally, in a peculiar but almost pathetically revealing point, Allen wanted his own title to be changed from Chief Visiting Surgeon to "Surgeon in Chief to Lakeside Hospital."

Mather discussed Allen's letter with trustee George Garretson before responding. "We reluctantly draw the conclusion that you have decided…not to again nominate Dr. Crile to the position on Lakeside Hospital surgical service that he has been holding," he ultimately wrote to Allen. "If this is true, we shall both regret it very much…." He then went on to warn Allen that if he did not renominate Crile, he would have to find "some other surgeon of equal…standing in this community" to take his place, because "we feel sure the trustees would be unwilling to leave your surgical wards in charge of your assistants during your absence."

Mather was scheduled to leave in just two days on an extended trip through Europe, however, and he concluded his letter by asking Allen to "let things remain status quo until after my return." In the meantime, Crile had been kept abreast of all that was happening, apparently by Garretson and other friendly trustees. While Mather was still out of the country, therefore, Crile took the opportunity to tell various board members of the numerous offers he had been receiving from institutions in other parts of the country. Then, in May, he sent to George Garretson what amounted to a memorandum for the record, a short letter detailing his own version of his arrival at Lakeside.

According to Crile, it had been Allen—"on his [own] initiative"—who had asked Crile to consider an association with him in the hospital's surgical service. Crile had been reluctant to accept, however, because the position would not allow him "sufficient accommodations for such private patients as could not afford to pay for private rooms" but who nevertheless sought Crile's services. Yet Crile had changed his mind and accepted the offer, and he explained his reasoning with unusual candor. He had, he wrote, harbored the belief that "in the future, with the natural changes that must come in the personnel of the staff, my position might be such that I could ultimately concentrate my work and efforts entirely upon Lakeside Hospital, as Dr. Allen is now doing." In other words, he had agreed to become Allen's associate because he fully expected eventually to be Allen's successor as chief visiting surgeon.

Crile went on to again express complete surprise at Allen's recent attitude, but he gave his "earnest assurance" of his "readiness to do anything reasonable that may help to preserve the equilibrium of Lakeside Hospital." In a cover letter to the memo, he wrote: "I need scarcely mention that I do not want a personal consideration in this matter, but

I do want to have such facts as seem to me important in your possession."

The conflicting versions of Crile's advent at Lakeside seemed to indicate that one of the two surgeons was either suffering from a serious memory impairment or was plainly prevaricating. Of course, it was indeed possible that each man simply remembered the events of 1900 differently. With Allen's documented passion for detail, however, it is hard to believe that he could have been so thoroughly mistaken about the intervention of Hickox and Garretson. On the other hand, why would either man concoct a story whose accuracy could so easily be checked? Of course, the answer may simply have been that both Allen and Crile genuinely believed that his own memory of the events was accurate.

The accumulated correspondence of the two surgeons did, however, go a long way toward explaining Crile's original motivation for wanting an affiliation with Lakeside. He had apparently decided that none of the hospitals with which he was affiliated at the time had adequate facilities for the caseload of paying patients he wanted to maintain. He recognized Lakeside not only as the largest and most fully equipped hospital in the city—an institution with sufficient resources to allow him to expand both his practice and his research—but also as a place that would welcome the many paying patients he could bring with him. Ultimately, of course, he could also position himself at Lakeside as the heir apparent to Allen's post.

From the start, then, Crile had seen his appointment as associate visiting surgeon both as a secure and stable short-term position and as a straight and easily traversed career path toward full control of Lakeside's surgical service. The Young Lion was, in effect, accepting a temporary subordinate position from which he could eventually inherent leadership from the aging leader of the pride.

In July, Mather returned from his European trip and met independently with Allen, Crile, and the board's executive committee, all to no effect. Still seeking to resolve the dispute by returning to the status quo, Mather wrote to Allen on July 12th to urge him to yield to the wishes of the board, which wanted both Allen and Crile to remain at Lakeside and to learn to get along with one another. Recounting his interview with Crile, Mather reported to Allen that the younger surgeon would "cheerfully change and modify his conduct and attitude" to suit the trustees' wishes and Allen's preferences, and that he had expressed "great respect and esteem" for Allen's "talents and character." But, Mather added, Crile had also insisted that giving up his other hospital appointments to come to Lakeside had been a great sacrifice, and that he never would have done so if he had not believed from the outset that the pivotal clause in his personal agreement with Allen—"Dr. Crile is to be nominated annually by Dr. Allen to his position as associate surgeon…"—had meant not that Allen had the *right* to nominate Crile annually but that he would *guarantee* his annual nomination. Mather naively concluded his letter to Allen with the hope that Allen would "agree with us in our conclusions"; that is, "unite with us and with [Crile] in doing all we can to further the best interests of Lakeside."

Allen reacted to Mather's letter as if he had been slapped in the face. He seemed to find in the board president's words evidence to support his suspicion that the trustees had, in effect, turned against him. Two days later he sent a terse reply to Mather, writing that it was his own "confidence [in] and respect" for the board that had led him to believe that "obstacles which at times have seemed insurmountable would ultimately be overcome. [But] possibly my point of view is wholly wrong." He repeated his assertion that Lakeside's surgical service as then conducted was not in "the highest interests of the hospital and certainly wastes the best efforts and reputation of its nominal head." And he ended his letter by saying that he had already suggested a possible solution to the problem, but that it was apparently being ignored by Mather, a situation he could not understand. "Since I seem to have entirely misapprehended my position in the hospital," he concluded, "I can only await your instructions."

A week later, Mather, ever the peacemaker, responded. "Our hope and desire to have the present status quo remain, with modifications to suit your wishes, has been fully expressed," he wrote. "To this expression of our wish you have not replied, but we should like to have you do so…." Apparently apprised of Crile's threat to take up one of the other offers he claimed to have received, Mather opined: "As to your suggestion that we should appoint Dr. Crile as Surgeon to the Private Room Service: I question very much—in fact I feel quite positive—that if you break the present agreement…and terminate his connection with Lakeside as associate surgeon, he will feel it necessary to terminate all connection with Lakeside and make other arrangements elsewhere."

Immediately after mailing off his response, Mather also sent copies of the three most recent communications between himself and Allen to Allen's father-in-law, trustee Louis Severance. In a cover letter he indicated his wish that Severance would "join with Dr. Allen's other friends [on the board] in bringing about a rapprochement" between the two warring surgeons.

Allen was out of the city for the rest of the summer and most of the fall, so it was not until late October that he drafted a reply to Mather. In a seven-page letter written in his characteristic stiff and formal manner, Allen recounted the details of his initial dealings with Crile, emphasizing that it was trustees Garretson and Hickox who had first broached the idea of bringing Crile to Lakeside. He reiterated the generous terms of his agreement with Crile, which allowed the younger man to retain his privileges at St. Alexis Hospital and provided him with a total of six Lakeside ward beds for his own admissions. He then dismissed Crile's claim of an agreed-upon "guarantee" to annual renomination as a figment of Crile's imagination.

"I can see no significance in retaining for myself as the head of a department the right to nominate my associate and assistants annually unless it also carries with it the power to decline to do so," he wrote, "nor would any man place himself in a position where he was obliged to nominate men whose services were not acceptable, harmonious and satisfactory."

Allen made plain that he considered himself to be working under "unjust conditions," and that his service had come to be "most unsatisfactory." It had become, he wrote, "increasingly difficult for me to control and satisfy my assistants, both in the hospital and in the dispensary. I question if it can long be done. When absent [from the city] my private interests are dissipated and the authority necessary to the successful conduct of my position ignored." He concluded by again recommending acceptance of his plan to separate Crile from the regular surgical service. And while he still wished to be guided by the desires of the trustees, he said, "It seems to me but just that, since I have relinquished all other positions and have been obliged by the terms of my contract to give up all private assistants, I should be sustained in my authority in the hospital."

Upon receipt of the latest installment in what was by then a nearly year-long correspondence, Mather was crestfallen. He immediately had Allen's letter delivered to George Garretson, along with a handwritten note asking Garretson to read the lengthy document and return it with his comments. "This is," he wrote to Garretson, "a disappointment. I had hoped he was going to let things remain in status quo."

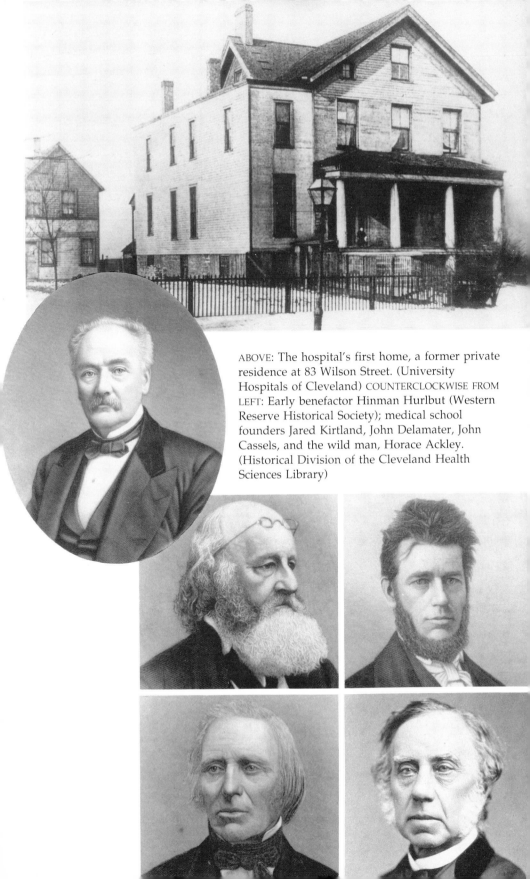

ABOVE: The hospital's first home, a former private residence at 83 Wilson Street. (University Hospitals of Cleveland) COUNTERCLOCKWISE FROM LEFT: Early benefactor Hinman Hurlbut (Western Reserve Historical Society); medical school founders Jared Kirtland, John Delamater, John Cassels, and the wild man, Horace Ackley. (Historical Division of the Cleveland Health Sciences Library)

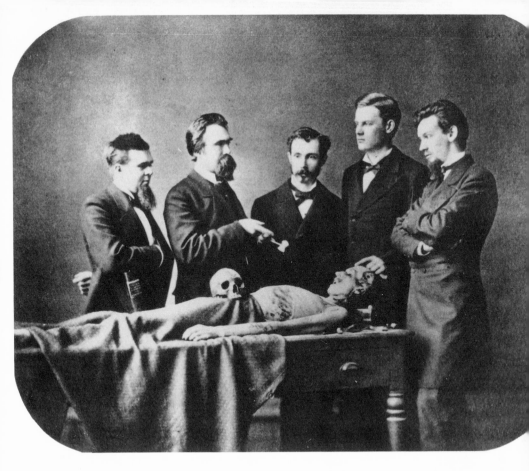

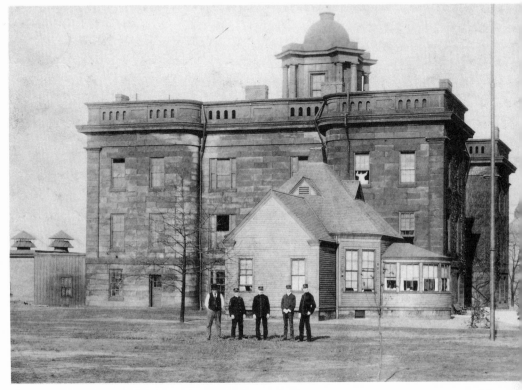

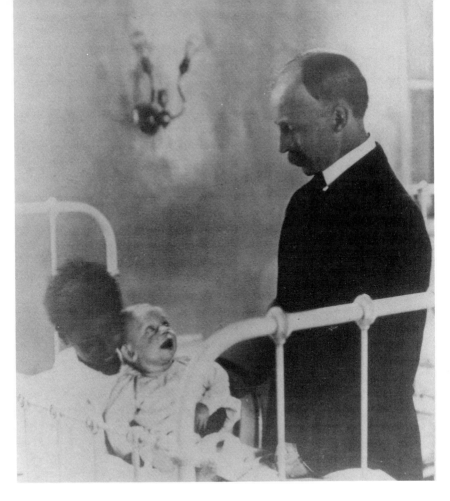

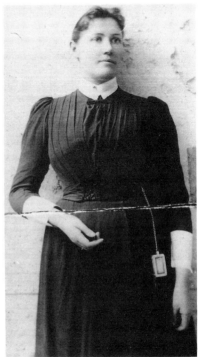

LEFT, TOP: The redoubtable Gustav Weber lecturing to medical students. (Historical Division of the Cleveland Health Sciences Library) LEFT, BELOW: The U.S. Marine Hospital viewed from the west, second home of Lakeside. (Cleveland Public Library) ABOVE: Edward Cushing, the city's most beloved pediatrician. (UHC) RIGHT: Nursing educator Isabel Hampton Robb. (Alan Mason Chesney Medical Archives of The Johns Hopkins Medical Institutions)

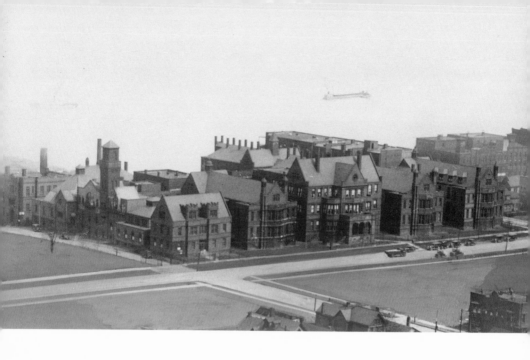

ABOVE: The magnificent new Lakeside, opened in 1898 just to the east of the Marine Hospital. (UHC) BELOW: The Johns Hopkins Hospital, model for the new Lakeside. (Alan Mason Chesney Medical Archives of The Johns Hopkins Medical Institutions) RIGHT: The man who made it happen, philanthropist Samuel Mather. (Cleveland Public Library)

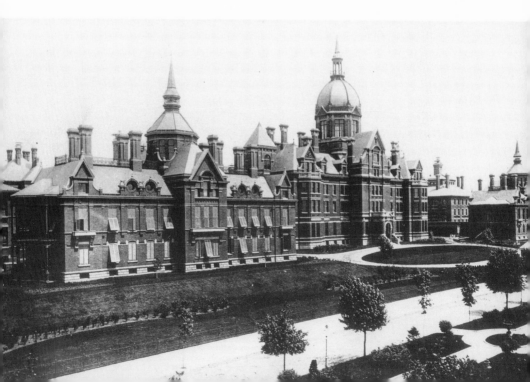

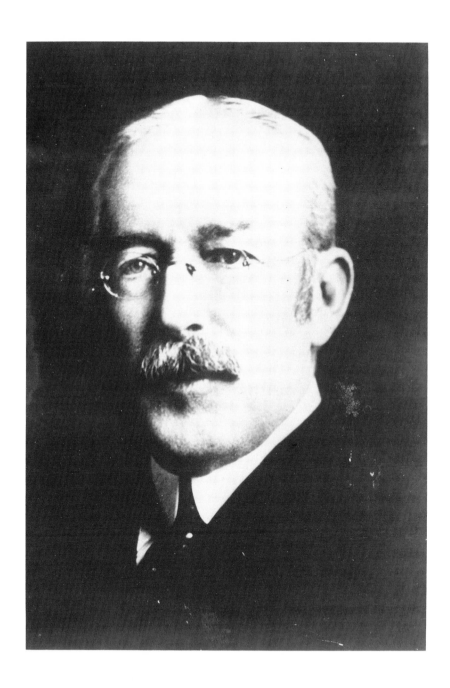

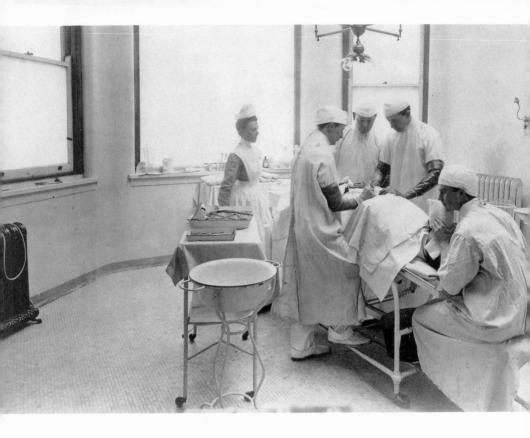

ABOVE: Surgery in the new Lakeside (note use of gowns, caps, and rubber gloves but absence of masks). BELOW: Lakeside's pathology laboratory. (UHC)

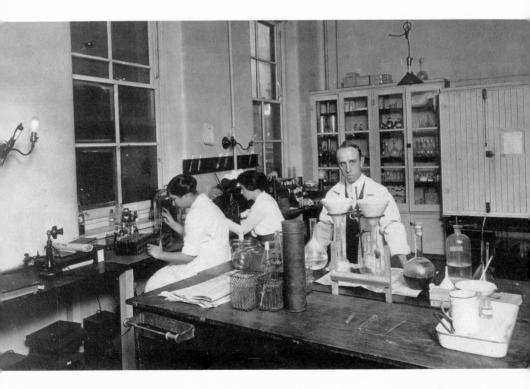

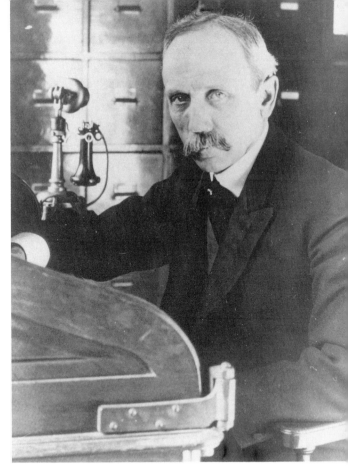

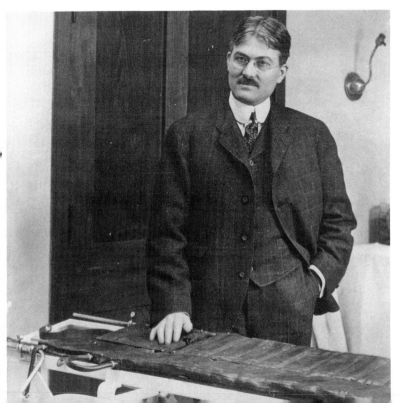

ABOVE: Chief
surgeon Dudley P.
Allen, who waged
a bitter war with
his younger rival
(left) George Crile.
(UHC)

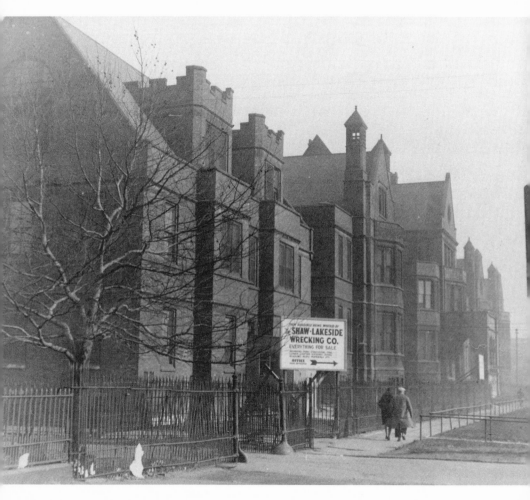

Death of the "new" Lakeside in 1931. The entire complex was eventually demolished, leaving no trace of its former glory. (Cleveland Press Collection/ Cleveland State University Archives)

By the middle of November, after Mather had apparently asked Crile to offer his own ideas for a solution to the contretemps, the young surgeon sent a carefully crafted six-page letter to the board president. He began the letter by defending himself, insisting that although he had never tried to preclude Allen's authority, Allen had "without notice or intimation to me of such intention" reneged on their agreement by refusing to renominate him. No longer promising to "cheerfully change and modify his conduct and attitude," Crile now refused to consider any attempt at reconciliation, noting that "the price in peace and comfort that I have paid for [my] relatively minor association with Dr. Allen has been so considerable that I am unwilling to increase the contact."

For the remainder of his letter, however, Crile boldly advanced his own plan for the reorganization of the surgical service within Lakeside, a plan that he had apparently been contemplating for some time. "If I may digress and take the liberty of making suggestions affecting the general policy of the hospital," he began coyly, "I will suggest the only solution that occurs to me by which the interests of the hospital may be promoted, future friction avoided and a relatively small expense incurred."

Crile would, as Allen had first proposed, relinquish his six beds on the open wards and confine himself to the private ward service. But he would do so only if the hospital were to radically alter its current assignment of space. Crile had noted that Cleveland's "exceedingly large middle class" was being denied access to private accommodations in the hospital because the cost of rooms—$15 a week and up—was simply too great for their limited means. "But these patients are self-respecting and have a certain pride and do not wish to accept a bed in the charity ward of a hospital," he believed, "[and] Lakeside has little to offer that this class can afford...or that their pride and self-respect could endure...."

Then, to ensure that Mather understood the full implications of what he was saying, Crile added: "As a practical policy, if a physician cannot find suitable accommodation at Lakeside for a patient of this class, he will send him to a hospital where such accommodations are provided, and where a physician sends one class of patients, he is quite likely to send all classes."

Changing the subject slightly, Crile relayed the complaints of his patients, many of whom found that their rooms in the private pavilion—the northernmost of the buildings in which patients were housed—were so close to the railroad right-of-way along the lakefront that the noise and dirt of the passing trains were immoderately disturbing. To illustrate his point, Crile referred to three patients who in the preceding month had refused to go to Lakeside for just this reason. And among those who "have felt this annoyance," he added, "there have been some of the hospital's loyal supporters and best friends."

Having heard no such complaints from patients in the open wards—the pavilions south of the long east-west corridor that connected the hospital's many separate structures—Crile concluded that the hospital should be rearranged "to place as many as is possible of the private rooms south of the long corridor." His proposal was to convert the second and third floors of the administration building—at the time the living quarters of the resident medical staff—into rooms for private patients. The northernmost single rooms in the private pavilion could then be converted to rooms accommodating two, three, and four beds each. These semiprivate rooms would carry weekly charges of only eight, nine, and ten dollars.

Ultimately, Crile implied, he would give his "earnest support" to Lakeside only if these changes and four other concessions were made. He should, he wrote, be allowed to admit to the semiprivate rooms "such charity or [partial-pay] patients whom I may personally send"; he should also be allowed to admit to the same rooms "railway, shop and other injured employees," these to be treated as his own private patients and looked after by "my own office associates and assistants"; third, the hospital should establish a mandatory retirement age of sixty for all members of the staff; and, most important, all concerned should understand "that this is a temporary arrangement to make a readjustment to satisfy the demands of Dr. Allen, and that my continuous support of the hospital be construed to mean that when a vacancy occurs at the expiration of the age limit, or otherwise, that if no disqualifying circumstances have in the meantime arisen, I shall expect the opportunity of filling the position of [Chief Visiting] Surgeon to Lakeside Hospital."

Crile attempted to ameliorate somewhat the predatory connotations of his proposal for a mandatory retirement age, saying "many hospitals have such regulations" and that they constituted "a dignified termination of one's hospital career." But then he made clear his true reasoning—and his true opinion of Allen—by remarking that a sixty-year age limit "protects the hospital against inefficient service of older and busier men, who likely are no longer interested in the more active problems of medicine...."

In effect, Crile was writing his own contract with the hospital. He was, to be sure, advocating changes that could alleviate the very real noise problem which aggravated precisely those patients the hospital could least afford to lose. But to accomplish that he proposed wholesale structural changes in the hospital, the potential cost of which no one knew. In recommending the move of private-pavilion patients to the space allotted to residents' living quarters, for example, he conveniently forgot to bring up the logical consequence of such a move: where, then, would the residents live?

Crile was also proposing the creation of his own surgical service, a service that—because it would include the remnants of his old industrial-accident practice, which he still maintained at St. Alexis, as well as responsibility for all private patients admitted to Lakeside by outside physicians—could over time become the largest in the hospital. Moving all of his patients to Lakeside would indeed bring more paying admissions to the hospital, but it would also save him valuable time by consolidating his work in one location. He would no longer have to oversee treatment of ward patients during Allen's absences from the hospital, and by agreeing to forego access to ward beds he was also avoiding the time-consuming chore of teaching. Ultimately, of course, he was virtually assuring himself the position of chief surgeon upon Allen's retirement.

Within a month, Mather and the trustees put before Allen a plan to resolve the stalemate between himself and Crile. Not surprisingly, the plan incorporated all of Crile's suggestions, with a detailed explanation of Crile's right to four private wards of six beds each, plus access to the new two- and four-bed rooms that would be priced at $10 per week and opened on the ground floor of the existing private pavilion. Contrary to Mather's earlier opinion, Allen would indeed be allowed to leave the care of his patients in the hands of his assistants during his absences from the hospital. And although the question of access to the hospital's operating rooms was not thoroughly resolved, the obvious implication was that the trustees would simply build Crile an operating suite of his own.

Allen quibbled over the number of beds allotted to Crile as well as some smaller elements of the new agreement, but eventually he endorsed all of its points—including the sixty-year mandatory retirement age, a subject that he and Mather had actually discussed and agreed upon some months before Crile's suggestion. Allen insisted, however, that he and he alone would have "control" of the surgical amphitheater, and his choice of words in making the argument revealed much about his state of mind.

"It seems to me," he wrote to Mather, "that to the chief of the surgical service, having in charge the official instruction in that department, should belong the *dignity* [emphasis added] of the direction of the amphitheater...."

By the end of January 1907, the war between Dudley P. Allen and George Crile was effectively over. Allen was the apparent winner, having succeeded in removing Crile from the hospital's regular surgical service and thereby eliminating what he perceived as a constant threat to his authority, not to mention his "dignity." Crile, however, received everything he had asked for in the way of beds, new operating-room facilities, assistants, and the like. And by denying Crile access to the open wards, Allen unwittingly freed the younger man from nonlucrative charity work and time-consuming teaching duties, thereby allowing him to concentrate on his research projects and on maintaining and increasing his private practice.

After six years of circumventing, undermining, and, ultimately, ignoring Allen's authority, Crile found himself rewarded with a near-perfect situation from which to pursue his interests. He was, in effect, given the opportunity to spend the remainder of the decade enlarging his practice, burnishing his reputation, and making himself altogether indispensable to Lakeside Hospital.

CHAPTER FIVE

Days of Empire

Just why the Lakeside trustees so quickly acceded to what were in effect George Crile's "demands" is not difficult to understand. For one, Crile's national reputation had already far outstripped that of his nominal chief, Dudley P. Allen, and even the most ardent Allen partisan would admit that the younger surgeon was a valuable addition to the Lakeside staff. Perhaps most importantly, however, Allen was by then perceived as a representative of medicine's old order—a fine clinician with a thoughtful, caring manner toward all of his patients, to be sure, but little more than that. Crile, on the other hand, was fully in step with the prevailing trend of medicine's new century. The laboratory, not the bedside, was fast becoming the arena of influence, and Crile's early and eager embrace of research marked him as a leader of the new order.

He had, of course, already experimented with dozens of new techniques and procedures, and his findings were widely published in journals and medical texts, both at home and abroad. He had, for example, successfully transfused blood directly from a donor to a patient, a process that involved suturing the cut end of the donor's radial artery to a vein in the recipient. And he had shown that injections of adrenalin could sometimes resuscitate otherwise moribund cases. Indeed, results of the latter procedure were often referred to in general-circulation newspaper and magazine articles of the time as "the miracle of resurrection," an unfortunate choice of words which conveyed the impression that Crile was capable of routinely raising the dead.

In addition, the Lakeside trustees had apparently begun to consider Allen as more of a liability than an asset. With their continuing concern over increasing the number of paying patients in the hospital, they could not have been pleased with Allen's diminishing practice or his long and frequent absences from the city. And his repeated complaints, behind-the-scenes maneuvering, and unending need to be reassured of his authority further eroded his position at the hospital. In truth, Allen was perilously close to becoming the very sort of man he had once abhored; for some time he had been displaying more and more of the personality traits of his old nemesis, Gustav Weber.

Not long after accepting the terms of his new agreement with Crile, however, Allen must have begun to realize that he was in effect a lame duck as chief visiting surgeon to Lakeside. But if he had a declining patient load and little incentive to begin long-term research projects, he was still vitally interested in medical education, and he soon threw himself into a project to study and recommend changes for the curriculum of the medical school.

Once before, in 1893, Allen had spearheaded a similar effort, and the result had been an extension of the academic year and the addition of a fourth full year of schooling to the degree requirements. Allen's expressed desire to improve the quality of medical education at Western Reserve was, in fact, one of the reasons he had enjoyed the backing of university president Thwing and some of the more progressive members of the school's faculty during the battle to unseat then-dean Weber. Now, between 1907 and 1908, Allen chaired a committee that eventually proposed a sweeping revision and reorganization of the curriculum. Course material was streamlined, classroom hours were reduced from forty-eight hundred to forty-one hundred, courses were rearranged into a more logical sequence, and a more balanced emphasis was given to each subject studied. The most radical of all the changes proposed by Allen's committee, however, was a new entrance requirement, to be instituted in the 1909 school year. From that point on, all incoming students would have to possess a bachelor's degree, a reform that made Western Reserve only the third medical school in the country—after Johns Hopkins and Harvard—to require a full undergraduate education for admission.

While Allen was engaged in the curriculum review process, Crile, who had been given the new title "Visiting Surgeon to the Private Ward," was already contemplating further requests of the Lakeside board, to meet the needs he saw arising from the wholesale structural changes in the hospital that his own earlier demands had inspired. In September of 1907, in a letter to Superintendent Ranney, Crile noted that, because of the "additions and alterations now being made in the hospital building and the change in the personnel of the surgical division," he would be responsible for patients in the new private rooms on the upper floor of the administration building as well as those patients in the semiprivate rooms being created in the northern end of the old private pavilion—both his own admissions and those of unaffiliated outside surgeons. Since there would be more than fifty new beds in his charge, and since he had already begun transferring "a large share of my support from St. Alexis to Lakeside," and since outside physicians were admitting more and more patients, Crile asked for permission to enlarge his own staff of assistants and to free them from any other possible duties in the hospital. In addition to adding his practice associate William Lower as assistant visiting surgeon to the private ward, Crile also asked for one resident, three interns, and a private anesthetist, the latter to be dispensary nurse Agatha Hodgins, whom he had already taught to administer nitrous oxide anesthesia and who was by then virtually his permanent anesthetist anyway.

When Crile had first outlined his proposal to alter the hospital in his 1906 letter to Samuel Mather, he had referred to the proposed changes as probably being accomplished at "relatively small expense." In the event, the bill for all the alterations, including the addition of a second story to the operating pavilion and the construction of a new residents' dormitory on the north side of the Lakeside property, came to more than $100,000. With additional incidental costs—the salary for a new nurse to handle Hodgins's old duties, for example—the final tally approached $105,000. Yet despite the expense that had been incurred in keeping Crile happy, the trustees were more than willing to take on the burden of further debt. They had chosen Crile to lead the hospital into the future, and the price of progress would simply have to be paid.

With increased bed space, two new operating rooms, a larger staff of visiting physicians and surgeons, an end to internal feuding, and a dispensary service handling more than thirty thousand visits annually, Lakeside was positioned to enjoy a period of renewed vigor as an institution. Yet 1907 proved to be a step backward for the hospital. Not only was there a new capital debt over which to fret (only about half of the cost of all the new construction had been subscribed by friends of the hospital), but another national bank panic and severe business depression in the latter half of the year, coupled with sustained increases in the cost of food and medical equipment, dealt a serious blow to the hospital's fiscal foundations. Even with patient revenue of some $70,000, guaranty-fund donations of $19,000, and endowment income of $58,000, Lakeside still showed a huge operating deficit for the year.

The problem of funding was further exacerbated in June of 1908, when Louis Severance, Dudley P. Allen's father-in-law, abruptly resigned from the board of trustees and even refused to fulfill his most recent subscription pledge of $25,000. Severance never commented publicly on the subject, but the reason for his resignation was widely believed to be his anger over what he considered the hospital's shabby treatment of his son-in-law.

Although he had been out of the country for much of 1906 and 1907, Severance apparently considered the other trustees lax in not attempting to consult him on either the sixty-year mandatory retirement rule or the expense incurred in the structural changes of the hospital buildings themselves. Board president Mather wrote to and met with Severance in an attempt to change his mind, but the longtime supporter of the hospital was adamant. Thereafter, Severance's name would be conspicuous by its absence from the annual lists of major donors to Lakeside.

Despite all the turmoil, rancor, structural changes, and financial reverses that disrupted Lakeside during the first decade of the new century, the hospital itself continued to serve without interruption the needs for which it had been built. And although much of the energy and attention of the trustees had been fixed on increasing the number of private paying patients admitted to the hospital, it was Cleveland's working class and poor who made up the bulk of the cases treated at the vast complex by the lake. For these people, so inordinately susceptible to illness and injury, Lakeside represented both the haven of first choice and the refuge of last resort.

For the trustees, however, there was a real and growing dichotomy between their public restatements of the historic "mission" of the hospital and the undeniable fact of the need for a steadier flow of income from a more stable base of wealthier patients. And in its least-disguised expression, the board's concern over the sheer bulk of free care provided was at least in part a tension born of differences in class and caste, as evidenced by an apparently generous donation offered early in 1909 by trustee Earl Oglebay.

The board's true perception of the hospital's charity patients could have been stated no more clearly than through Oglebay's offer to underwrite the cost of constructing a "lodge" on the eastern side of the hospital, essentially a one-story waiting room in which visitors to patients in the charity wards could wait in relative comfort for visitation hours to begin. The new lodge would indeed provide shelter for the families and friends of patients on the wards, but it would also serve to segregate charity-ward visitors from the rest of the hospital, keeping them out of sight of both the pay-ward patients and their visitors. And when the trustees discussed details of the actual construction of the lodge, they further revealed their opinion of the charity population of the hospital by insisting that the new structure was to be "so built that it could be washed out with the hose daily, and thoroughly aired."

§

As the first decade of the century came to a close, the ranks of Lakeside trustees and friends began to be depleted with alarming speed. From among the old guard of longtime supporters, Louis Severance was, for his own reasons, the first to depart, in 1908. Then, in January of 1909, Flora Stone Mather, wife of the board president and long an active and generous supporter of Lakeside, succumbed to breast cancer, despite what her surgeon, George Crile, called the "most extensive and thorough operation" he had ever performed. Three months later, former board president Lee McBride died, followed not long after by Ralph Hickox and Mrs. Hinman Hurlbut, who with her late husband had been so much a part of the birth of the hospital more than forty years before. Then, in April of 1910, Isabel Robb was fatally injured when she was crushed between two streetcars while attempting to help a friend out of the way of that newest threat to urban safety, a "speeding" automobile.

Finally, on August 6, 1910, in a single-sentence letter to Samuel Mather, Dudley P. Allen tendered his resignation from the hospital, two full years before Lakeside's mandatory retirement provision would have forced him to relinquish his post as chief visiting surgeon. Allen gave no reason for his decision, but anyone who knew his personality and the hospital's internal politics might have predicted that he would not wait to be forced out by so undignified a means as an age limit imposed through the influence of his younger rival.

The war with George Crile and its aftermath, the resignation of his father-in-law as a hospital trustee, his apparent loss of favor with other members of the board—all no doubt weighed heavily on Allen's mind at the time. And there were other indications that he must have construed as meaning that his time was past. Nearly two years before Allen's resignation, for example, when Flora Mather's cancer was first diagnosed, Sam Mather had not even consulted with the man who was, after all, the hospital's chief surgeon. Instead, William Halsted was brought from Johns Hopkins to give his opinion of the case, and George Crile was asked to perform the necessary surgery. Then, in November 1909, Howard Hanna made a donation of $250,000 toward the medical school's $1 million endowment-fund drive. Hanna, a trustee of both Lakeside and Western Reserve University, provided the generous gift with but one stipulation: that his "friends" Edward Cushing and George Crile should serve as "an advisory committee upon the use of the income of [the] fund."

For Allen, who had always been a more enthusiastic educator than Crile and who had just devoted more than a year to revising the school's curriculum, the provisions of Hanna's gift must have seemed not only a cruel irony but yet another indication that he had lost favor with at least some of the trustees. Of course, other factors no doubt played a part in his early retirement. He was, in fact, fifty-eight years old, and his own health and stamina had always been problematic. In truth, he was probably growing tired of the daily grind of hospital routine, and he might well have wished to spend more time pursuing his other interests, such as collecting fine art.

In January of 1910 he resigned his seat on the adminstrative council of the Cleveland Medical Library Association, an institution that for years had been a consuming passion. Later in the year he donated his own collection of medical volumes to the library, a clear indication that he was about to leave the profession. When his retirement was finally announced, therefore, it was only mildly surprising to many at the hospital. As Superintendent Ranney later wrote to Sam Mather, he had "felt quite sure that [Allen] would hand in his resignation to the trustees some time before the expiration of his age limit...."

Newspaper articles at the time of Allen's resignation contained speculation about the reasons for the surgeon's early retirement, many commenting on his 1906 battle with Crile. Officially, according to Mather, Allen had resigned "because of ill health on the part of his wife and himself, and in order to be away for a year [on a round-the-world trip]." But the newspapers also commented on the "strong probability" that George Crile would succeed Allen as Lakeside's chief surgeon, and before long the suspicion was proved correct. In October, just three weeks after Allen's resignation had at last been formally accepted, a lengthy article in the *Leader* appeared under the eye-catching headline, "Johns Hopkins To Have Rival Here."

The *Leader* article announced what everyone in the city's medical community already knew: George Crile, "one of Cleveland's most celebrated surgeons," would in fact succeed Dudley P. Allen as chief visiting surgeon at Lakeside. But the article went on to trumpet a genuine piece of news. The hospital's trustees planned to make Lakeside "one of the greatest centers of medicine and surgery in the land, placing it eventually on a par with Johns Hopkins University."

Quoting an unnamed Lakeside "official," the article revealed the decision of the trustees to make "an important change in the policy of the institution." The change would mean a "new era" for the hospital, a radical departure from its old direction that would take it from being simply "an institution where the afflicted and indigent may secure the highest medical and surgical attention possible" to "the greatest source of medical knowledge and progress in the land."

The nature of the new policy was described by Crile himself, who acknowledged that while the "first aim" of the hospital was to provide care to all who required it, "upon that foundation a higher superstructure... should now be raised." It was Crile's belief that Lakeside could in ensuing years produce "a set of men who are not only fine practitioners themselves but who would be able to give the world the best thought and make themselves recognized as the highest authority on medical affairs in the country."

Crile's idea was simply to emulate Johns Hopkins (which itself had emulated the great German hospitals and universities) by providing promising young physicians with guaranteed incomes after their residencies were completed. Such a scheme would allow the younger doctors to remain at the hospital to pursue extended research projects, rather than following the standard course of immediately entering private practice.

In effect, Crile was advocating the restructuring of Lakeside with a plan to transform what was at heart a community hospital into something more closely resembling an academic medical center. And although he took pains to mention that the "present aim of the hospital would in no way be lost sight of by such a course," it was obvious that at the very core of his plans was a diminished emphasis on clinical medicine and a new position of importance for the laboratory. "I can," Crile concluded, "conceive of no higher aim for any medical institution...."

Crile's statements, made publicly and without fear of contradiction from the hospital's trustees, clearly defined a turning point in Lakeside's history. His own abiding interest in research happened to coincide perfectly with the major trend in medicine of the era, and he was able to convince the members of the board that the hospital should be an active and leading participant in that era. Knowing that the medical school then enjoyed its largest endowment to date—a good portion of which was under his virtual complete control, thanks to the stipulations of Howard Hanna's gift—he could confidently show the hospital's trustees that an expanded definition of Lakeside's role was both timely and proper, and that he, Crile, was the man to chart the institution's new course.

Indeed, the "official" quoted in the *Leader* story revealed Crile's true place in the hospital hierarchy when he inadvertently referred to him not merely as the new chief of the surgery department but as the new "head of Lakeside." And in an even more suggestive line, the article reported that the hospital's new direction was "one of Dr. Crile's great ambitions for Lakeside, a subject to which he had given great attention long before there was any suggestion of Dr. Allen's retirement."

With Allen removed from the scene, Crile was free to pursue his own agendas, a situation he had longed for since first coming to Lakeside a decade before. And to Crile's partisans both locally and nationally, Allen's retirement had been no less desired. Indeed, one of the most remarkable congratulatory letters Crile received at the time came from Harvey Cushing at Johns Hopkins, who was well acquainted with both Allen and Crile and who had followed the progress of their war through dispatches from his brother Edward.

Referring to the *Leader* article, a clipping of which had been sent to him in Baltimore, Cushing lauded Crile as a "generous and forgiving soul" for having praised Allen in print. "No one except the few who have been aware of what you have gone through would guess but that every-thing has been smooth and Allen has made a dignified retirement and it's well that it should be so.

"Now for you, dear boy," he continued. "You have a clear field and the freedom from irritations which would have maddened anyone with a less sweet disposition. And it will mean a lot to Ned [Edward Cushing] and the others [at Lakeside] who have longed for this occasion probably much more than you have ever done. And so God bless you. May you long remain the very top of our heap."

Not long after assuming his new post, Crile became known at Lakeside simply as "The Chief," a sobriquet used not only by hospital personnel but even by his own wife. In full control of the hospital's surgical service, he embarked upon one of his most productive periods, an era that, like similarly happy times in his life, he sometimes later referred to as the "Days of Empire."

To ensure a steady supply of anesthesia, for example, he asked for and received a nitrous oxide plant, which was built on the hospital grounds and paid for by his friend, trustee Howard Hanna. Thus supplied, he was able to draw up personal surgical schedules that could include up to twenty separate procedures each day, from appendectomies, skin grafts, and thyroidectomies to hernia repairs, excisions of carcinomas, and even dilation and curettage. According to his schedule, none of the procedures required more than forty-five minutes to complete.

His large private practice, research work, and frequent consultations outside the city left him with little time for the mundane chore of monitoring ward patients, so he was allowed to delegate that job to one of the surgical service's senior assistants (a privilege the trustees had denied Dudley P. Allen when he first suggested it for himself). The trustees even went so far as to reimburse Crile secretly for the purchase of the new surgical instruments he deemed necessary to his work, a substantial perquisite offered to no other Lakeside surgeon. One of the rare occasions on which the board denied a Crile request came when he asked for "electric hoists" to raise and lower window shades in the teaching amphitheater. At a projected cost of $1,250, the hoists were deemed something of an extravagance, and Crile was asked to endure raising the shades by hand.

In the laboratory he continued his experiments on dogs, setting for himself the rather formidable goal of attempting to isolate "the basis of all life and emotion." Although such a statement might have been interpreted by some as an indication of overweening hubris, it was nevertheless accepted widely, bathed as it was in the glow of his brilliant reputation. Amy Rowland, a laboratory assistant who worked for Crile for years and who was devoted to "The Chief," once described such pronouncements as nothing less than evidence of Crile's "prophetic vision."*

---

*Some years later, Rowland would provide one of the few eyewitness accounts of Crile's work habits in the laboratory. In an unwittingly candid portrait that she intended as a fond remembrance of "The Chief," Rowland described a man whose mind "leaped over the routine necessities of research to what he believed to be the inevitable findings of that research, and usually he was right. [But] as a consequence of this characteristic, he was often impatient with the need for repeated experiments. He would often discourage his associates

§

The emergence of medical research as a priority of Lakeside Hospital and the medical school of Western Reserve University was a bold step for the institutions, but it was far from an isolated incident. The new direction taken in Cleveland was mirrored by similar phenomena at a growing number of institutions around the country. And although the reasons for the new point of view in American medicine were many, two incidents at Lakeside at the time serve as compelling illustrations of at least one of the factors that influenced the thinking of the medical establishment.

The first incident was the case of an Austrian immigrant who, less than an hour after his arrival in Cleveland, suffered a minor cut on his thumb. Ten days later he lay dying in Lakeside with a case of lockjaw so far advanced that even the relatively new and effective tetanus antitoxin could not save him. Then, not long after, a six-year-old boy who had fallen three and a half stories out of a tenement window was brought to the hospital by ambulance. The boy's mother, however, begged the Lakeside doctors to allow her to take the child home. Despite her son's injuries, she firmly believed that a hospital was the last place he should be.

Such stories indicated that the old fear of hospitals as houses of death still lingered in the minds of many—so much so that one gravely ill patient would delay seeking treatment of his condition until he was beyond help, and one concerned mother would prefer to care for her seriously injured child at home rather than allow him to be treated by a group of mysterious strangers who operated behind the forbidding walls of a fortress-like structure. The general public's confusion over and distrust of medicine (*and* doctors) still existed to a great degree, a holdover from the decades of quackery, ignorance, and false cures that had been so much a part of the profession in previous years.

But as the generation of doctors who had come of age in one of medicine's darker periods began to be supplanted by a new generation of physicians untainted by many of the old ideas and prejudices, there was a growing recognition of the need to build medicine on a more reasoned and scientific footing. Longstanding theories were being disproved

---

by jumping to a conclusion from a single experiment and being even angry with anyone who desired further confirmation of the results secured."

through experimentation, new ideas were put to the test of more rigorous review, and research followed by publication of results was coming to be the new path to success.

Ironically, as a direct result of just the sort of advances the laboratory had begun to provide, physicians faced a whole new set of problems with the public's perception of their craft. Medicine had in fact achieved remarkable progress over the preceding two decades, and to many individuals, the ability of a doctor to deal successfully with disease and injury was already taken for granted. Patients grew to expect more from their physicians. They wanted to believe that modern medicine was capable of relieving all suffering and that doctors themselves were nothing less than demigods of healing. As one well-known physician and educator of the time wrote, however, no matter how alluring they found their new status, physicians would ultimately be ill-served if they allowed the public to consider medicine as an "exact science." Realizing the profession's limitations and the vast areas of ignorance that still existed, it would, he thought, be far better if the practice of medicine were to be "compared rather with farming or gardening."

The choice between being viewed as a gardener or a demigod was just one symptom of the era of change with which physicians had to contend. At an almost frenetic pace, some of medicine's most cherished beliefs were being discarded and replaced by new concepts that been tested and proved in the laboratory. The revolution that had begun in the famous hospitals and universities of Europe was spreading rapidly across the Atlantic, and although it would not immediately find a foothold in all corners of the country, it would soon be aided by a most persuasive domestic agent.

In 1909, Abraham Flexner, a graduate of Johns Hopkins University and a former schoolteacher in Louisville, Kentucky, was commissioned by the Carnegie Foundation for the Advancement of Teaching to compile a report on the then-current state of medical education in North America. One of a series of investigations of various aspects of education conducted by the foundation, "Bulletin #4: Medical Education in the United States and Canada" would come to be considered a watershed document in the history of American medicine.

With no formal training in medicine (although two of his brothers were physicians), Flexner surveyed and evaluated each of the one hundred and fifty-five medical schools then extant in North America. The results of his investigation proved shocking: most "medical schools," for example, had entrance requirements no more stringent than either a high school diploma or "the rudiments or the recollection of a common school education." Only sixteen schools required at least two years of college as an entrance requirement, and of these, Johns Hopkins, Harvard, and Western Reserve were still the only ones to require an undergraduate degree. Indeed, at the time only about fifteen percent of individuals awarded diplomas at medical schools had first earned bachelor's degrees.

Many institutions were nothing more than updated versions of the old proprietary schools, where no applicant with sufficient funds to pay his tuition was turned away. Doctors often paid large sums to obtain their professorial "chairs" in such schools, because in addition to dividing up tuition payments for their salaries they also earned valuable prestige in their communities and lucrative consultations from grateful former students.

As a Johns Hopkins alumnus (and the brother of another), Flexner was already biased in favor of his old school. But he was sincere when he recognized the import of the Baltimore institution's academic-medical-center concept, and he pronounced it "admirable," the highest accolade in his lexicon. He noted that third- and fourth-year students in the Johns Hopkins medical school were "made a factor in the conduct" of the Johns Hopkins hospital by serving as clerks and surgical dressers. Rather than presenting four years of uninterrupted lectures, the Johns Hopkins curriculum gave students hands-on experience by assigning them patients on whom they would, under supervision, perform many routine procedures. And students were expected to follow their cases from admission to discharge—and even, when the case warranted it, to autopsy.

"Nowhere else in the country has so consistent a scheme been so admirably realized," Flexner wrote in his report. "There is no insuperable reason why several other medical schools should not take advantage of a fortunate relation to hospitals to bring about an equally effective organization...."

Although Johns Hopkins represented his ideal, Flexner also singled out the Medical Department of Western Reserve University for its praiseworthy admission standards and facilities. The factor that truly impressed Flexner, however, was the degree of cooperation exhibited between Western Reserve and Lakeside Hospital, both private, independent entities. "The enlightened action of [the university's] trustees," he wrote, "is rapidly perfecting the connection between the admirable Lakeside Hospital of Cleveland and Western Reserve University."

Flexner referred to Western Reserve as "already one of the substantial schools of the country," and he went so far as to suggest that its relationship with Lakeside constituted "a precedent worthy to be generally followed" in such larger cities as New York, Chicago, and Boston. "Western Reserve and Lakeside," he concluded, "thus prove the feasibility of a smooth working connection between a university department of medicine and a private hospital...." In fact, Flexner was so taken with the arrangement in Cleveland that even before publication of his study he wrote to Western Reserve president Charles F. Thwing to say that, in his opinion, "The Medical Department of Western Reserve University is, next to Johns Hopkins..., the best in the country."

Flexner was not, of course, the first observer to note the efficacy of a wholly contained medical "campus" such as Johns Hopkins had created. Nor was he the first to see the potential advantage of affiliations between private hospitals and private universities. But "Bulletin #4" gave form and substance to the new ideal, and because the Carnegie Foundation carried so much weight with university and hospital administrators and trustees, Flexner's findings provided much of the impetus needed to at last force the country to cast a critical eye over its system of medical education.

The combination of patient care, teaching, and research as exemplified by Johns Hopkins was, to Flexner, the proper model for the rest of the nation to follow. And what soon came to be known as "The Flexner Report" served to emphasize that point and disseminate it widely. The report also spurred the medical profession to eliminate entirely the virtually worthless proprietary schools, and it reemphasized the need to consolidate marginal university operations. Indeed, in April of 1910, the Carnegie Foundation suggested and facilitated the consolidation of the Medical Department of Ohio Wesleyan University—the last incarnation of Gustav Weber's original Charity Hospital Medical College—with the Medical Department of Western Reserve.

But the high praise that Abraham Flexner heaped on Lakeside and Western Reserve came at time when both institutions were beginning to feel pinched by their own successes. The medical school building—once considered a state-of-the-art structure—was, even at the time of Flexner's visit, already proving inadequate to the demands of modern medical education. As for Lakeside, the hospital was becoming even more isolated amid the noise and dirt of the nearby lakefront railroad and the spreading decay of its immediate neighborhood. (By 1910, a Lakeside nurse wishing to walk to the center of the city could do so only with a male escort because the route lay directly through Cleveland's rowdy and dangerous Tenderloin district.) And the same sandy substrate that had originally delayed construction of the hospital was now causing damage to the structures built atop it, necessitating expensive repairs and reinforcement of the northernmost buildings on the site.

In addition, new wards for the care of children and of maternity cases were longstanding and as-yet unmet needs. At the time, three independent institutions in Cleveland provided a measure of care for children and maternity cases, but each was too small and inefficient to make a dramatic impact on the abysmal conditions encountered by the city's poorest residents. The Maternity Hospital of Cleveland, for example, had been in operation since 1891, but it was housed in a small, aging two-story residence in the center of the city. An independent charity supported by private donations, the Maternity Hospital was never adequately staffed or operated in its earliest years and had no formal ties to any Cleveland medical schools or hospitals.

The hospital relocated three times in its first two decades, gradually increasing its bed capacity from half a dozen to about sixty. It remained a marginal operation for some time, however—so much so that students in Lakeside's nursing school were sent to maternity hospitals in other parts of the country to receive their required three months of obstetrical training. Indeed, even well into the twentieth century only about ten percent of all babies born in Cleveland were delivered in a hospital setting.

The Medical Department of Western Reserve had started an outpatient obstetrical service of its own in 1906, but it was essentially a one-man operation for its first three years. Arthur Bill, then an assistant in obstetrics at the medical school, worked virtually alone, making hundreds of home visits to the poor to provide prenatal care and to perform deliveries. In 1909, however, Bill convinced the medical school to rent a residence on East 35th Street for use as a maternity dispensary. In that same year, the university entered into an informal working arrangement with the Maternity Hospital of Cleveland, whereby Bill was named obstetrician in charge and medical students were assigned to assist in the work.

Facilities for the treatment of children were also in short supply, although two private, independent efforts were proving to be effective within the constraints of their limited resources. The first, Rainbow Cottage, had been founded on Thanksgiving Day in 1887, when nine young women—Mary Cary, Mary Chisholm, Bella Cooke, Lucia Edwards, Helen

Morley, Marion Parsons, Marguerite Pechin, Mary Root, and Charlotte Tod, all daughters of well-to-do Cleveland families—met to create a local chapter of a national women's charitable organization known as the King's Daughters. Calling themselves the Rainbow Circle, the women set out to establish and maintain a permanent convalescent facility for the sick, malnourished, and crippled children of the city.

In the poorer sections of Cleveland, even when hospital or dispensary treatment for children was sought out, the patients were, of course, ultimately returned to the same environment from which they had come. Without follow-up professional care attending to improved nutrition, regular changes of surgical dressings, adjustments of braces, splints, and the like, a convalescent's chance for full recovery was severely diminished.

The women of the Rainbow Circle attempted to break that cycle by creating a place where children could convalesce in clean and comfortable surroundings, with ample fresh air, nutritious food, and professional attention to necessary follow-up measures. After four years of planning and fund raising, the nine young women obtained a lease on a two-story frame house on a chicken farm located at the northernmost end of what would later be called East 105th Street. Situated on a bluff overlooking Lake Erie, the new facility, named Rainbow Cottage, opened in May of 1891. In its first year it housed a total of thirty-two children, most of them crippled by either disease or injury. Ten years later, Mrs. William L. Harkness donated $25,000 for construction of a new and larger Rainbow Cottage, a three-story brick building in the eastern suburb of South Euclid.

By 1905 the Rainbow Circle had successfully raised sufficient funds to purchase a nearby property and its three frame buildings, which nearly tripled the original cottage's bed capacity. Two years later, Rainbow obtained a formal affiliation with Lakeside Hospital, whereby convalescent children could be admitted to the cottage only through the hospital or its dispensary. The same agreement stipulated that Rainbow's medical staff would be appointed only from the staff of Lakeside dispensary assistants. One of their number, Chauncy Wyckoff, was named the institution's first resident physician.

Rainbow Cottage successfully addressed one otherwise overlooked aspect of Cleveland's medical system, but some of the most egregious deficiencies of the city's health-care apparatus affected much younger children. Infants and newborns in particular died in astonishing numbers; at the time, roughly half of all deaths recorded in Cleveland each year were of children under the age of five, and the city's infant mortality rate was nearly twenty percent. The latter figure actually constituted an improvement over previous years. In 1889, the infant mortality rate had been *thirty-three* percent.

Squalid living conditions, poor nutrition, contaminated food products (pasteurized and tuberculin-tested milk was not widely available to poorer families), lack of proper hygiene, parental ignorance—all combined to produce shockingly high incidences of anemia, rickets, pneumonia, tuberculosis, and other diseases and conditions. Many children died of common diarrhea, which, unchecked, resulted in fatal dehydration.

The first attempt to address the problems of children occurred in 1904, when a small Infants' Clinic was established in a neighborhood settlement house called the Friendly Inn. The clinic was created by the Visiting Nurse Association of Cleveland and the Milk Fund, the latter a private charity that had been founded in 1899 by Edith Dickman, the daughter of an Ohio Supreme Court justice. Dickman had no medical training, but she was wise enough to understand that safe milk, provided free or at nominal cost to poor mothers, would go far toward reducing the appalling rate at which Cleveland children were dying.

In 1906, Lakeside's Edward Cushing spearheaded a drive to create the first independent infants' hospital in the city. The son and grandson of physicians, Cushing had always shown himself to be an unrepentant anachronism, a doctor whose career was distinctly anomalous in medicine's era of change. Even as specialists began to dominate the clinical scene, and as investigators in the laboratory were being accorded the status of medicine's new "heroes" (as one contemporary writer put it), Cushing steadfastly remained a generalist.

He was, in the opinion of many, eminently qualified to be a player on the national stage, either as physician or surgeon, yet he maintained a family practice throughout his career. And although the families he attended were for the most part among the city's elite, he spent a large part of his time providing medical services to the poor and indigent as well. A gentle and genuinely caring man, he worked harder than any other local physician to improve the level of care available to Cleveland's infants and children. Indeed, one colleague expressed a widely held belief when he referred to Cushing as "the foremost man in Cleveland," adding that "no man has been so useful in the life of this community...."

With the cooperation of the Visiting Nurse Association and the Milk Fund, and with the assistance of Lakeside physician John Lowman (son of one of the hospital's founders) and a young assistant professor in the medical school named Henry J. Gerstenberger, Cushing founded the Babies' Dispensary and Hospital in 1907. The new facility was housed in a former residence on East 35th Street, not far from the Western Reserve maternity dispensary. Gerstenberger, himself a graduate of Western Reserve, was placed in charge of the infant dispensary, which in its first year treated some two thousand cases, with more than four thousand home visits by the facility's physicians and nurses.

The Babies' Dispensary became the first such institution in the country to provide medical advice to parents of well children—in effect, practicing preventive medicine even before the term was coined. Visiting nurses fanned out into the shanty towns and slum neighborhoods of Cleveland, instructing immigrant mothers on the proper ways to feed and handle their babies. (With only fifteen individuals, the Visiting Nurse Association nevertheless managed to make more than thirty thousand home visits in its first year working out of the Babies' Dispensary.) The dispensary even printed an instructional brochure on infant care in five languages—English, German, Italian, Slovak, and Yiddish—and distributed copies throughout the city.

By 1910, Cushing had raised enough money to build a new and larger home for the dispensary. An elaborate fund-raising campaign, broadcast citywide through Cleveland's daily newspapers, had exhorted citizens to "Save the Babies" by conjuring up images of grief-stricken mothers and "little empty cradles." One particularly effective article urged readers to consider the plight of "the poor, skinny, half-starved little chaps that come into the world of alley tenements, hoodooed at the start and standing little or no chance to finish anything better than cripples, invalids, or criminals." The new Babies' Dispensary and Hospital opened in 1911 on the site of its predecessor, but even as the new building had been under construction, Edward Cushing was already looking beyond it. Cushing planned something even more ambitious: a full-fledged hospital of fifty beds, the first in Cleveland to be devoted solely to the care of infants and children. Just one month after the opening of the new Babies' Dispensary, however, in March of 1911, Edward Cushing died of cancer at the age of forty-eight.

A newspaper editorial of the time noted that, while many fine physicians had "come and gone" from the Cleveland scene over the years, none had provoked "the sense of loss that Dr. Cushing leaves." But in addition to the personal bereavement felt by hundreds of Clevelanders, the sudden death of Edward Cushing had a further, more painfully practical effect. Without his leadership and guidance, the drive to build the babies' and children's hospital was postponed indefinitely.

The death of Edward Cushing proved to be a loss for all of Cleveland, but the loss was experienced no more keenly than at Lakeside Hospital. And the hospital's trustees—as if they felt the institution could not continue to function without a member of the Cushing tribe practicing medicine there—soon offered a post to Edward's brother Harvey, by that time the chief surgeon at Johns Hopkins. What no one at Lakeside knew, however, was that Cushing had just accepted an offer to go to Harvard, where the new Peter Bent Brigham Hospital was being built, essentially for him, at a cost of $1 million.

At the time, Harvey Cushing was already generally considered to be the foremost neurosurgeon in the world. Unlike his late older brother, Cushing had chosen the high-profile path of specialization, winning renown as a skillful operator in the hitherto inaccessible region of the human brain. His addition to the Lakeside staff could only have further enhanced the hospital's reputation—not to mention attracting private patients from around the world—and would have raised Cleveland to the level of such other international centers of medicine as London, Paris, and Berlin. Cushing's decision to turn down an offer from Lakeside for the second time was, therefore, no small blow to the hospital's aspirations.

The Lakeside trustees could not afford to mourn the loss of the Cushing brothers for too long, however. Their most immediate concerns centered on the deterioration of the hospital's physical plant and its surrounding neighborhood. Despite the obvious drawbacks of the hospital's location, the trustees could not very well abandon their $600,000-plus investment little more than a decade after the hospital had first opened its doors. And although a completely new hospital in a better location would have been the ideal solution to their problems, no one at the time seriously entertained such a possibility. Thus, early in 1911, when Lakeside was at last in a position to think seriously about building its long-delayed maternity ward-*cum*-children's facility, the trustees could only consider how best to locate the structure in proximity to the existing hospital buildings.

As the *Leader* reported, however, the Lakeside trustees did not plan to expand the hospital complex onto the extra parcel of land that had been purchased for just such an eventuality some fifteen years before. They were instead attempting to procure a large piece of property directly across the street from the hospital, on the south side of what was by then known as Lakeside Avenue. The reasons for this apparent contradiction of previous policy were twofold: buying the new land across the street would effectively eliminate the slum housing there, one of the area's chief drawbacks; and the trustees had entered into serious negotiations for the sale of their extra parcel to the Gund Brewing Company, which had continued to evince an interest in the land even after the brewery's initial overtures were rebuffed in 1902.

In December of 1911 the sale to Gund was consummated, bringing to the hospital a substantial profit that was used to pay for repairs and alterations to its existing buildings.* Although funds sufficient to erect a new maternity and children's pavilion were still not in hand, the trustees were confident that the necessary contributions would be forthcoming shortly. In fact, Superintendent Ranney boasted to the *Leader* that work on the hospital's expansion would doubtless begin within the year. Before long, however, the notion of simply expanding the hospital would be abandoned in favor of a more ambitious scheme.

The Medical Department of Western Reserve having long since outgrown its aging home, the school's faculty and the university's trustees had come to agree that a new, larger, and more adequately equipped building would be necessary if the school were to maintain the level of quality that had so impressed Abraham Flexner in 1909. (Ironically, Flexner's praise of Western Reserve in his Carnegie Foundation report probably contributed to the school's growing pains by attracting more potential students than the existing facilities could possibly contain.) Knowing that the hospital was proposing to expand onto new property on the south side of Lakeside Avenue, the school's administrators began to consider the possibility of building their own new structure in closer proximity to Lakeside. Pushed along primarily by Howard Hanna, a trustee of both institutions, who thought that placing the medical school next to

---

*Ever mindful of their role as guardians of the hospital's moral landscape, the trustees insisted in their contract with Gund that the land was to be used solely for office and storage facilities for a period of twenty-five years, and that no buildings erected on the property could exceed sixty feet in height. Storage facilities facing the hospital's eastern side could not have windows. Buildings used for office space could be fenestrated, but only with windows that opened "in such a way that the inmates of the office shall not be able to see into the windows of the nurses' [residence]."

the hospital would result in "better accommodations for effective and combined work," informal discussions between members of the faculty and both boards began. And by the end of 1912, an agreement in principle was reached.

In January of 1913, the university officially changed the name of its medical department to the Western Reserve University School of Medicine. Shortly thereafter, a formal meeting of the medical faculty and the trustees of the university and Lakeside voted to purchase jointly about seventy thousand square feet of land on the south side of Lakeside Avenue, directly opposite the hospital. The property, it was agreed, was to be used solely for a new medical school building and the hospital's proposed new pavilion.

Howard Hanna and Samuel Mather together pledged $80,000 toward the total purchase price of the required land. But with the characteristic bad luck that dogged Lakeside whenever the hospital planned new construction, the country was even then entering what would prove to be a year-long recession, a profound economic slowdown that was precipitated in part by the introduction of the nation's first federal income tax. As the availability of further contributions became more problematic over the course of the year, both hospital and university trustees began to explore alternative sources of funding for their proposed projects. Ultimately, they settled on the idea of holding a joint conference at the Union Club in the fall of 1913, to which they invited two potential saviors: Dr. Wallace Buttrick, secretary of the Rockefeller Foundation's General Education Board; and Buttrick's new first assistant, Lakeside's old admirer, Abraham Flexner.

Although no record of the Union Club conference was made at the time, later events revealed that both Buttrick and Flexner approved of the plan to build a new medical school on the hospital's "campus." Unfortunately, neither man could promise that the foundation would make funds available for the project. But if the meeting produced no concrete commitments from the Rockefeller Foundation, it did engender a provocative new proposal, a plan that bore all the earmarks of a Flexner-inspired idea. Consequently, the old notion of building a small children's pavilion on the newly acquired land across from the hospital was scrapped. In its place was a new program, one that would, by bringing together a number of disparate elements in one location, move Lakeside even closer to Flexner's ideal, Johns Hopkins.

By December, a Joint Committee on Hospital and Medical School

Buildings was formed to investigate the feasibility of erecting not only a new medical school contiguous to Lakeside but also a full-fledged babies' hospital, the fulfillment of Edward Cushing's dream. The committee met for the first time just a few days before Christmas to vote on the elaborate new plan that had been shaped by its members: from Lakeside, Samuel Mather and George Crile; from Western Reserve, university president Charles Thwing and professor of pharmacology Torald Sollmann; and from the Babies' Dispensary, medical director Henry Gerstenberger and board member Arthur D. Baldwin, a prominent local attorney and co-founder of Cleveland's Legal Aid Society.

Crile presented the committee's "general scheme for cooperation and development of the university medical school and university hospital," the first time the latter phrase had been used in regard to Lakeside. In addition to a list of requirements for the new medical school building itself, the plan included the concept of reorganizing the Babies' Dispensary as a babies' and children's hospital, with its own free-standing facility to be built on the south side of Lakeside Avenue. The new hospital was to be closely tied to the medical school as its pediatric department, the university having already paved the way for this move by withdrawing the subject of pediatrics from the Department of Medicine and making it an autonomous department, with Gerstenberger as its chief.

As for Lakeside, one of Crile's own longstanding pet notions was to be implemented. Lakeside's existing buildings were to be rearranged to accommodate medical, surgical, obstetrical, and "psychopathic" wards, with a possible combined ward for such "secondary specialties" as dermatology and "nose and throat." All of the hospital's private patients would then be moved to a new private pavilion, to be built on the grounds of Lakeside's former home, the United States Marine Hospital. Although the Marine Hospital was still a functioning entity, Crile had been eyeing the site for months. He considered it an ideal location for a grand new private pavilion that he would, of course, control. In fact, he had begun his attempts to negotiate the lease or purchase of the property from the federal government even before the rest of the "scheme for cooperation and development" had been assembled or even conceived.

Focused on the prospect of creating a medical "campus" along the lines of the prestigious Johns Hopkins, the members of the Joint Committee managed to ignore some of the more obvious drawbacks of their plan. Lakeside itself, for example, would still be subject to the vagaries of its shifting foundations; all of the buildings, both old and new, would still be enveloped in the smoke and dirt of the area's industries; and some of the city's worst neighborhoods would still be virtually at the doorstep of the complex. Yet despite these objections, the members of the committee had clearly decided even before the first official meeting that they would expand Lakeside and erect a new babies' hospital and a new medical school building, all in the same location. And even though the country was still in the midst of a deep recession—and there was little hope of receiving outside funding for the project from the Rockefeller Foundation—Sam Mather announced at the committee meeting that he and Howard Hanna had already begun to secure options on several parcels of the land they would need to realize their plan.

Within a month, the Joint Committee met again, this time to choose a temporary consulting architectural firm to "draw up the necessary block plans." Sam Mather had already discussed the subject with, among others, Harvey Cushing, and Cushing's advice echoed that of many others: the firm to secure was Boston's Shepley, Rutan & Coolidge, designers of, among other buildings, much of the Harvard Medical School's new campus. Mather also reported that at least some of the landholders on Lakeside Avenue, having learned of the hospital's interest in their property, were asking unreasonable prices for their parcels. This unexpected complication affected not only Lakeside, the university, and the proposed babies' hospital, but also two additional institutions. The Western Reserve Dental School was by then expressing an interest in becoming a part of "the group," and the Research Committee of the National Association of Dentists was seriously considering the site as the location for their new national laboratory. What had started as a relatively small expansion of Lakeside Hospital was becoming, on paper at least, a true medical center.

By February of 1914, the architects were in Cleveland to discuss the Joint Committee's ideas and to tour the hospital and medical school buildings, as well as the proposed site of construction. The committee asked its architects to produce preliminary drawings as soon as possible, as if there were already complete unanimity of purpose among the many players involved in the process of creating the university hospital group. Yet at a committee meeting not long after, Sam Mather himself offered the first hint that at least one member of the committee was still weighing other options.

Ironically, the president of the hospital's board of trustees had for some time been thinking the unthinkable, and he was at last ready to raise the issue in a disturbingly straightforward question. Would it not be wise, Mather inquired, to consider tearing down Lakeside and building an entirely new hospital on another site? A lengthy discussion of the question ensued, during which the numerous drawbacks of the existing hospital buildings were weighed against the estimated $1 million cost of erecting a new structure at a new location. Although no definite decision was "reached or asked for" at the meeting, it was clear that Mather was not convinced that the lakefront was still a viable location for the hospital or its prospective new adjuncts.

Although Mather's sudden questioning of the lakefront location appeared to be spontaneous and unprovoked, it was in fact a reasoned response to circumstances at the time. By the date of the committee meeting, the City of Cleveland was already entertaining proposals to expand the railroads along the lakefront, creating a deeper right-of-way with additional tracks for more traffic—particularly freight trains—and establishing freight houses along the road. There were also proposals for the creation of expanded dock facilities, as well as growing sentiment in favor of building a passenger terminal on the lakefront. If even half of the proposed projects were to be realized, therefore, the increased industrial usage of the area would inevitably result in even more noise, dirt, and unsavory surroundings for Lakeside.

In addition, Mather, in his capacity as a trustee of Western Reserve, had been investigating the price of land in the vicinity of the school's campus as early as May of 1912. With an eye toward potential expansion of the university, Mather had explored two large properties in the area of the city known as University Circle. The first, owned by Jeptha Wade, president of the Western Union Telegraph Company, was situated on the north side of Euclid Avenue, directly across the street from Western Reserve and running north along East Boulevard to Bellflower Road. The second property, owned by Horatio C. Ford and his family, consisted of three parcels totaling some eleven acres that filled most of the block between Adelbert and Abington Roads, just east of the university. At the time, the Wade land was valued at about $300,000, the Ford land at $240,000.

Mather knew that the then-current proposals for lakefront development might, if all were to be implemented, prove disastrous to Lakeside Hospital. He also knew that many of the city's wealthier residents were moving out of Cleveland proper and into the burgeoning eastern suburbs, all of them much closer to University Circle than to the lakefront. Even as he and Howard Hanna continued to accumulate parcels for the hospital on Lakeside Avenue, therefore, Mather kept the University Circle properties in mind. Indeed, in April of 1914, a local real estate consultant retained by Mather reported to university president Thwing that both of the University Circle tracts were still available, although the Ford property had the disadvantage of being in the path of what Thwing once referred to as the "peril of the Sicilian invasion"—a potential influx of Italian residents from their nearby neighborhood enclave.

Just one month later, Mather formally requested the members of the Joint Committee to express their opinion of the feasibility of moving away from the lakefront to the vicinity of the university. In written responses, most of the members agreed with Henry Gerstenberger, who favored the move because it would "bring together and into touch all of the various factors that are instrumental in developing the theoretical and practical sides of medicine..."—that is, hospitals, medical school, and university. Moving to University Circle would, said Gerstenberger, give them the opportunity to create an academic center on a par with Johns Hopkins, a far better goal than merely to build "another and better Lakeside on the ruins of the present one."

The only voice of dissent among the committee's members was that of George Crile, who for reasons of his own argued strenuously against the move. Crile dismissed the current hospital's drawbacks almost cavalierly, calling the sooty discharge from passing trains, for example, merely "a housekeeping problem," and adding that "no one has been able to show that any material ill health results from smoke." In fact, Crile insisted, the "smoky haze" that hung over Lakeside most of the year was actually an asset for patients in the hospital, because it enhanced "the beauty of the sunsets over the lake."

Moving to University Circle—whose environs he described as "dull and stupid"—would cut off the hospital from the rest of the city, because of the limited streetcar service entering the area. Being situated close to only one poor neighborhood—"the Italian"—would also reduce the amount of clinical material available in the wards. And nothing would be gained "by a closer relation between the hospitals and the academic interests" of the university.

Coming from the same man who just three years before had stated publicly his ambition to turn Lakeside into the Johns Hopkins of the Midwest, Crile's opposition to a move that could have been the first step in the creation of a true academic medical center seemed inexplicable. His reluctance was not, however, as out of character as it appeared. Toward the end of his response to Mather, Crile revealed his principal reason for fearing the move to University Circle, and in doing so he also revealed much about his personal goals and priorities. "If we should remove to the university site...and if the present hospital should be purchased by the city...and become strongly efficient," he concluded, "then our hospital would easily be forced into second place and kept there...."

Despite Crile's alarm at the possibility that Lakeside could lose its position of preeminence among Cleveland health-care institutions, a new location for both the hospital and the medical school seemed inevitable. In June of 1914, the school's dean, Carl Hamann, polled the medical faculty to determine which of nine potential sites around town they preferred. Of the nine, three were in the downtown area, one was on the lakefront at East 105th Street, one was midway between downtown and the university, and four—including the Ford property—were in the immediate vicinity of the university.

Most members of the faculty believed that proximity to the university was preferable, although there was no consensus on the actual site. Almost all raised the point of access via streetcar, however, insisting that the school and hospital should be "accessible to the districts from which charity hospital patients would be largely derived." Conversely, a few—thinking about the comfort of their private patients—feared a potential conflict, noting that "to be surrounded by slums and immoral districts decreases the number of people who would otherwise go to the institution."

Predictably, George Crile argued that the "whole group should be developed with the hospital and its interests at its center." The new hospital should, therefore, remain in the heart of the city, while laboratory buildings for the medical school could "go out to the university...." But the concept of relocating to University Circle was also approved by the staff and management of Lakeside Hospital, and the combined weight of opinion of those in favor of the move proved overwhelming.

A secondary question in Hamann's poll of the medical faculty sought opinions on another and arguably more momentous change for the school and the hospital. Again following the lead of Johns Hopkins, which had taken a similar step the year before, Western Reserve's school of medicine now contemplated a major internal realignment: conversion to what was known as the "full-time" system of teaching.

In a "full-time" school, the heads of clinical departments gave up most of their private practices to devote the bulk of their time and attention to teaching and research. As full-time professors, they were employed by and received salaries from the university, salaries much larger than their normal remuneration from the school, to make up for the income lost when they reduced their patient rolls.

A hugely expensive undertaking, the full-time system had been initiated at Johns Hopkins the year before only with the help of an Abraham Flexner-inspired endowment grant of $1.5 million from the Rockefeller Foundation. Western Reserve as yet had no such endowment, but a strong majority of the medical faculty approved the idea of exploring the full-time plan. Two notable exceptions, however, were George Crile and his close associate Frank Bunts, the latter of whom went so far as to describe the scheme as a "fatal mistake."

As with his opposition to the move to University Circle, Crile's antipathy toward the full-time system seemed incongruous for someone who already spent a great deal of his time with research work. But in a spirited defense of the system, professor of histology Frederick C. Waite offered his own explanation of Crile's point of view when he described the typical "fractional-time man" as "a utilitarian, a materialist and, in a preponderating degree the country over, a commercialist, using the school as a means to his personal ends.... Ultimately we must come to the condition where the clinical departments will be controlled by full-time men, but I doubt that men who have grown up with the other ideals can change quickly...."

Crile's opposition notwithstanding, there were clear mandates in favor of both the move to University Circle and the adoption of the full-time plan, two elements fundamental to the creation of Cleveland's first true academic medical center. By the end of June 1914, therefore, Samuel Mather and Jeptha Wade, acting for all of the parties involved, obtained an option on the Ford property on Euclid Avenue. The way at last seemed clear to begin the lengthy task of raising funds to implement the ambitious plans of the medical school and its affiliated hospitals.

Of course, at the time no one knew that the realization of the medical center dream would be postponed for more than a decade. Because no one knew that even then an ardent Serbian nationalist in a city called Sarajevo was aiming a loaded pistol at the heart of an Austrian archduke.

CHAPTER SIX

Greater Than the Whole

In truth, the war in Europe that began in August 1914 had little immediate impact on Lakeside Hospital, save for the temporary loss of George Crile's services. Just three months after the outbreak of hostilities—with the United States still a neutral party—Crile petitioned the hospital's trustees for a leave of absence to staff an operating room and ward in the American Ambulance Hospital in Paris. His intention, he stated at the time, was simply to "lend a hand" to the French medical services.

Regarding the European war as a "human laboratory" on an enormous scale, Crile convinced the board that France would be the perfect arena in which to give nitrous-oxide anesthesia and his own shockless surgical method a "thorough and practical test" under extreme conditions. He wished, he explained, to take advantage of "this unparalleled opportunity to study the effect of emotion and exhaustion" on what he referred to as the "human material" of war. Crile asked for and received permission to take four of Lakeside's surgical residents and four nurses, all volunteers, for a three-month tour of duty in France, and before the end of the year the small expeditionary force was overseas.

If the earliest stage of the war had a minimal impact on the day-to-day operations of Lakeside, its effect on the creation of Cleveland's "university hospital" group was more pronounced. The first consequence was felt in October of 1914, when Samuel Mather recommended that Abraham Flexner be invited in from New York to give his "expert and unbiased judgment" of the new hospitals' proposed University Circle location. (Although Mather himself had first suggested the University Circle site, he thought that a confirming opinion from Flexner would alleviate any fears that Cleveland parties might still be harboring about the move east. It would also keep Flexner himself—who represented the Rockefeller Foundation, a potential source of funding—involved in the process.) By the end of the month, however, even Flexner's approval would become a moot point.

In the midst of an ongoing deep recession that was only aggravated by the uncertainties engendered by the outbreak of war, board members from the medical group's member institutions would not risk sizable commitments to acquire land or erect new buildings. In fact, the university's trustees even decided not to renew their option on the Ford property. And despite a later upturn in the economy, for nearly a year thereafter virtually no progress was made toward the goal of establishing a university hospital group. Indeed, the year 1915 proved to be one of stagnation and frustration for Lakeside, the medical school, and the nascent Babies' and Children's Hospital.

The new year would also be one of loss for all of Cleveland's medical community. On January 6th, after a brief illness, Dudley P. Allen died of pneumonia in his suite at the Ritz Carlton Hotel in New York. Just three days later, on the date of Allen's funeral, his old friend Hunter Powell died at his home in Cleveland. And one year to the day after Allen's death, local newspapers carried the obituary of Benjamin Millikin, Allen's longtime partner.

Although all three men had long since retired from the profession, the deaths of Allen, Powell, and Millikin constituted the symbolic closure of an era in Cleveland medicine. The passing of three of Lakeside's most prominent former division chiefs marked the true end of the nineteenth century for the hospital, because with Allen, Powell, and Millikin went virtually the last vestiges of nineteenth-century attitudes and modes of thought. Just as the World War itself would eventually sweep away America's longstanding isolationism and usher in its new international role (not to mention changing the country from a debtor nation, which it had been since its founding, to the world's largest creditor nation), the war years would set the stage for Lakeside's full emergence into medicine's new century. It would be an era dominated by change, and much of what was new would come from physicians who spent more of their time in the laboratory than on the wards.

Typical of the new era's changing attitudes was the 1915 initiative that extended the training of Lakeside's surgical residents. The trustees approved a plan requiring candidates for the post of head resident to first undertake six months of work in the pathology laboratory and six months in the Laboratory of Experimental Medicine.

A 1906 gift of Howard Hanna and Oliver H. Payne, the experimental-medicine lab was itself an example of the shifting focus of health care at Lakeside. Although it had been in operation for just a few years, its researchers were already on the verge of radical breakthroughs. David Marine, for example, the associate professor of experimental medicine, had come to the medical school a decade earlier as a mere demonstrator in pathology. Yet by 1915 he was well along in a pioneering study of simple goiter, a condition so prevalent in the entire Great Lakes region that the area had become known as the "Goiter Belt" of the country. Even then Marine was preparing to begin a large-scale test of a group of schoolchildren in the nearby city of Akron, which would ultimately prove that the cause of goiter was iodine deficiency and that its prevention could be effected by the addition of iodine to the diet. Ultimately, Marine would be remembered as the father of iodized salt.

In the pathology department, Howard Karsner, who in 1914 had succeeded the hospital's first true pathologist, William T. Howard, was establishing himself as one of the country's most innovative investigators and most exacting teachers. In addition to his duties as resident pathologist of Lakeside and professor of pathology in the medical school, Karsner also found the time to write. His *Human Pathology* would for years be considered the definitive textbook on the subject, ultimately being reprinted in eight editions.

But if the successes in the laboratories of both Lakeside and the school of medicine were of great value to medicine as a whole, they did nothing to advance the progress of Cleveland's planned university hospital group. The long delay was in fact less a question of science than of economics—the lingering effects of the recession that had begun in 1913. By the fall of 1915, however, the nation's economy had begun to respond to the stimulus of wartime production orders from France and Britain, and earlier fears about the duration of the recession began to dissipate.

To Western Reserve University president Charles F. Thwing, it seemed a propitious time to reintroduce the subject of acquiring the Ford property in University Circle. His desire to see the massive medical-center project at least begun if not completed before his retirement was obvious, but Thwing was also feeling some urgency to move openly on the land purchase for a different reason. In addition to his longstanding fear of a potential "invasion" of the area by residents of the nearby Italian enclave, Thwing wrote to Sam Mather to express his further alarm at recent reports that "the Roman Catholics are looking for a site for a cathedral… and they wish for one in this neighborhood."

Mather, too, was impatient to begin the project, yet he wisely counseled Thwing against even raising the issue at an upcoming university board meeting. "We do not want to buy that land except for medical college and hospital purposes, and that means several million dollars, as you know," Mather wrote from New York, where he was traveling on business. "So I think we should [privately] secure as long an option from Ford as possible—several months, six if we can—by paying him something for it, so as to have time to get [architectural] drawings, 'pictures,' estimates of cost, etc."

Only when they were fully prepared to explain and defend their plans —when "we know what we are talking about and can show prospective [contributors] that the scheme has been well thought out"—would they make known their intentions. Then they could take the proposition to the likes of Howard and Leonard Hanna, Jeptha Wade, and Mather's own half-brother, William, as well as to New York, to "see what the Flexner crowd will do."

"While delays are risky in one sense," Mather concluded, "yet each month now brings nearer the time when men like [these] will feel safe in counting on the business improvement being a genuine and permanent thing—and we shall need the generous aid of such men and others like them."*

Mather's slow and careful approach to fund raising proved to be the wisest course. Less than two months later, with more concrete plans in hand, he was able to convince Jeptha Wade to participate in a land-acquisition syndicate, and together the two men contributed a total of $75,000 as a down payment on the Ford property. Just as he had prophesied, Mather then went on to successfully promote the assistance of his brother, as well as that of Howard and Leonard Hanna. Together the five men eventually purchased the Ford property outright for some $423,000 and donated it to the hospital group.

Early in 1916 Mather at last had the opportunity to bring Abraham Flexner to Cleveland, to confer on the hospital group's proposal to create a medical center "campus" contiguous to the university. Flexner, whose

---

*An astute judge of character, Mather further explained his reasons for delay by cleverly interpreting a casual comment that Howard Hanna had once made about John D. Rockefeller. "When 'H.M.' spoke at our last meeting about 'J.D.R.' being human and wishing only to be associated with successes," Mather explained to Thwing, "he spoke, I am convinced, of his own viewpoint fully as much as of J.D.R.'s!"

ideal continued to be the pioneer medical center of Johns Hopkins, was favorably impressed by the Cleveland group's project. He encouraged both hospital and medical school trustees to apply for assistance from the Carnegie and Rockefeller foundations to implement their plans. Unfortunately, neither foundation was forthcoming with grant monies.

The problem of funding construction of the new hospitals was exacerbated by rising building costs as the year went on; nationally, costs were already up some fifty percent over those of 1915, and conditions in Cleveland reflected the national trend. The boards of the medical-group institutions therefore instructed their architects—Coolidge and Shattuck for the medical school and the new Lakeside, Abram Garfield for the babies' hospital—to postpone further work on drawings for the complex.*

In addition to their obvious fears about exorbitant building costs, many of Cleveland's most generous philanthropists were hesitant to make pledges to the medical-center capital drive because many were still paying off earlier commitments to the medical school's endowment-fund campaign. Although the projected total cost of building the medical school and its two affiliated hospitals was at the time only $3 million (an estimate that would ultimately prove laughably inaccurate), few of the medical community's longtime supporters were anxious to begin discussing further contributions at the time. By the beginning of 1917, however, Sam Mather would decide to break the logjam on his own.

Because architectural drawings for the new medical school had been virtually completed even before the 1916 postponement, the only factor that had been preventing immediate groundbreaking was the lack of sufficient pledged funds. At the end of January 1917, therefore, Sam Mather transferred ownership of some $300,000 worth of stock to the university, with the proviso that the equities should be used as the nucleus of a building fund for the new medical school. Characteristically, Mather, who was in New York on the day of the transfer, wired President Thwing to remind him: "Should desire of course to keep [news of the gift] from the papers."

Under ordinary circumstances, a major contribution from Mather

---

*Ironically, the additional delay only created a new money problem: the university faced the possibility that the Ford parcels would be subject to local property tax, since they were only being held, not used, by the tax-exempt Western Reserve. In an inspired suggestion, President Thwing managed to avoid assessment of the property by ordering the university's baseball team to use the otherwise empty Ford land as its official practice field.

would have spurred at least a few additional donations from some of the medical community's other benefactors. But the German navy's ongoing policy of unrestricted submarine warfare was urgently threatening American neutrality, and the possibility that the country could be swept into the European conflict proved too grave a fear for other potential donors to overcome.

When the United States did in fact declare war on Germany on April 6th, therefore, the medical school building-fund account still totaled only $300,000. And with a war to fight, the creation of a medical complex in Cleveland became just another domestic project to be postponed "for the duration." Ironically, the first uniformed Americans to arrive in France, on May 25th, were the physicians and nurses of "Base Hospital #4," a medical unit that consisted primarily of volunteers from Lakeside Hospital. And the unit was commanded by Major General George W. Crile.

§

As the rest of the country mobilized for war, Lakeside found itself dealing with a growing shortage of both physicians and nurses. In addition to Crile and his group of volunteers, the hospital soon began to lose more and more of its trained personnel to enlistment and the draft. By October the ranks of staff physicians were so depleted that senior medical students from Western Reserve were thrown onto the wards to serve as interns.

New students for Lakeside's Nurses' Training School were heavily recruited, following War Department warnings of an impending severe shortage of qualified nurses. In addition, the loss of much of the hospital's visiting staff severely curtailed the number of paying patients entering Lakeside. The reduced number of paying patients adversely affected the hospital's income for the year, but the shortfall also allowed an entire floor of the private pavilion to be converted for use as a residence hall for the new and larger class of nursing students.

As the fighting dragged on in Europe, the War Department sponsored Lakeside-based research projects on such problems as the effects of chemical warfare and the optimal design of gas masks. Physicians and researchers by the dozen arrived in Cleveland from Washington and other parts of the country. The sudden influx transformed the earlier personnel shortage into an acute housing squeeze, however, and a number of residents, lab technicians, and housekeeping employees were soon pushed out of the hospital proper and temporarily housed in refurbished residences in the immediate vicinity of Lakeside.

But if the war and its attendant support activities on the homefront occupied the attention of most of Cleveland, planning for the new medical center at University Circle still managed to continue. Indeed, by November of 1917 another institution had been added to the list of those already committed to building new homes on the proposed medical campus.

The Cleveland Maternity Hospital, which in its earliest years had been the poor sister of the city's charitable hospitals, had been improving steadily through the second decade of the century, both in terms of its operational efficiency and the quality of the care it provided. The improvements at Maternity were due largely to the efforts of the hospital's then-new superintendent, Calvina MacDonald, who had been brought to Cleveland from Boston's Lying-In Hospital in 1908 by Edward Cushing. Cushing had only been looking for a qualified individual "to assist him in the nursing of his obstetrical patients," but before long the full range of MacDonald's abilities were recognized and put to use. As superintendent of Maternity, MacDonald ran what one observer called "a first-class course and training." Indeed, by 1914, the Lakeside nurses' training school was able to discontinue the practice of shipping its students to other cities for instruction in obstetrical nursing, sending them to the revitalized local facility instead.

Early in 1917, Maternity Hospital director Arthur Bill engineered the extension of teaching privileges at the hospital to the faculty of the School of Medicine of Western Reserve. He also began to seek a formal designation of his facility as "the affiliated teaching obstetrical hospital of...the medical school." This was a somewhat stickier question, however, because although the hospital's care of patients and training of nurses had improved dramatically, nothing had been done to upgrade its crowded and wholly deficient physical plant. Indeed, the Maternity Hospital was still housed in two aging former residences so small that to make space for delivery rooms and a laundry it had been necessary to adapt an adjacent horse barn.

Although hobbled by its inadequate facilities, the Maternity Hospital nonetheless boasted a fairly sizable endowment and only a minor operating deficit. The obvious solution to its one overriding dilemma was construction of a wholly new hospital facility, and in November of 1917,

Bill and several members of his board of trustees proposed to university president Thwing and his trustees that a new Maternity Hospital be included in the plans for the medical-center group at University Circle.

The obvious need for a new facility, as well as the potential benefits of a combined fund-raising campaign among all the participating institutions, made the Maternity proposal attractive to all of the parties involved, and an agreement was soon reached. Still, the fact of the war precluded any action on the process of raising funds or actually beginning construction. Indeed, so remote was the possibility of achieving real progress on the project that in the spring of 1918, in the interests of furthering homefront causes, the fallow Ford property was "loaned" to employees of the Halle Bros. department store, for cultivation as a huge vegetable garden.

Meanwhile, the patient population of Lakeside, as well as those of most other hospitals around the country, exploded as the influenza pandemic that had started in Europe spread across the world. In excess of five hundred flu victims were admitted to Lakeside alone during 1918, and more than a quarter of them succumbed to either the disease itself or its resulting complications. Because the vast majority of the influenza patients at Lakeside were poor or indigent, the hospital experienced additional erosion of its annual income. But at year's end, the city's Red Cross chapter commended Lakeside for having done "more than any other [local] hospital" to meet the needs created by the epidemic.

Despite occasional shortages of equipment and supplies, those Lakeside physicians who remained stateside continued their work, both in the wards and in the research labs. Henry J. Gerstenberger, for example, was well on the way to successfully concluding a project that had consumed him since 1913. With fellow pediatrician Harold Ruh and chemist William Frohring, Gerstenberger was attempting to create a viable infant formula as a substitute for mother's milk, and by 1915 the research team had hit on the specific ingredients of a mixture they called "Synthetic Milk, Adapted," or S.M.A.

It took another four years of testing and refining before Gerstenberger could apply for and receive a patent on S.M.A. Eventually, he signed over all royalties from the commercial sale of the product to the Babies' Dispensary, to create a fund for teaching and research.

Gerstenberger's great triumph came, however, in the wake of an unsettling event on the children's ward of Lakeside: the unexpected death of a child in his care. The young patient had already been treated and cured of the complaint for which it was first admitted, but Gerstenberger apparently kept the child in the hospital through June of 1918, to include it in an experiment he was then conducting. When some members of the house staff brought criticisms of Gerstenberger's conduct to the attention of the trustees, board president Mather ordered the full visiting staff to investigate the case. A staff committee ultimately absolved Gerstenberger "from the charge of willfully subjecting children under his care to hazardous experiments...."

Early in July, however, the hospital's attorneys reported to the trustees that Gerstenberger was being sued for malpractice by the dead child's mother, who had retained a flamboyant local personal-injury litigator by the name of Harry Payer. Gregarious, witty, and well liked by even the most hidebound members of the city's establishment, Payer was a gifted courtroom performer who was genuinely feared by his opponents before the bench. He was not only the most effective attorney in Cleveland at the time, but he was also acknowledged by his peers to have obtained more favorable verdicts and won larger dollar awards for his clients than any other practicing trial attorney in the United States.

Lakeside's law firm learned that Payer had in his possession "practically all the facts" of the case, and that he would "be able to show very convincingly before a jury that Dr. Gerstenberger had been at fault in keeping this child in the hospital for experimental purposes...." This information, combined with Payer's reputation as a genius of courtroom oratory and the trustees' obvious desire to keep the case from the newspapers, undoubtedly influenced the board's decision to settle the Gerstenberger case out of court.

The attorneys recommended that the hospital accept a proposed settlement with the parents amounting to less than $4,000, which effectively ended the case. And although Sam Mather urged all members of the hospital's medical staff to "realize the seriousness...of any one of their number attempting research work without some check or control," he nonetheless expressed his "confidence" in Gerstenberger. As had been true with the secret firing of Lakeside's former superintendent, James Knowles, not a word appeared in print about the case of Henry J. Gerstenberger.

The Gerstenberger incident highlighted a number of serious deficiencies within both Lakeside and the medical school: the lack of formal constraints on the actions of medical personnel engaged in research; the near-absolute power of departmental and division chiefs within their domains; the unwillingness of physicians to censure their colleagues, even when the facts warranted such a move; and the further unwillingness of trustees to allow their institutions to be the object of negative publicity, even when that, too, was warranted.

The potential for abuse of departmental power had, of course, always existed. Indeed, Gerstenberger's rule of the pediatric service was reminiscent of the excesses of the hospital's first autocrat, the formidable Gustav Weber. (And in later years, Gerstenberger would, if anything, grow even more highhanded.) Perhaps the prime example of an all-powerful division head was George Crile, who over the years had been able to run a virtually autonomous service with the blessing of the board of trustees. Aside from being denied the electric window-shade hoists he had once requested, Crile was given numerous unprecedented privileges, and he had been essentially free to operate without constraints since being named chief of surgery in 1911.

During his wartime duty overseas, however, Crile came to believe that even his privileged position at Lakeside did not afford him sufficient autonomy. At Base Hospital #4, he worked with a small team of specialists, each member of which was available to lend his particular expertise to a situation immediately, without first clearing measures through administrative entanglements or levels of authority. Accountable only to themselves, the team members of Base Hospital #4 considered their time in the war as one of the most productive periods of their lives.

After the armistice of November 11, 1918—which was, coincidentally, Crile's fifty-fourth birthday—Lakeside's chief surgeon began to consider a new path for himself, a situation that would include the best of his experiences in France with the best ideas of his friends the Mayo brothers, whose "group practice" clinic in Minnesota he admired. With minimal overseer authority above them and the ability to make decisions on the spot, the Mayos seemed to Crile to enjoy the perfect medical practice. And upon his return to Cleveland, in 1919, he immediately began to explore the possibility of creating a similar paradise for himself.

§

Although a new home for Lakeside was still years away, by the first month of 1919 the hospital's visiting staff was meeting with the rest of the medical school's faculty to reiterate for the record their desire to see a "permanent affiliation" of the new hospital and the university. Of course, the meaning of this statement had less to do with the eventual physical proximity of the two institutions—already an established premise—than with a much more radical proposition: the faculty's formal acceptance of the long-debated "full-time" system of teaching.

"We believe," concluded the hospital's visiting staff, "that the heads of [Lakeside's] larger clinical departments should have their chief interest in the work of the hospital as a university institution...." Thereafter, clinical chiefs would give up most of their private practices to devote full time to their roles as educators and researchers. And the staff further endorsed the full-time concept by specifying that the "selection of patients for [Lakeside's] open wards should be with a view primarily to teaching and investigation."

When implemented, these two provisions would constitute the culmination of the revolution that had begun at Lakeside at the turn of the century. The hospital was, in effect, changing its self-designated role in the community, redefining itself to become but one element in a larger institution—an academic medical center, whose purview would include increased emphasis on laboratory research and medical education.

Lakeside could no longer be precisely the institution its founders had envisioned, a hospital that was "free to all, the most needy being considered the most worthy." To choose ward patients "with a view primarily to teaching and investigation" would mean that patient care itself, once the sole focus of the hospital, would be subsumed within academic medicine's wider focus. What had originally been merely the haven of poor Clevelanders seeking medical care would become a true university hospital, and as such it would follow the course charted by the trendsetters of American medicine, Johns Hopkins and Harvard.

Of course, even with the admirable goal of becoming part of an academic medical center, Lakeside continued to serve its patient population much as it had always done. But if the hospital maintained its reputation as one of the city's most valued assets, the quality of the patient care it provided soon came into question.

A citywide hospital and health survey conducted during 1919 by the Cleveland Hospital Council was released as a published report the following year, and the results of the investigation proved disturbing to say the least. Overseen by the council's director, Dr. Haven Emerson, the survey was a thorough assessment of each of the city's hospital facilities and its role in the provision of health care to the community. Not unlike Abraham Flexner's landmark 1909 survey of medical schools, the Emerson investigation uncovered numerous instances of laxity and incompetence, shocking waste, duplication of effort, and outright stupidity among the physicians and administrators of Cleveland's hospitals.

Although it was not the site of the most egregious deficiencies uncovered by the survey, Lakeside came in for its share of criticism. And many of the problems encountered at the hospital were directly attributable to Lakeside's growing emphasis on its commitment to teaching and research.

Through interviews with former patients, the survey investigators learned that Lakeside physicians had a disquieting tendency to adopt a cavalier attitude toward the suffering of charity patients. Routinely failing to provide adequate explanations of a patient's condition, the typical Lakeside physician would discharge a ward case without giving the patient sufficient instructions for steps to be taken during convalescence at home. Charity patients also deeply resented the fact that the hospital's teaching physicians often referred to them—in their presence—not as individuals but as mere "interesting cases."

Paying patients in the lower-priced semiprivate wards also expressed dismay at what they considered the hospital's overemphasis on monetary concerns. Many complained that upon discharge, the last representative of the hospital they encountered was a bookkeeper, who wished them good luck in returning to work quickly so that they could soon begin paying their hospital bills.

The Emerson investigators made numerous recommendations to the city's hospitals about redressing their problems, including a recommendation that Lakeside run all its own ambulances, rather than continuing the practice of hiring out ambulance service from local morticians. The latter suggestion had sprung from the story of one man who was frightened out of his wits when, after being rendered unconscious in an automobile accident, he regained his faculties in the back of the hearse that was conveying him to Lakeside.*

But if the Emerson report brought to light a host of problems at the hospital, it also praised the proposed medical center project that would

---

*In recalling the incident later to a Hospital Council investigator, the unfortunate victim summed up the experience by saying, "I don't *never* expect to get over *that* wake-up."

bring together Lakeside, the School of Medicine, and the new babies' and maternity hospitals. The report even included a recommendation that the new facilities be erected in the order in which the community most needed them: the medical school first, followed by the babies' and maternity hospitals. (Infant mortality in Cleveland, although far lower than in most American cities of comparable size, was still quite high at the time, and according to Abraham Flexner, maternal mortality in the United States was the highest in the world.) Only after all the other components of the group were in place, said the report, should the new Lakeside be erected.

The unstated message of the Emerson report was that Lakeside would do better to resolve its internal problems before it addressed the task of building a new home. Coincidentally, the hospital's superintendent had resigned just weeks before, and the board was thus afforded the opportunity to install a new man to oversee the remedial efforts called for in the report. At the urging of Samuel Mather, the trustees chose for the job a forty-year-old locally trained physician named Robert H. Bishop.

A native of Kansas, Bishop grew up in Oxford, Ohio, where his great-grandfather had been the first president of Miami University. A graduate of the Western Reserve School of Medicine, Bishop first made his mark in medicine in the field of public health, as one of the founders of the Anti-Tuberculosis League and, later, as Cleveland's wartime health commissioner.

In 1914 Bishop married Constance Mather, the only daughter of Lakeside's board president, but no one would have suggested that nepotism played a part in his appointment at the hospital. Bishop's long experience in public health and his proven administrative and managerial talents made him a more than credible candidate for the job of Lakeside superintendent. And as events were to transpire, his role in the shaping of not only Lakeside but the entire medical center group would prove to be pivotal.

At the time, however, organization of the long-delayed medical group was still moving forward at only half speed. Early in January of 1920, for example, representatives of the university and all of the hospital members of what was then being called "The Associated Hospitals and Medical School of Cleveland" met to discuss the findings of a committee investigating the cost of erecting a central power plant for the new medical group. The disturbing committee report indicated that the price of one coal-burning plant that could supply steam heat and distribute purchased electric power to all of the buildings of the complex would alone be more than $700,000. And no one even cared to speculate as to what the plant's annual operating costs might be.

The rate of inflation continued to rise unabated—the phrase "the high cost of living" was just entering the idiom at the time—and potential price increases for virtually all goods and services mitigated against embarking on major construction projects. Of course, postwar inflation was not the only obstacle in the path of the new medical center: designs for the individual hospital buildings, not to mention the configuration of the group as a whole, were still being revised.

In the wake of the postwar inflation, yet another severe recession further eroded the confidence of potential donors, and even the much-needed new medical school was still no more substantial than a set of drawings in the Boston offices of architects Coolidge and Shattuck. Within so uncertain an economic climate, it was not surprising that for more than a year virtually no constructive action was effected on any of the projects within the group.

It was not until June of 1921 that Sam Mather would again attempt to set an example to be emulated by boldly making a $500,000 cash contribution to the medical school building fund. At that point, Mather's total gifts for the school's building fund—exclusive of his share of the cost of the Ford property itself—amounted to $800,000. As had happened after his first major donation, however, none of the other old friends of the university followed Mather's lead.

Meanwhile, Lakeside itself was experiencing an embarrassment of riches. In a three-month period early in 1921, the hospital saw a thirty percent increase over the number of operations performed in the same period the previous year. Much of the increase was attributed to George Crile, who had developed a high-speed technique of performing surgery on patients in their own beds, on both the charity and semiprivate wards. Crile's method was to attack an entire floor with lightning speed, moving from one patient to the next as a team of assistants closed incisions in his wake.

While the increased number of surgical patients benefited the hospital's revenues in the short term, one unfortunate consequence of Crile's mass-production technique was that Lakeside's nursing corps found itself taxed to the limit, both physically and mentally. Although the number of nurses available for duty in the hospital on any given day was substantial, the nursing corps was never meant to be sufficient to handle operations on the wards themselves.

Before long a nurses' revolt in one of the semiprivate wards was brought to the attention of the trustees, who were informed that, due to the "constantly increasing number" of Crile's in-ward operations, the nursing service was "in a fair way of breaking down completely." The Lakeside board's executive committee was asked to intercede with Crile on behalf of the nurses, but the trustees promised only to suggest to the chief surgeon that he consider slowing his pace somewhat.

Crile was indeed working at a furious pace, and he was doing so because he had a pressing incentive to collect as many fees as possible. Indeed, even as Lakeside's trustees spent some $8,000 to fulfill Crile's most recent request—alterations and new equipment for his operating room—Crile himself was spending his own money on a project outside the walls of Lakeside: the construction of his own autonomous health-care facility, an institution that he would call The Cleveland Clinic.

During their wartime service in Base Hospital #4, Crile and his longtime colleagues Frank Bunts and William Lower had seen the efficacy of bringing together specialists of different disciplines to work together as a team. The Mayo brothers had already shown that a civilian group practice—in which each of the member physicians gave up his private practice to work together in a clinic setting, deriving income as a salary from the clinic rather than as fees from patients—could function successfully. Now surgeons Crile, Bunts and Lower joined with local internist John Phillips to create a Cleveland version of the Mayos' Minnesota clinic.

In October of 1919, Crile and his colleagues took the first formal steps toward creating their new group practice, pooling their resources to fund construction of their own clinic building. By the time of the nurses' revolt at Lakeside, Crile was committed to delivering nearly $7,000 a month to the Clinic building fund, which was one of the reasons he attacked with such urgency the cases of paying patients on the semiprivate wards.

In February of 1921, The Cleveland Clinic officially opened in a new building on Euclid Avenue, less than a mile from the proposed location of the university medical center. The trustees of Lakeside, while congratulating Crile on his bold new venture, also sought reassurances from him that a working relationship could exist between the hospital and the clinic. But by the end of July, trustee Frank Scott reported to the board's executive committee that after continuing attempts at dialogue with Crile, as yet no progress had been made in determining just what if any formal relationship would exist between the two institutions.

Puzzled by this response, the executive committee urged Scott to press

Crile more strongly. Less than a week later, Scott announced to the trustees that Crile had "no suggestions" as to a possible relationship between the Clinic and Lakeside. Sam Mather relayed this information to university president Thwing by letter, with a handwritten notation in which he remarked that Crile's behavior was "a great surprise to me and to us all...."

Despite his apparent lack of interest in formalizing a relationship between the Clinic and Lakeside, Crile's status within the hospital remained unaffected. Early in 1922, for example, he successfully renominated Lower as associate visiting surgeon in charge of Lakeside's genitourinary service over the strenuous objections of Robert Bishop, who thought Lower had not demonstrated "any marked interest...in the development of his department."

Bishop argued that Lower—who was also chief of surgery at another Cleveland hospital—spent more time with patients at the Clinic and elsewhere than he did guiding the interns and residents of his service at Lakeside. Although Crile ultimately had his way and saw Lower renominated, Bishop had sounded an early and prescient warning about the inevitable competition that would develop between the Clinic and the University Hospitals group, of which Lakeside would soon be a member.

§

By February of 1922, it was obvious to everyone concerned with Cleveland's proposed medical center complex that, in terms of funding at least, the outlook for the massive project was unremittingly bleak. Speaking with unusual bluntness, Sam Mather told a university board meeting that despite his earlier hopes, he was now convinced that there was "no prospect" of securing funds from a public subscription campaign to build a new medical school and power plant, the first elements of the University Hospitals group.

After making this funereal pronouncement, however, Mather proceeded to inform his fellow trustees that he would nonetheless "authorize the building committee to go ahead" with construction of the new school. "And," he added, "I will pay for it."

Within six months of Mather's stunning announcement that he would personally underwrite the entire cost of both the medical school and the power plant, construction of the first stage of the mammoth medical center project began at last. Not long after, Robert Bishop resigned as director of Lakeside to assume the new post of executive secretary of the medical group's executive committee. Bishop's job included oversight of construction of the complex in University Circle and coordination of the full-scale fund-raising campaigns that at some point would have to be undertaken if the rest of the hospitals in the group were ever to be built.

Architect Abram Garfield had virtually completed his drawings for the babies' and maternity facilities, and the only impediment to actual construction of the two hospitals was the absence of funds. The new Lakeside, however, was as yet no further advanced than a rough rendering of its possible appearance, a sketch that had been exhibited publicly in the April 1922 issue of the Cleveland Academy of Medicine's monthly bulletin.

The drawing of the proposed new Lakeside revealed that the hospital's trustees were again thinking in monumental terms, just as they had done in 1893, when conceiving the original Lakeside. Their new hospital was slated to be a huge, thousand-bed facility, located between Adelbert and Abington Roads, with its main entrance facing Euclid Avenue. A central corridor with eight connecting wings of four stories each would run straight back from a main three-building cluster for more than half the depth of the parcel on which it would stand. Directly south of Lakeside would be the babies' and maternity hospitals, and behind the latter would be the new medical school.

So large a hospital would be monumentally expensive both to build and to operate, but the trustees were buoyed in their optimism by the knowledge that $2.5 million had already been pledged to their building fund. In addition, Lakeside's permanent endowment by then totaled some $4 million, most of it in the form of blue-chip stocks and high-yield bonds from such enterprises as New York's Interborough Rapid Transit Company and even the Dutch East Indies Company. Indeed, at that point the hospital's endowment was some fifty times the amount that had been held in trust in 1898, when the first "new" Lakeside opened its doors.

Even as the trustees dreamed of creating a grandiose medical facility for the future, however, they could not ignore the ongoing difficulties of maintaining their current home. And before long they would be faced with a personnel problem of overweening importance: finding a successor to George Crile.

By the provisions of the same mandatory retirement clause he had engineered in 1906, Crile would be forced to retire as chief surgeon in 1924, when he turned sixty. Although it may have seemed to some that he had been hoist with his own petard, Crile expressed no misgivings about leaving Lakeside at the time; the Cleveland Clinic was already thriving, and Crile's plans for the institution included the creation of its own full-fledged hospital facility.

By the spring of 1923, therefore, Lakeside's trustees were hard at work searching for a new chief for the surgical service. Not surprisingly, their first choice was the same man they had been trying to bring back home for nearly a quarter of a century: Cleveland native Harvey Cushing. In the face of Cushing's long-established relationship with Harvard and its Peter Bent Brigham Hospital, however, even the prospect of a wholly new Lakeside building proved to be insufficient inducement for the noted neurosurgeon to return to his native city.

In turning down the Cleveland post, however, Cushing offered a piece of advice that would change the trustees' thinking about their proposed new hospital. In a letter to the board, Cushing advised against building the thousand-bed hospital that the trustees and their architects had been contemplating since the inception of the project. Instead, Cushing recommended a hospital of some three hundred beds, with a large outpatient department that could function as a "feeder" for the wards.

"If you have a whale of a hospital with a great private ward," Cushing warned, "you may do some good work for a lot of people, but as an academic institution nobody will ever hear anything of you. The other big hospitals [in Cleveland will] have to do the rest of the work [because] it cannot be thrust on the shoulders of your teaching staff."

Cushing's own Brigham Hospital, he explained, had but thirty-eight private rooms, and he urged the Lakeside board to consider a similar division of bed space in their new edifice. "If you do this," he concluded, "you will make a great name for yourselves and for Cleveland."

The Lakeside trustees took Cushing's advice to heart and begin to revise the existing plans for the new hospital. At the same time, construction of the new medical school had begun, and plans were being finalized for a fund-raising campaign for the two other hospitals in the medical group. Chaired by Babies' and Childrens' board president Arthur D. Baldwin, the campaign to raise $2.5 million was scheduled to be held over an eight-day period in the second week of May 1923, a period chosen because it coincided with the occasion of Mother's Day.

The combined campaign to fund construction of the Maternity and the

Babies' and Children's hospitals was run along roughly the same lines as previous campaigns for Cleveland's Community Fund, an overseer entity which raised funds for the annual operating needs of roughly one hundred member charitable agencies and organizations. (Community Fund monies were apportioned by a sister organization, the Welfare Federation of Cleveland, which served as a planning agency for the Fund's charities.) Not coincidentally, Sam Mather had initiated the practice of combined fund-raising in November of 1917, when he chaired Cleveland's first "War Chest" drive, a $4 million campaign that was the immediate precursor of the later Community Fund drives.

For the 1923 hospital-group campaign, a small army of volunteer fund-raisers was enlisted from among the city's business and industrial leaders. Local newspapers served as unofficial cheerleaders, helping to publicize the campaign with free coverage—including front-page editorial cartoons—throughout its duration. A local public relations firm produced publicity materials for the campaign, with a suitably emotional logo that became ubiquitous on posters, billboards, theater-lobby placards, and streetcar advertisements throughout the city.

A masterpiece of salesmanship, the logo depicted a destitute mother clutching an infant in her arms while another, older child stood clinging to one of her sleeves. Hovering above this group stood a nurse with arms outstretched, and behind them all in the distance were representations of the two new hospitals. The illustration was accompanied by the slogan, "Give Them a Chance."

Other slogans were advanced over the campaign, including "Save the Babies," "Will You Help Them a Little?" and "Give It For Mother." Each new line was accompanied by suitably sympathetic photos of waifs and urchins. Most of the city's major department stores and other large advertisers included the campaign logo in their newspaper promotions during the week, but perhaps the cleverest use of the fund-drive logo appeared in an ad for a vaudeville house. ("Two Big Things You Should Attend To This Week," read the ad. "Help The Baby Hospital...and See The Great Show at B.F. Keith Palace Theatre.")

Accounts of each day's take were duly reported in the papers, in articles of unrelenting cheerfulness. Toward the end of the campaign, however, the newspapers began to run stories under such headlines as "Leaders Alarmed at Day's Showing," a transparent ploy designed both to maintain interest in the campaign and to startle slackers into making their own contributions.

As the fund drive wound to a close, the trustees of Lakeside Hospital arranged to transfer to the campaign the more than $100,000 in its own Edward F. Cushing Fund, an endowment originally created by Howard Hanna for the "care of mothers and babies" at Lakeside. Jeptha Wade contributed $150,000, an individual donation second in size only to the $172,000 gift of Sam Mather. Finally, on the last day of the campaign, the $2.5 million goal was met and exceeded thanks to a $100,000 contribution from Edward Harkness. The son of the Standard Oil partner, Harkness lived in New York but was always willing to donate to worthy causes in his boyhood home. Indeed, having already solicited his contribution, the campaign's organizers held the Harkness gift in reserve to cover any possible shortfall on the last day of the drive. But the final tally of the fund drive showed that more than $2.6 million had been raised in just eight days.

§

At the end of the first month of 1924, with George Crile's retirement from Lakeside imminent, the trustees of both the hospital and the medical school at last settled on a choice for the post of chief visiting surgeon. Elliott Cutler was only thirty-five years old at the time, but he was already an associate in surgery at the Peter Bent Brigham Hospital and director of the laboratory for surgical research at the Harvard Medical School. Recommended highly by his own teacher and colleague, Harvey Cushing, Cutler genuinely impressed the search committee from Cleveland. Charles Hoover, director of Lakeside's Department of Medicine and himself a renowned diagnostician and educator, praised Cutler with one of his highest accolades when he described him as being "endowed with the ideals of a teaching man."

(Cutler was not, of course, the first man considered for the post; in addition to the initial offer to Cushing, the trustees had also approached Western Reserve School of Medicine Dean Carl Hamann for the job. But the dean, whose imperious manner and insistence on strict discipline as the school's longtime professor of anatomy and clinical surgery had earned him the nickname "King" Hamann, turned down the offer, primarily because he wanted to retain his connection with Charity Hospital, where he was already chief of surgery.)

With a new chief surgeon assured, the Lakeside trustees had one more piece of internal business to take care of before they could turn their full attention to planning for their new home. In February, the board officially recommended the merger of the Lakeside Nurses' Training School into Western Reserve's newly endowed School of Nursing.

Just two months before, Frances Payne Bolton, the wife of state senator Chester C. Bolton, had offered a $500,000 endowment to Western Reserve to turn the school's Department of Nursing into a distinct college within the university. A longtime friend of the Cleveland medical community, Bolton was deeply interested in bettering the profession of nursing and promoting higher education for women. She was also disturbed at what she perceived as the condescending attitude of Lakeside's doctors toward the hospital's nurses, who were often viewed as infringing on physicians' professional prerogatives. Indeed, in a letter to Sam Mather at the time of the merger, Bolton objected strongly to a widely held view among Lakeside physicians that the hospital's nurse training school was "over-educating" its students. She also expressed her disgust at what she saw as a lack of "reverence for their fellow beings" among the hospital's medical staff, some of whom she labeled as downright "boorish."*

The Lakeside board agreed that merging the hospital's school into Western Reserve's new college of nursing would provide "university value" for nurse training, thereby helping to attract as candidates "some of the young women seeking entrance to colleges." (At the time, Western Reserve was still one of only a small number of universities in the country that admitted women.) And the elimination of the hospital-run nursing school would be but one more example of the increasingly close ties between Lakeside and the university, ties that had originated in the first agreement to make Lakeside the official clinical arm of the medical school.

But if the hospital's teaching relationship with the university was applauded as an important element of medical education in Cleveland, it also proved a source of recurring difficulties for Lakeside. In the spring of 1924, for example, the Welfare Federation of Cleveland conducted a survey of hospital operating costs, one result of which was a reprimand

---

*Bolton was pleased, however, at the choice of Elliott Cutler as chief surgeon, because Cutler was known to her as "a cultured gentleman and a real scholar."

to Lakeside for what were deemed excessively high charges related to, among other things, its teaching component.

Since the Welfare Federation in effect spoke for the Community Fund, a much-needed source of operating funds for the hospital, the trustees were forced to consider ways to cut costs while maintaining what the Federation called the hospital's "high type of service." Some months later, therefore, the board hired a consultant—one of the men who had compiled the federation survey, in fact—to "inject into the hospital a person whose viewpoint is predominantly that of the businessman." It would not be the last time that third-party funders would pressure the hospital to somehow reign in its operating costs without cutting services.

Costs were not, however, one of the factors with which the trustees groped as they worked at redesigning the new Lakeside. The board had long since rejected the proposed massive structure against which Harvey Cushing had argued so forcefully and had begun to consider a scaled-down version. The new plans called for only about one-third the number of beds of the first proposal, and of these, roughly two-thirds would be devoted to charity cases. The remaining third would be divided between private and semiprivate rooms, despite the fact that such a division would increase annual operating costs by more than $250,000 and, in one trustee's words, "reduce hospital revenue materially."

The decision to follow Cushing's advice would inevitably widen the gap between operational costs and revenues at the new Lakeside, but it was the only path to follow if the hospital were to be taken seriously as an element of a true academic medical center. And as Robert Bishop pointed out, a smaller hospital with fewer private rooms would also make easier the task of raising the funds necessary to actually build the new Lakeside.

Bishop's scheme to raise the capital to build the new hospital entailed what he called a "quiet campaign" among Lakeside's friends, from whom he thought roughly $1 million could be secured before a public campaign was even initiated. When combined with an additional $1 million from the nearly $2.5 million already in the building fund, a "wing for private and semiprivate patients" could be built. Then, when it became necessary to raise the remainder of what was projected to be a total cost of some $7 million in a general campaign among the public, the hospital could truthfully say that "the appeal would simply be for the open [charity] wards and dispensary accommodations."

To forego a large number of private rooms, however, put the hospital at a distinct disadvantage in the citywide competition for paying patients. And that disadvantage became even more pronounced as of June 14, 1924, when George Crile officially retired from Lakeside and opened his new Cleveland Clinic Hospital, all on the same day.

Although the Lakeside trustees marked the end of the Crile era with a resolution praising his "fine talents and great energy" and by offering their "sincere good wishes," it must have been obvious to them that, as of that moment, Crile was nothing less than a full-fledged competitor. And if in the future they might decry the number of private patients who chose Crile's Cleveland Clinic over Lakeside, they would have to remember that they were themselves partly to blame.

If in 1906 the trustees had sided with Dudley P. Allen rather than with Crile during the great war of the two surgeons, it is not inconceivable that Crile might have left the city to look for greener pastures elsewhere. Then, instead of a thriving Cleveland Clinic less than a mile from Lakeside, there could easily have been a Boston Clinic, a Chicago Clinic, or a Pittsburgh, Milwaukee, or St. Louis Clinic, none of which would have posed any threat at all. But in 1906 the trustees had chosen to cast their lot not with the older, established Allen but with the brash young Crile, the man who to them represented dynamism and progress. At the time they were, no doubt, right to do so, believing as they did that Crile rode the wave of modernity that was then breaking on medicine's shores. Ultimately, however, with the clarity of hindsight, they may well have questioned the wisdom of their actions.

§

The new home of Western Reserve's School of Medicine, the first element of Cleveland's academic medical center, was dedicated and opened for public inspection on October 9, 1924. For the first time in its history the medical school was located far from the center of the city, on the extended "campus" of the university itself. And with nearly two hundred thousand square feet of floor space, the new building provided three times the usable area of its aging predecessor on East 9th Street, whose multistory amphitheaters had become anachronisms just a few years after opening.

Along with the steam- and electrical-power plant at the southernmost edge of the University Circle property, the new medical school had been built at a total cost of $2.6 million. And like the earlier school building, a gift of benefactor John Lund Woods, all of the money for the new facilities had come from one donor: Samuel Mather.

Just one year after the opening of the medical school, on October 28, 1925, the new Maternity and Babies' and Children's Hospitals were also completed. Despite an unseasonably intense snow and sleet storm, hundreds of Clevelanders turned out to hear Abraham Flexner, by then secretary of the Rockefeller Foundation's General Education Board, make the principal address at the dedication ceremonies. The two new hospitals, constructed at a total cost of some $3.5 million, were opened for two days of guided tours, so that the people of the city could see how their donations in the 1923 fund-raising campaign had been put to use.

Together the two buildings formed an L-shaped complex just north of the new medical school. Each had six floors with open seventh-story "sun" wards for patients who might require "the benefit of sunshine and outdoor treatment." The hospitals were connected at basement and sub-basement levels by subterranean tunnels, extensions of which would eventually connect all of the buildings of the medical center.

The emblem of the babies' hospital, located directly above the front entrance, was a design modeled after an Andrea della Robbia terra cotta frieze at the Foundling Hospital in Florence. It showed an infant in swaddling clothes with its arms outstretched, and the Biblical phrase, "A small one shall become a great nation." Inside, a bronze plaque indicated that the hospital was dedicated to the memory of Edward F. Cushing, "the devoted friend and physician of babies and children."

The new children's facility boasted a capacity of one hundred fifty beds, each floor having two eight-bed wards in which each bed could be separated from its neighbors by glass-walled partitions. There were also sixteen private rooms, all of them with southern exposures and each sporting French doors that led out to individual sun porches. On the fifth floor was a small surgical ward for infants under the age of one month (older children requiring surgery would be sent to Lakeside), as well as a special ward for children requiring what was called "mental training," a euphemism that covered both retardation and mental illness.

The new hospital included a suite designed solely to provide dental care, while premature babies would be housed in a temperature- and humidity-controlled room with seven basinettes. In an innovation unique in the country, an entire ward on the second floor was segregated for the use of contagious-disease cases, with access available only from a separate elevator in the basement. The basement also housed the hospital's own milk laboratory, to ensure a steady supply of pasteurized, tuberculin-tested milk. Other laboratories, as well as living quarters for the resident physicians and a medical library, were on the sixth floor.

The subbasement of the Maternity Hospital housed a kitchen large enough to supply meals to the occupants of both buildings. Of approximately the same size as its sister institution, the maternity facility featured two-bed "wards" surrounding central nurseries on most floors, while the entire fifth floor was given over to private rooms. On the sixth floor were the delivery and operating rooms; occupying the ground floor were a prenatal clinic, physicians' living quarters, and the requisite waiting room where expectant fathers could pace back and forth in relative comfort.

The superintendents of both new hospitals were registered nurses: Gladys Sellew at Babies' and Children's, and Calvina MacDonald at Maternity. From the start, Sellew won the appreciation of parents by instituting liberal visiting hours and encouraging parental involvement during recuperation. She also told her nurses to learn from parents as much as they could about the habits and needs of their charges, in order to recreate as closely as possible elements of their home environment. Sellew's innovative policies resulted in additional work for the hospital's nurses, but they proved beneficial for the children and earned the nursing corps the respect of the entire community.

As a manager, Calvina MacDonald was already a proven success, having brought the old Maternity Hospital—once a failing institution—into legitimacy during her decade of service there. Her work contributed substantially to the improvement of the hospital's seven citywide dispensaries as well. Indeed, thanks in no small part to MacDonald, Cleveland's infant mortality rate had dropped to just 6.6 percent, at the time the lowest rate among the country's ten largest cities.

With the opening of Cleveland's two new hospitals, a holding company was created to oversee the operations of all of the medical center's member institutions. On January 1, 1926, "University Hospitals of Cleveland, Incorporated," officially took over administrative control of Babies' and Childrens', Maternity, and Lakeside Hospitals. Although each institution maintained its own board of trustees and retained control of its own endowment funds, all were answerable to the University Hospitals corporation and its board of trustees, which included representatives from each of the hospitals.

Sam Mather was elected chairman of the new corporation's board, and Dr. Karl H. Van Norman, a Toronto native and graduate of Johns Hopkins, was hired to serve as director of administration of the hospital group. Two months later, the first tangible expression of the new working agreement among the parties of the University Hospitals group federation came in the most mundane of ways: Lakeside began to do the laundry of both of its sister hospitals.

By the fall of 1926, with the need for a new home of its own more pressing than ever, the Lakeside trustees entered into a secret agreement to sell their lakefront property through an intermediary to the Pennsylvania Railroad. The sale price—$1.5 million—resulted in a tidy profit for the hospital, monies that would be put toward the construction of the new Lakeside in University Circle.

Indeed, a joint planning committee to create a fund-raising drive for the remainder of the needed funds was already being formed, with trustees from all of the University Hospitals institutions represented. Robert Bishop was asked to lead the fund drive, and his first task was to head by train for Thomasville, Georgia, the principal wintertime retreat of Cleveland's elite, to attempt to sign up early pledges.

By February of 1927, the members of the joint committee announced publicly that in May they would attempt to raise funds to build, equip, and endow a new Lakeside and related nurses' and resident physicians' dormitories, as well as a new Rainbow Hospital to replace the old facility in South Euclid. These buildings would be the final elements of what was by then being called "The Medical Center," a name that would be used in all of the campaign's advertising and promotional literature. They would, they announced, attempt to raise $6 million, the largest sum ever sought in Cleveland for a single charitable entity.

The Medical Center campaign was modeled after the successful 1923 effort for the Maternity and Babies' hospitals, which itself had been patterned after Sam Mather's ingenious Community Fund drives. First, a goal was established and announced publicly. Then, prominent individuals were brought in as captains of fund-raising "teams" assigned to cover specific territories and individuals. Finally, the newspapers were enlisted to provide daily coverage and to act as cheerleaders for the drive. Everyone in town knew that the bulk of the donations would come from the city's wealthiest citizens, but it was still deemed important to enlist all Clevelanders in the process, no matter how small their donations might be. Although a private entity, The Medical Center was to be thought of as a community asset.

Early in April, both Samuel Mather and Edward Harkness pledged $1 million donations to the campaign, providing a solid base on which the fund-raising teams could build during the formal drive, which was scheduled to begin on May 16th and to run for five days. A local public relations firm created a slogan for the campaign—"The Medical Center: Where Science and Mercy Meet"—and produced publicity materials and stories to be supplied to the newspapers throughout the week.

Abraham Flexner, the guru of medical modernity, was enlisted to write the foreword to an informational booklet the fund-raisers handed out to prospects. ("The success of your development," wrote Flexner, "will make Cleveland a model to the rest of the country.") And in a well-publicized letter to new Western Reserve University president Robert E. Vinson, William Welch of Johns Hopkins said that Lakeside and the medical school were in the "front rank" of health-care institutions in the country, having "advanced the science and art of medicine...in the most eminent degree."

A huge billboard for the campaign was erected on one wall of the Cleveland Trust bank building, in the very heart of downtown. The billboard depicted Moses Cleaveland, founder of the city, having his blood pressure taken by a nurse. The amount of money pledged to the fund drive was indicated by the level of the mercury reading on the sphygmomanometer, which rose steadily each day of the campaign.

Almost a carbon copy of the 1923 pledge drive, the Medical Center campaign was accompanied by daily newspaper accounts of donations, from thousands of dollars to handfuls of pennies. There were the requisite heartwarming stories of widows and orphans donating small sums even as Cleveland's titans of industry pledged hundreds of thousands of dollars. The same manufactured suspense was built toward the end of the week, with intimations that the goal might not be met. One major difference between the two campaigns, however, was evident in the newspapers' emphasis on how the new Medical Center would not only provide health care but also serve to "advance medical science" as a "modern coalition against disease," thus making Cleveland—the fifth-largest city in the country at the time—a national center of medical research.

The denouement of the week was also reminiscent of the 1923 effort, although two unexpected donations added an element of surprise to the campaign's conclusion. On the last day of the drive the goal of $6 million was not only exceeded by more than $500,000, but two additional major gifts were announced: Frances Payne Bolton, who had already endowed the School of Nursing, donated an additional $750,000 to build a separate home for the school and a group of dormitories for student nurses; and the widow of Leonard C. Hanna and her son, Leonard, Jr., donated $750,000 to erect a building exclusively for Lakeside's private patients—in effect, a very large private pavilion. After just five days, therefore, the combined total of funds raised actually exceeded $8 million.

With the capital drive a success, the Lakeside trustees set to work with their architects to finalize plans for their new hospital. No longer the "whale" of a building that Harvey Cushing had warned against, the new, more compact structure accommodated only about three hundred beds and was to be constructed in the shape of a large letter "H," with its main entrance fronting not on Euclid Avenue but on Adelbert Road. At the same time, construction began on the new Rainbow Hospital in suburban South Euclid, which, although separated geographically from the University Circle campus, would officially join the University Hospitals group that year.

Because Medical Center campaign pledges were to be paid over a thirty-six-month period, it was another year before sufficient funds were in hand to turn the first shovelful of dirt on the construction site. On October 14, 1928, however, ground was at last broken for the final elements of the University Hospitals complex. At about the same time, the new Rainbow Hospital for Crippled and Convalescent Children was being completed; its formal dedication took place on December 4th.

To the doctors and nurses at the old Lakeside, work on the new facility had begun none too soon. The lakefront complex was operating virtually at capacity, seeing more than seven thousand patients a year in the by-then crowded and decidedly obsolete set of buildings spread out along Lakeside Avenue. And maintenance problems were again draining resources, just as they had when Lakeside had operated out of the former Marine Hospital next door. Few if any members of the staff would have agreed with the Cleveland Hospital Council's opinion that, among all the proposed construction of health-care facilities in Cleveland, a new Lakeside was actually of the lowest priority.

In addition to their difficulties with the hospital building itself, the Lakeside staff also faced the problem of finding a new chief of medicine, someone to replace the respected Charles Hoover, who had died in June of 1927. The two-year search by the visiting physicians and the rest of the medical school faculty came to fruition in July of 1929, when Joseph T. Wearn began his tenure as professor of medicine in the medical school and head of Lakeside's Department of Medicine.

Wearn came from his alma mater, Harvard Medical School, where he had been teaching for six years. Considered a brilliant instructor and investigator, he met all the criteria by which a member of the faculty of an academic medical center could be judged. Indeed, Wearn was so determined to push Lakeside and the medical school further along the path of progress that he actually endangered his own appointment. In his negotiations with the hospital and medical school trustees, he insisted as a condition of employment that wholesale changes be made in the layout of the new Lakeside—which was, of course, already under construction.

With backing from Robert Bishop, who understood the importance of the new chief's recommendations, Wearn lobbied successfully for installation of the Laboratory of Experimental Medicine on the third and fourth floors of the hospital, in areas that had previously been allocated to resident staff housing. It was a measure of the value placed on a teacher of Wearn's caliber that Lakeside's trustees ultimately spent an additional $500,000 to refit those floors, and they did so without qualm. During the next quarter century, it would prove to be one of the wisest investments they could have made.

But investments of a different order were soon to be preoccupying the trustees of Cleveland's new medical center. On October 31st, the Lakeside board convened at the downtown headquarters of the Union Trust Bank to discuss progress on the construction of their new facility. Although the minutes of their meeting included only references to the business at hand, it seems unlikely that the industrialists and financiers of the board would not have talked among themselves about the debacle that had transpired on Wall Street just two days before. Ironically, one shock wave emanating from the stock market crash of 1929 would soon be felt in the very building in which the Lakeside trustees were meeting. Because within just a few short years the Union Trust Bank—devastated by the Great Depression—would be faced with the prospect of closing its doors for good.

And before long, so too would University Hospitals of Cleveland.

CHAPTER SEVEN

Intensive Care

Early in October 1929, the trustees of University Hospitals expected construction of the new Lakeside—the last element of Cleveland's vast medical center complex in University Circle—to be completed within exactly one year. Blissfully unaware of the financial firestorm about to break over the entire country, they were optimistic about the future, and their optimism was only heightened by the October 7th dedication of the medical center's new Institute of Pathology, an addition to the complex that had not been included in the project's original plans.

Designed by architect Abram Garfield to complement his other buildings on the medical campus, the new institute was the product of a prodigious lobbying effort on the part of pathology chief Howard Karsner, the city's preeminent laboratory man and one of the most dedicated educators in Western Reserve University's School of Medicine. Karsner had come to Cleveland from Harvard in 1914 to fill the post vacated by the departing William T. Howard, at a time when Lakeside was still the only hospital in the city with a resident pathologist. Within just a few years, however, Karsner-trained pathologists would be working in virtually all of Cleveland's major hospitals.

As the importance of pathology within the medical curriculum had grown, and as the inadequacy of the laboratory facilities at Cleveland's medical school had become more and more apparent, Karsner itched to have a building of his own. Not long after the successful 1923 capital campaign for the Maternity and Babies' and Children's Hospitals, Karsner approached Abraham Flexner of the Rockefeller Foundation and attempted to convince him that Cleveland's proposed medical center would not be complete without a separate building to house a vastly expanded group of pathology laboratories. Over a period of years, and virtually on his own, Karsner promoted $750,000 from the foundation's General Education Board to build the Institute of Pathology—in which, ultimately, Karsner himself would reign supreme for the next two decades.

With the opening of Karsner's building, the University Hospitals board foresaw no obstacles to impede the scheduled completion of the new Lakeside. Even at the end of October 1929—in the wake of the great stock market crash in which some $30 billion in the real value of equities had simply disappeared—almost every medical center trustee still believed that Lakeside's scheduled completion date of October 1930 could be maintained. It was not until the first months of 1930 that the enormity of the financial debacle that had occurred on October 29th was widely understood, as the initial effects of what would be known as the Great Depression began to be felt.

It was an inauspicious time to be dunning contributors for the balance of their pledges to the Lakeside capital campaign, and as the flow of money slowed, so too did the pace of construction. And even as the scheduled completion date passed with no end to the work in sight, additional problems began to arise. A larger than normal new group of interns, for example, found itself stranded, in effect, in the old Lakeside. Slated to begin work in the new building in University Circle, the interns were instead trapped in the old Lakeside with nothing to do, no space in which to be housed, and no opportunity to attempt to start a residency elsewhere. To deal with the problem, department heads arranged to place a portion of the newcomers in research positions in the pathology laboratories, while others were given temporary "fellowships" with which to visit major hospitals and labs, both in the United States and abroad.

Then, as work continued on the new hospital through the summer of 1930, the old Lakeside buildings began to show more signs of decay. Some areas of the hospital were weakened structurally by the irremedial problem of shifting foundations, and at one point a major portion of the ceiling in the children's ward actually collapsed. For a time it looked as if the city would shut down the hospital as unsafe, but emergency bracing of walls and ceilings kept the buildings open and functioning.

The need for a new facility was becoming acute, but as had happened every other time the trustees attempted to purchase or build a new home, a nationwide financial calamity again hampered their efforts. Lakeside had actually become one of the country's most accurate economic indicators: the mere mention of plans for new construction seemed inevitably to be followed by frenzied bank panics, lengthy recessions, or outright depressions. And by the end of 1930, the "Lakeside Effect" was clearly in evidence, as nationwide more than one thousand banks had failed and some six million people had lost their jobs.

Early in 1931, however, a small but measurable improvement in the economic environment led many people—including the trustees of University Hospitals—to believe that the worst of the hard times were over and that a recovery had begun. Although the hospitals' new director of administration, Frank Chapman (a former superintendent of Cleveland's Mt. Sinai Hospital), submitted a budget for the year that included an estimated $165,000 reduction in annual income from the endowments of the hospital group, this figure was looked on as merely a one-time, short-term loss. The board decided to procure loans from local banks for each of the hospitals in the medical group—$10,000 for the Rainbow Hospital for Crippled and Convalescent Children; $35,000 each for Maternity and Babies' and Children's; and $120,000 for Lakeside—the funds to be used as working capital which would, in the words of one trustee, "in a very large measure solve the problem of the University Hospitals in this emergency."

In its naiveté, the board advised Chapman to institute only minor cost-cutting measures for the year. Ultimately, he would eliminate most of the free meals served to employees and the practice of reimbursing the expenses of staff physicians traveling to conferences in other cities. (Chapman also curtailed the serving of milk and crackers to nurses in mid-morning and mid-afternoon, an amenity that he said entailed "considerable expense.") Only one board member seemed to recognize the true potential for disaster that lurked in the shadows of the January economic recovery. Arthur D. Baldwin urged that "every item of expenditure" be monitored closely, because the hospitals' depressed revenues, combined with a growing demand for free service, were creating the "grave danger of a retrenchment in activities."

Fears about the future of the national economy were temporarily forgotten at the end of January, however, as the new Lakeside at last neared completion. On January 26th, the new hospital's dispensary department opened, and less than a week later, on February 1st, ward patients were moved from the old lakefront complex to the elaborate new facility on the medical center campus in University Circle.

Formal dedication of the new hospital was held one day after the School of Medicine's graduation ceremonies in mid-June, by which time the dispensary was already seeing five hundred patients a day and most of the nearly four hundred beds available in Lakeside and its contiguous private pavilion, Hanna House, were occupied.

As with previous dedications, the public was encouraged to tour the new hospital buildings, which had been furnished and decorated under the aegis of the Ladies' Advisory Committee, successor to the old Board of Lady Managers. And the public was suitably impressed with the nine-story monolith of steel and stone, which was, as its predecessor on the lakefront had been in its day, the very embodiment of modernity and up-to-date "scientific" thought.

Starting at the subbasement level, visitors were shown the inner workings of the new hospital, the steam and electrical lines that ran from the medical center's power plant building through the subterranean corridors that connected all of the structures on the campus. The subbasement also housed a special room for the storage of radium for the X-ray department, a room for storage of gas anesthesia, and even lockers and squash courts for the house officers.

At the basement level were an emergency admitting suite, three emergency operating rooms, and a dispatch center that served as the nexus of the pneumatic-tube message system that carried charts, prescriptions, and other written materials between floors. On the first floor, the dispensary was located near the hospital's Abington Road entrance, while the administrative offices were clustered along a hallway near the main entrance that fronted on Adelbert Road.

The medical and surgical clinics and the X-ray department were found on the second floor, along with twenty-eight private and semiprivate rooms. One floor up were clinical laboratories, medical staff offices, an eighteen-bed isolation unit, and additional clinics. The fourth floor housed the medical department's two male and two female wards, each with twenty-five beds, as well as numerous small labs for both medicine and surgery. The fifth floor was given over to the two-story surgical amphitheater, with eighty ward beds for surgical cases.

The sixth floor was also designated for surgical cases, while the seventh floor consisted almost entirely of operating suites. Special surgical suites segregated for use by the eye, ear, nose, and throat specialists were on the eighth floor, while the ninth floor "penthouse" was actually the location of the hospital's ventilating facilities and vaults for the storage of old X-ray films.*

---

*The decision to store films on the highest floor of the building had come about in large

The smallest of the medical center's new buildings—the four nurses' dormitories erected just north of Lakeside—had been in use since September of 1930, when they had been dedicated to the memories of four longtime local contributors to and backers of the profession: Flora Stone Mather, Isabel Wetmore Lowman, Kate Hanna Harvey, and Isabel Hampton Robb. (Robb House would keep its name even though it had already been given over for use by the resident medical staff, which had been displaced when chief of medicine Wearn moved the Cushing laboratories into Lakeside.)

At the formal dedication ceremony itself—held just across Euclid Avenue in Severance Hall, the home of the Cleveland Orchestra—the invited guests of the hospital heard an address by Hans Zinsser, professor of bacteriology at the Harvard Medical School. As if he had been scripted by the medical center trustees themselves, Zinsser confirmed the judgment they had made more than a decade before—that the adoption of the "full-time" faculty program and the creation of a genuine academic medical center had made the hospital group a pacesetter in teaching, research, and patient care. Indeed, asserted Zinsser, Cleveland's new health campus was exemplary of "the beneficent change which has come with the reorganization of medical education" in the United States, a reorganization that had been led by such schools as Western Reserve. The affiliation and close ties of the medical school and the hospitals, he added, could only serve to further lift medicine "out of the storm and strife of the last twenty years"—a message that brought no small measure of gratification to the friends of the medical center assembled that day.

§

Buoyant from the public reception of the completed medical center, the University Hospitals trustees would nonetheless be brought back to earth in less than a month. On July 9th, the hospitals' able administrative director, Frank Chapman, died suddenly after a short illness, and once again

---

measure because of the May 1929 Cleveland Clinic disaster, in which nitrocellulose film stored in a basement room spontaneously decomposed, releasing deadly fumes up through the entire clinic building. More than one hundred and twenty people died in the disaster, including John Phillips, one of the Clinic's founders.

Robert Bishop was called upon to shoulder the responsibility of day-to-day management of the medical group. Then, the hospitals' midyear financial report revealed that revenues were down nearly $150,000 from budgeted projections, with a further loss of $44,000 in earnings from endowment funds. In addition to a substantial decrease in the number of paying patients at all of the University Hospitals member institutions, Lakeside and Maternity were both providing vastly more days of free care than would have been considered normal. And Community Fund contributions were also down more than $30,000, which only added to the concern over a possible $300,000 deficit by the end of the year. The board was therefore forced to consider not only layoffs (in the trustees' words, the elimination from the payroll of "extra people"), but also cutbacks in service.

At Lakeside, Sam Mather—who had just celebrated his eightieth birthday—initiated a study of possible cutbacks, asking medical chief Wearn and head surgeon Cutler to find ways to lower operating expenses without interfering with teaching and research in the hospital. For three days Cutler and Wearn poked at the problem, but neither wanted to eliminate beds from his own department and neither could come up with a strategy that would not seriously hamper the hospital's ability to attract quality candidates for internships and residencies. Ultimately, their only recommendation to Mather and the board was the time-honored fallback position of all doctors facing the cost-cutting ax: they suggested that the size of the nursing staff be reduced.

The Lakeside trustees decided to postpone any radical internal changes until a reevaluation of the situation in October. Meanwhile, the Outpatient Department was being swamped with cases, recording a daily attendance of some five hundred patients, with as many as eighty percent of them being treated on a charity basis. As a stopgap measure, Robert Bishop suggested raising from twenty-five to fifty cents the established per-visit fee for those patients who could afford to pay, because after the first six months of the year the department was already $30,000 in the red.

Part of the reason for the large number of free-care patients at the hospital's dispensary was, in the opinion of the Cleveland Academy of Medicine, laxity on the part of the Lakeside staff. As they had been doing for years, many members of the Academy were again complaining that individuals who might easily afford the services of a private practitioner were slipping undetected into the hospital as charity patients. The Academy's mounting displeasure forced Bishop to hire three additional social workers whose sole job would be to check the eligibility of patients applying for charity aid.

By the agreed-upon reevaluation date at the end of September, however, it was obvious that nothing short of wholesale cuts in spending would bring Lakeside and the rest of the medical center's hospitals even close to their targeted budgets. Robert Bishop therefore proposed an across-the-board salary and wage cut of ten percent. All eleven hundred people on the University Hospitals payroll would be affected, from those making thousands annually to those earning less than $100 a month.

In addition to the salary cuts, Bishop also recommended that some one hundred employees be furloughed, a suggestion that seemed to shock the members of the board. Apparently still unconvinced that the national "economic reversal" was anything more than a temporary setback, the trustees were loath to take the drastic step of actually cutting adrift members of the hospitals' "family." Bishop, however, understood clearly the gravity of the country's financial predicament, and he pressed for the layoffs despite the irony inherent in his recommendation (i.e., the city's newest, largest, and most fully equipped hospitals were being forced to cut their staffs merely to keep operating). In the end, the trustees acceded to the inevitable, but only after recommending that Bishop "consider every means to provide at least part-time work for as many people as possible."

The salary cuts and employee layoffs were an emotionally charged issue for the board to absorb, but their significance paled in comparison to the blow that was sustained just three weeks later. Shortly after midnight on Sunday, October 18th, Samuel Mather suffered a fatal heart attack at his lakefront home, where he had been confined for the preceding two weeks due to failing health. Only four months after the triumphant dedication of the last elements of the city's ambitious new medical center, the man most responsible for the success of the project was dead.

On the day of Mather's funeral, flags above government buildings in the city were lowered to half-staff, and hundreds of people stood in a driving rain outside Trinity Episcopal Cathedral during his memorial service. The man who was called the "first citizen of Cleveland" had touched the lives of virtually every member of the community through both his business and his philanthropies, and the community seemed to feel the need to pay its last respects.

Of course, nowhere had Sam Mather's influence been felt more profoundly than at the University Hospitals medical center. More than any other individual he had fostered the growth of both the hospitals and the university with which they were affiliated. Through gifts amounting to some $10 million over half a century (beginning with his first donation—$10—in 1874), and through the vast amounts of time and energy he had devoted to the boards of both institutions, Mather had been the leader without whom—in that era, at least—no such endeavor could have survived. And as the medical center board noted in its offical message of condolence to his family, Sam Mather had sought for himself no gratitude or public approbation for his efforts. Instead, he had been content simply to wear "duty's iron crown."

Mather was so powerful a symbol of generosity in the community that, during citywide fund-raising campaigns for various charitable efforts, local newspapers urged Clevelanders to "Give as a Mather Gives." He was even the subject of occasional editorial cartoons that pictured him as a kindly, ethereal presence who hovered watchfully over the city. Indeed, once, during a testimonial dinner for Mather at the conclusion of the Community Fund's annual campaign, one of the evening's speakers offered an opinion that was widely shared in Cleveland: on the day when death finally claimed the great philanthropist and he approached heaven's gate, he would be met by a broadly smiling St. Peter, who, the speaker had no doubt, would tip his halo in a gesture of respect reserved for those occasions when one saint greeted another.

Sam Mather's interest in the medical center institutions had been genuine and abiding, a heartfelt desire on his part to bring the hospitals, the medical school, and Western Reserve University as a whole to positions of leadership, not only in the city but in the country at large. Over the decades his personal involvement had, if anything, grown deeper, his commitment even stronger.

Ironically, medicine had in many respects failed him miserably over the years. The death of his mother at a young age, the lingering disability from his own early accident, the premature demise of his wife—all might have been prevented or alleviated if the medical care available at the time had not been so painfully inadequate and ineffective. Indeed, his own experiences with medicine's failures may well have been one of the forces that moved him to devote so much of his time and his fortune to improving the science. Whatever were his reasons, his interest in the world of medicine never flagged, even as he approached the end. On the very night of Mather's death, a member of his family noticed that the book he had been reading just a few hours before was a history of the Boston City Hospital.

The death of Samuel Mather marked the end of another era for the hospitals of Cleveland's new medical center. Never again could they rely on the leadership of the city's most influential man, and never again could they call on the generosity of a single individual to retrieve them from the brink of calamity, as they had done so often when he was alive. If Mather himself was gone, however, another member of his family was already coming to the fore within the medical center, at a time when the hospitals were facing their most dire crises. Much of the responsibility for guiding the medical center through an uncertain future devolved upon Mather's son-in-law, Robert Bishop, and the new director of administration soon proved himself up to the task.

§

As the year 1931 wound to a close, the University Hospitals group took what at the time must have been considered Draconian measures. In addition to the ten percent wage and salary cuts already instituted, new provisions were advocated by Robert Bishop as the only possible remedial actions to keep the medical center within sight of its budget projections. The board at last agreed to making genuinely drastic cutbacks throughout the hospitals by pulling out of service two divisions in Lakeside and shutting down entire floors in Maternity, Babies' and Children's, and Hanna House, the private pavilion.

With the loss of so much bed space in the hospitals, the outpatient clinics quickly became even more flooded with cases, most of them seeking free care. Indeed, the clinics were so overcrowded that a committee was formed to study and recommend changes in their operating policy. Under Bishop's chairmanship, the committee began its work by asking a fundamental question about the "province" of the hospitals, a question that in earlier times would have been unthinkable: "Shall we continue to render an unlimited amount of free service...or shall we make an effort to limit the number of patients accepted for care to a figure consistent with our financial limitations and needs for teaching purposes?"

After a period of study and discussion, the committee recommended the latter course, a policy that was already in place at other large hos-

pitals around the country. The full board ultimately agreed, implement-
ing a seven-point plan to reduce costs by winnowing out those patients
who could be treated more appropriately somewhere other than at an
academic medical center. The policy required judgment calls that under
ordinary circumstances the hospitals could have avoided, but in light of
the nation's ongoing economic catastrophe, they were choices the hospitals were now prepared to make.

Foremost among the new guidelines was a stricture against burdening
the clinicians with "the routine care of numberless cases presenting little
or nothing in the way of teaching value." Free care would be provided
only to those individuals living on relief payments from the Community
Fund, to emergency patients, or to cases "of great scientific or teaching
interest." Clinic admission fees would be raised, and charges would be
levied for X-rays and prescription drugs.

For the first time a running tally of the actual costs of free services
would be maintained. After reaching the annual limit of the funds provided to the hospitals for such care by the Community Fund, no further
free cases would be accepted. The new policy would, it was thought, "go
far toward dissipating the prevalent conception that dispensary and hospital service facilities are unlimited and without cost." And its correlative
effect would be, in Bishop's words, to "educate the community to the fact
that medical care is something which should be paid for and that health,
while perhaps intangible, is an individual's greatest asset."

As a sop to the city's private practitioners, all outpatient charity
admissions would be prescreened by "financial interviewers," who would
establish each individual's eligibility for services. All new applicants who
had at any time during the preceding five years visited a private practitioner would be referred back to that physician, either to obtain paid
care if they could afford it or to get a release from the doctor allowing
them to be admitted to the hospital as a charity patient.

Although the members of the committee wholeheartedly recommended
the changes to the full board, none of the trustees was unmindful of the
effect the new rules might have on the public's perception of the new
medical center. But if, as the committee's report concluded, "such policies
...are contrary to the traditions of the units now comprising the University Hospitals," the value of maintaining those traditions still had to
be weighed against the constraints of economic necessity. And "economic
necessity" was by then a concept not to be limited to the current period
of national depression: the report specifically mentioned the urgent need

to alter the "growing public conception that dispensary care is something which will be given free of charge to anyone for the asking."

To a large degree, the actions of the board constituted the most radical steps away from the historic missions of the hospitals since their inception. More than merely an extension of the principles adopted in the 1919 "full-time" faculty decision—when for the first time all of the hospitals affiliated with Western Reserve's School of Medicine would actively attempt to limit charity admissions to those cases that provided good teaching "material" for the academic medical center—the new guidelines were a response to a widespread change in the very meaning of health-care delivery.

From the latter half of the nineteenth century right up until October of 1929, medical care had been dispensed to the masses with something approaching abandon, the gracious gift, in effect, of the grandees who had established and who maintained hospital facilities in cities around the country. But the devastating effects of the Depression made clear to the managers and administrators of those hospitals that the largesse of the upper classes could not be counted on forever, and that medical care, especially for the poor, would thenceforth be provided within a wholly new environment. For a man like Robert Bishop, who was the principal author of the committee report, it was abundantly clear that University Hospitals could never return to the days when the institution functioned within the simple, rose-colored mores that the founders had delineated as long before as 1866. The new strictures might have seemed callous and unnecessarily harsh to someone of Samuel Mather's sensibilities, but the fact was that the hospitals simply had to change if they were to survive.

If further proof of the severity of the ongoing crisis were needed, it was to come early in January of 1932. The Welfare Federation of Cleveland informed all its member institutions that they should plan on appropriations from the Community Fund being fifteen percent smaller than those of the previous year. In addition, dividends were being cut on many of the stocks in the hospitals' endowment funds, which further reduced the budgeted income for the year. Western Reserve University, which had usually been able to reimburse the hospitals more than $100,000 annually for teaching expenses, was suddenly unable to pay even half that amount. And the value of the stocks and bonds bequeathed to the medical center by Sam Mather had been so severely eroded by the market crash that it would have been folly to attempt to liquidate them at the time to get much-needed capital.

The possibility of a complete collapse of the hospital group was, therefore, not only thinkable but imminent. More cuts in service were made immediately. The roof wards of the Babies' and Children's Hospital were closed; responsibility for pre- and postnatal field nursing was shifted from the Maternity Hospital nursing corps to the city's Visiting Nurse Association; and fifteen more Medical Center employees lost their jobs. A savings of $400 a month was effected by using Lakeside's kitchens to prepare meals for Hanna House patients, and the same expedient was soon implemented for Maternity patients as well. Contingency plans were readied in case it became necessary to close four more Lakeside wards, which would reduce the hospital's usable bed capacity to just one hundred and eighty-five. The fortunes of the hospitals were being affected so intensely and so rapidly by the economic crisis that the board took the extraordinary step of creating a new Fiscal Control committee, a group charged with reviewing the hospitals' operating budgets not on a yearly basis but every thirty days.

In the midst of the turmoil, chief surgeon Elliott Cutler tendered his resignation and announced his intention to return to Harvard to succeed the retiring Harvey Cushing as surgeon in chief at the Brigham Hospital. Although faced with near-daily monetary crises, the hospitals' board of trustees had to turn its attention to the task of recruiting a replacement for Cutler. Surprisingly, they formed a search committee whose mission was to "canvas the entire country" to find the best available surgeon for the job, no matter what the cost might be. Despite the obvious need for fiscal constraint in all corners of the medical group, the trustees realized that to maintain the hard-won reputation of University Hospitals, a first-class surgeon who demanded a first-class salary would have to be found. They decided, therefore, that any "financial question" that might arise would be resolved by special individual donations from among their number.

The decision to ignore the cost of procuring a top-flight surgeon even as cutbacks were being effected all over the hospitals was one measure of how seriously the trustees perceived the question of maintaining the institution's standards. Such a degree of idealism, however, was rapidly becoming a luxury that the medical center simply could not afford, because as early as March of 1932 the hospitals were again facing projections of a huge deficit for the year.

One suggested stopgap measure was to set up a salary "reserve," withholding five percent of every employee's wages until the end of the year, at which time the money would be paid out only if the hospitals were not running a deficit. Robert Bishop thought the reserve might prove disastrous for morale, however, coming as it did after the earlier ten percent pay cut and the discontinuance of free meals for employees. He suggested instead that if at least one free meal a day were to be provided, an even higher reserve of ten percent might be instituted without harm. After due discussion a compromise plan was worked out, and beginning in April a seven percent reserve would go into effect.

The only member of the university medical group still operating at a surplus at the time was Rainbow Hospital, so no salary reserve needed to be implemented there. No matter what the size of the reserve for the other hospitals, however, it quickly became obvious that further personnel cuts would also have to be initiated. And the cuts would include not just service personnel but also the staff of residents, which would eventually be reduced from eighty-six to sixty-five.

Additional wards were closed in April, with the hope that the stringent austerity measures might actually result in a small surplus by the end of the year. But by the middle of May, after computing balance sheets for the first four months of the year, it was found that the hospitals had still been bleeding money all along, and that the deficit stood at more than $42,000, with no end in sight. Further personnel cuts were then made among housekeeping staff, elevator operators, social service workers, and the like, but these necessary reductions ultimately proved to be futile gestures.

In July, assistant director of administration John Mannix created a new form of payment plan called a "flat rate" scheme, under which patients were charged a fixed fee per day rather than a group of charges for the various services—no matter how many—that were provided during their stay. Available only on payment of cash in advance, the flat rates actually increased the income of the hospitals for a time, while producing a side benefit of reducing some of the workload in the accounting department.

The cash-flow problem continued unabated, however, with the trustees going so far as to postpone publication of the hospitals' annual report, merely to save the minuscule $600 printing cost. Such minor economies would be forgotten by September 1932, however, when Robert Bishop reported to the board that the salary reserve had already been wiped out and that the hospitals would probably finish the year with a deficit of roughly $100,000. And Bishop's projections for 1933 were even darker: a potential deficit of nearly $400,000. The only possible solution was to implement three major cutbacks: reduce salaries by an additional ten percent; further cut the size of the resident staff; and, most radical of all, close the Babies' and Children's Hospital and move its remaining patients onto the sixth floor of Lakeside.

The cost of operating University Hospitals remained higher than that of any other hospital in Cleveland by all measures—cost per patient, per meal, and even per cubic foot of space. In his report to the hospital board, Bishop called the outlook for 1933 "grave," noting that standards and volume of work could not be maintained if further expense reductions were to be required. "If it becomes necessary to take another $100,000 or $150,000 out of the picture next year," he told the assembled trustees, "you must be prepared to sacrifice some of your ideals."

Indeed, the ideals to be sacrificed could well include the principal motivation for founding the hospitals: to provide virtually unlimited free medical care to the poor. By December, Bishop was investigating a proposal of the Cleveland Hospital Council to create a "finance corporation," a pool of funds contributed by all local hospitals from which patients could borrow to pay their medical bills. Designed to be repaid in installments, the loans were actually intended, in Bishop's words, as "a psychological approach to the problem of securing a realization on the part of the general public that hospital service should be paid for as any other commodity...."

In Lakeside's earliest days, many indigents had actually shunned the hospital, seeing it as merely another "pest house" in which the sick poor were placed to die. Now, Lakeside and the other institutions of University Hospitals were so encumbered with patients unable to pay for their care that the entire medical group found itself on the verge of collapse. The Hospital Council's "finance corporation"—an absurd idea, in terms of short-range economics—was nonetheless studied seriously by the medical center's trustees. Their most immediate need was for more paying patients—even if the payments themselves would be measured in cents, not dollars, and even if much of the money involved was merely the same funds being recirculated among the city's hospitals.

But the longer view inherent in the council's proposal, a view that Robert Bishop perceived most astutely, was that the delivery of health-care services in hospitals had long since ceased to be a largely eleemosynary undertaking. The process that had begun at Lakeside years before with the recognition of the importance of maintaining a large and steady population of paying patients was, at the end of 1932, reaching its logical conclusion. The hospitals that had been founded by the city's wealthiest families as expressions of their religious and charitable impulses were now largely business enterprises, sustained more by their own service-generated income than by the beneficence of their rich patrons. And during a period of business reversal, healthy revenues derived from the patient population were more important than ever.

§

The medical center enjoyed relative stability as 1932 ended, actually concluding the year with a small surplus of funds, after having reduced annual expenses by some $400,000. And in December, a replacement for Lakeside's departing chief surgeon, Elliott Cutler, was at last named. After a nationwide search, the Lakeside board had settled on someone from its own backyard—Carl Lenhart, a graduate of Western Reserve who had also taken his medical degree in Cleveland.

A research-oriented physician who had done much of his experimental work in collaboration with George Crile, Lenhart had been clinical professor of surgery at the medical school and chief surgeon at the City Hospital since 1930, when he filled the posts left vacant by the death that year of Carl Hamann. Although not as famous as his erstwhile research collaborator, Lenhart was widely known and respected within the profession, and his appointment was applauded at the time. He had not, however, been the hospital's first choice. Incredibly, the Lakeside search committee had first offered the job to Harvey Cushing, the very man whose retirement from Harvard had prompted Elliott Cutler's departure from Cleveland. For the fourth time in three decades, however, Cushing had turned down an offer to practice in his native city.

Early in 1933, the financial health of the hospitals took another turn for the worse. Lakeside in particular faced a severe cash shortage, with patient revenues down more than fifty percent. The hospital's trustees were forced to commit what in their own eyes must have been a cardinal sin: they penetrated the principal of the Lakeside endowment, selling bonds and using the proceeds as "temporary" operating funds, not only for Lakeside but for the entire medical group.

At the same time, a wave of fear was sweeping the country's financial system as bank panics and runs began to occur in various cities. At the end of February, Cleveland banks instituted a blanket limitation on the amount of money that could be withdrawn from accounts, in effect impounding more than $100,000 of the hospitals' funds that were earmarked for operations. Early in March, many banks closed their doors—some temporarily to stop runs, others (like Cleveland's insolvent Union Trust and Guardian Trust) permanently. Then, on March 6th, newly inaugurated President Franklin D. Roosevelt declared a national bank holiday, closing all financial institutions for a week-long cooling off period during which some semblance of order might be returned to the system.*

The medical center now faced not just financial difficulties but a full-blown operational crisis. Such old stopgap measures as discontinuing the nurses' afternoon milk and crackers seemed pathetically inadequate in retrospect, because the time had come to effect genuinely drastic cuts. Indeed, the only possible solution to the budget problems was advanced in a board meeting held on the first day of the bank holiday: not only would the Babies' and Children's Hospital have to be closed, but so too would the Maternity Hospital, with the patients of both facilities being transferred to those areas of Lakeside and Hanna House that had previously been mothballed.

Robert Bishop worked out the details of the transfer, which by his calculations would save more than $12,000 a month in expenses. All chiefs of service were asked to discharge immediately any patients who might safely be returned home early. New admissions—unless they could pay cash in advance—would be limited to emergency cases, although all obstetrical patients would be reclassified as emergencies for the sake of maintaining good will in the community. But hospital personnel were instructed to cut the use of X-rays, drugs, and other supplies to bare minimums. The Outpatient Department was closed two days of the week, and a five-day, forty-hour work week was instituted throughout the medical group, to help absorb on a part-time basis many of the employees of the two closed hospitals. Within weeks, however, a waiting list of prospective

---

*The impoundment of University Hospitals' funds was not the first such incident in the annals of Cleveland medicine. In 1854, state money provided for the construction of an insane asylum was withheld by a local bank until the trustee of the funds, backed by a court order and a band of sheriff's deputies, broke through the bank's outer wall with a sledge-hammer and began to attack the main vault. Before further damage could be done, the bank released the money in question to the trustee, a fairly well-known local surgeon by the name of Horace Ackley.

patients—most of them surgical candidates—had grown to more than three hundred names.

Despite the cutbacks, by April even the Lakeside/Hanna remnant of University Hospitals was found to be running a first-quarter deficit of roughly $70,000. That same month, Western Reserve University announced that it could no longer even partially fulfill its longtime obligations to the hospitals. The university asked to be forgiven its normal payment to offset the costs of teaching in the hospitals.

In the midst of retrenchment and the devastating new round of cutbacks, however, Robert Bishop made an extraordinary proposal. At a meeting of the Fiscal Control committee, Bishop presented his thoughts on a subject he had been investigating for months: the need for "an organized publicity and educational program for the University Hospitals," a program to be run out of the hospitals themselves by personnel hired specifically for the task.

Having already cut the medical, nursing, and service staffs to the bone, Bishop nonetheless proposed that new people be hired immediately to create an ongoing advertising and public relations campaign for the hospitals. "In large measure," Bishop argued, "the future of the hospitals depends upon their ability to keep [news of] their work before the general public."

With the generation of most generous "saints" dying off, and with the remaining family fortunes in the city being depleted by the effects of the Depression, Bishop knew that an entirely new crop of "friends" for the medical center would have to be cultivated if even some remnant of the hospitals' endowments were to be maintained. In addition, he understood the growing competitiveness within the local hospital community and what it would eventually mean in the struggle for paying patients. Having seen the positive results of two carefully orchestrated publicity campaigns during the 1923 and 1927 fund-raising drives, he was ready to embrace the techniques of public relations to increase the patient population of the University Hospitals group.

More sanguine than most of his colleagues on the board, Bishop attempted to allay the fears of some of the more conservative trustees by deliberately noting in his proposal that the advertising he foresaw would only be used "in a thoroughly ethical way." "I think there is much that can be done in acquainting the public…with the professional work that is carried on in this great institution," he urged. "This, in turn, will bring us patients and support." And, he implied, the publicity would also serve to further the cause of educating the public to the notion of paying for health care.

To buttress his case, Bishop mentioned that the majority of crippled children living outside the city were bypassing Rainbow and going to a similar hospital in Elyria, a city some thirty miles to the southwest. "At the time [the Elyria] institution was started there was much publicity given to it, and that publicity has been kept up through the medium of the Rotary Club," Bishop explained. As a result, "every Rotary Club throughout the state of Ohio is pulling for that institution and cases are going through Cleveland to get to Elyria.... [But] there is no reason why we should not have more of this business for the benefit of the University Hospitals."

Bishop was asking for only $150 a month to establish what he called an "educational department," but the rest of the committee decided that the ongoing financial situation was so grave that it might be wise to wait before broaching the idea with the full board. Although the subject was not raised at the time, at least some of the committee's members no doubt still harbored doubts about the ethical question of hiring anyone, let alone publicity brokers, while the hospitals were laying off more important personnel.

The financial situation was indeed deteriorating rapidly, as by the end of April the deficit had grown to more than $100,000. In June, the trustees of Lakeside again dipped into the principal of the hospital's endowments to raise operating funds, even though the sale price of the stocks and bonds yielded some $13,000 less than their book value. In fact, the true worth of the hospital's entire investment portfolio had already fallen to $4.5 million, nearly $3 million less than its book value. The market crash and subsequent Depression had so devastated equities across the board that almost forty percent of the value of the hospital's endowment investments had simply evaporated.

As the year ended, the deficit reached $423,000 before a Community Fund reimbursement payment of some $300,000. Once again, the salary reserve was used to defray the deficit, leaving a $15,000 debt for the year. The cash shortage was so severe that early in 1934 the board vetoed as extravagant Robert Bishop's request to replace the Maternity Hospital's two aging Plymouths—used by the staff to make home visitations—with two new Plymouths, each priced at $605. The board would, however, authorize Bishop to purchase two Chevrolets at $556 each, thus effecting a net savings of exactly $98.

Then, suddenly, revenues began to increase in the new year, as demand for private and semiprivate rooms grew. And the hospitals foresaw even further revenue increases from a recently signed contractual agreement with a newly formed private insurer, the Cleveland Hospital Service Association. The association's "periodic payment plan" was nothing more than a pool of funds—accumulated from monthly payments by subscribers—that was tapped to cover the expenses incurred by those subscribers during their stays in member hospitals. The prospect of a steady supply of patients whose bills were guaranteed to be paid, albeit by a third party, imbued the trustees with sufficient confidence to loosen the reins on fiscal control. Before long they had given back to the hospitals' employees a small portion (in most cases $5 a month) of the wages that had been cut so severely over the preceding years.

At the same time, the good will that had been engendered when maternity cases were classified as emergencies and admitted irrespective of financial status now began to bear unexpected fruit. A crush of potential paying obstetrical patients allowed the trustees to consider reopening the Maternity Hospital. Even so expensive a suggestion as Arthur Bill's request for a $25,000 wing to be added to Maternity—to at last put the gynecology and obstetrical services in the same building, as almost every other maternity hospital in the country had already done—was considered, despite a projected deficit of nearly $20,000 for the entire medical group. Just how to go about raising the funding for the new wing, however, was never fully discussed.

Robert Bishop addressed the question of outside support early in 1935, when he recommended the creation of a publication to be called *University Hospitals Illustrated News*. The newsletter would contain "news items furnished by the directors of service and department heads," and would serve to keep all personnel "informed of what is going on in the hospitals...." Initially, the *Illustrated News* would be sent to all employees and patients, but Bishop also saw the paper as a valuable tool to use in developing new sources of funds for the hospitals' by-now severely diminished endowments.

Indeed, Bishop specifically mentioned to the Fiscal Control committee that he planned to "build up a mailing list of...people who at one time or another had contributed to the development of the organization, or who might be interested in contributing to it." In other words, the newsletter would be an updated but only slightly more subtle version of the old naked pleas for funds that had been inserted in previous years' annual reports. With the demise of so many members of the hospitals' family of the faithful, Bishop recognized the need for a more modern method by which to coax support from a broader base of Clevelanders. And although the yearly cost of printing up to five thousand copies of the bimonthly newsletter would be some $2,500, he deemed it a small price to pay in light of the potential rewards that could accrue from the exercise.

The more immediate task to be faced, however, was the reopening of the Maternity Hospital as quickly as possible, with or without a new gynecology wing. Fortunately, by midyear more private patients were returning to the hospitals, thanks in large measure to the Hospital Service Association insurance coverage which so many Clevelanders of moderate means could afford. The infusion of revenues allowed the trustees to at last open Maternity, whose second floor was given over to the gynecology department.

In August the Babies' and Children's Hospital also reopened, freeing forty beds in Lakeside for conversion to private or semiprivate paying status, a response to the Fiscal Control committee's dictum that "as much [as possible] of the space and facilities of the University Hospitals group [should be converted] into revenue-producing space." With due recognition of the importance of maintaining those areas "provided for the care of staff cases necessary in the development of our teaching and research program," the committee members nonetheless stated emphatically their belief that "from now on every effort should be made to build up our earnings from patients."

The committee's wholehearted endorsement of a concept so antithetical to the historic mission of the hospitals bore the earmarks of Robert Bishop's acuity. Bishop saw that the future health of the entire hospital group was inextricably bound not to the fortunes of the city's leading families, as had been the case in previous years, but to the sheer numbers of paying patients that could be admitted. Samuel Mather, the quintessential nineteenth-century patrician, had provided the moral and monetary leadership for the hospitals when they were still nothing more than the embodiment of Calvinist responsibility to the less fortunate. Now Mather's son-in-law, a decidedly twentieth-century man, would help to chart a new path for the hospitals as they attempted to respond to the cold, hard realities of economic necessity. The world had in fact changed drastically in just the few short years since Mather's death, and a man of Bishop's particular genius was the only type who could respond successfully to the challenges of the times.

And those challenges arose frequently throughout 1936, even as private occupancy in the hospitals continued to grow. Admissions to the babies' hospital, for example, improved so dramatically that the hospital's work force, which was still maintained at drastically reduced levels, was stretched to the breaking point. And because salaries remained some twenty-five percent lower than those of 1931, employees—especially general-duty nurses—began to leave in droves for positions at better paying institutions. At one point during the year, the corps of fifteen nursemaids at Rainbow Hospital actually refused to report for duty unless something were done about their overly heavy workload and their $15-a-month wages.

With the ongoing improvement in revenues at the medical center, the board finally instituted modest pay raises for the nursemaids and other hard-hit employees, while at the same time ordering long-delayed repairs to some of the medical center's buildings. (The trustees also renamed the Maternity Hospital in honor of former superintendent Calvina Mac-Donald, who had retired in 1933 after devoting her professional career to improving the quality of health care available to Cleveland mothers.) But even with the improvement in revenues, fixed expenses were also growing, and the year ended with yet another operating deficit of well over $100,000.

The same trend prevailed in 1937, as income from patients rose more than $100,000 over the previous year's while expenses grew by some $150,000. In addition, an audit of patients covered by the Hospital Service Association group insurance plan revealed that the hospitals were actually losing money on every patient admitted, to the tune of about $1,000 a month. And pathology chief Howard Karsner pointed out that the medical center was writing off a whole class of potential patients to the Cleveland Clinic because University Hospitals had no facilities or personnel to conduct even routine tests in endocrinology, which he rightly called a "rapidly growing field." Karsner asked to start such a service in-house at a projected cost of $1,000 a year, and despite the addition to the deficit that the expenditure represented, the board had little choice but to agree.

In an attempt to slow the new cash hemorrhage, Robert Bishop informed the director of the Hospital Service Association that University Hospitals would consider refusing admission to the insurer's subscribers unless a new, higher reimbursement rate could be negotiated. The association reluctantly raised its payment rate slightly, but at the same time it insisted that the hospitals reduce expenditures, asking for limitations on the use of even such necessities as X-rays.

In June of 1938, despite the highest level of patient income ever recorded, the hospitals faced ever-rising deficits. A new round of layoffs was initiated, temporarily eliminating the jobs of more than forty service workers, with an additional drastic cut in the number of paid sick-leave days allowed for each employee. The savings that would be effected from the cutbacks amounted to some $10,000 a month.

By fall, however, with the prospect of a $70,000 deficit even after all of the new cuts had been made, the hospitals considered again closing some of their charity wards. The annual expense of providing unreimbursed care had risen to $90,000, and even though Cleveland's City Hospital had itself recently closed nearly two hundred beds, thereby shifting even more of the burden of free care onto the medical center, the trustees saw no other way to at least temporarily slow the rising tide of red ink.

But an argument against further bed reductions was voiced in the hospitals' board room, and it came from a most unexpected source—the medical center's fiscal director, Frank Scott. Although best known as a hard-nosed businessman who routinely made difficult bottom-line decisions, Scott openly expressed his fear that University Hospitals was in the process of forgetting its *raison d'être*.

"We must not lose sight of the fact that...it was in support of a program of teaching and research and care of a certain number of indigent sick that the community gave several million dollars a few years ago," Scott reminded his colleagues on the board. "We have a certain obligation to the community to carry on this work as promised and not cut beds simply because we find ourselves in a difficult financial situation."

In addition to arguing against further reductions, Scott was inadvertently delineating what was increasingly the central dilemma of the medical center. An institution whose member hospitals had been conceived and built as havens for the destitute was, of economic necessity, now being forced to consider first not the need of a potential patient but his ability to pay for care. If University Hospitals were to maintain at least some part of its historic mission, therefore, it would have to reshape its goals to take into account a working environment that the hospitals' founders could never have imagined.

Early in 1939, for example, Robert Bishop actually threatened to refuse a contract with the state's industrial commission unless the reimbursement rate provided for worker-injury cases cared for at the hospitals—$6 a day, a figure unchanged since 1920—were to be raised. In a situation emblematic of the internal struggle taking place between old ideals and the bottom line, the hospitals ultimately signed their contract with the commission even though they had not won an increase. The business of the hospitals—caring for the sick and injured—would, in this instance at least, take precedence over the need to "build up our earnings from patients."

Midway through the year, however, the question of retaining ward beds again arose, and this time economic necessity prevailed. A budget cut of some $40,000 for the remainder of the year necessitated not only additional salary reductions but also a reduction of services in the Outpatient Department and in the areas of teaching and research. Ward beds ordinarily reserved for "teaching material" were converted for use by paying patients, of whom there were now larger numbers than ever before, thanks to third-party payers such as the Hospital Service Association and other private insurers. Indeed, at the end of 1939 the hospitals discovered that income from patient fees for the year exceeded $1 million, the largest amount ever earned. Unfortunately, the year still ended with a $20,000 deficit.

Other problems also beset the hospitals, all of them tied to Adolf Hitler's blitzkrieg into Poland on September 1st and the declaration of war on Germany by Great Britain and France two days later. The cost of food rose steadily, as did the number of employees leaving for more lucrative jobs. American industry, newly revived by the demand for war materiel from overseas, was hiring workers at good salaries for the first time since 1929. Men and women who in the lean years of the Depression would accept any job were suddenly in demand again, as factories fired up to fulfill orders for President Roosevelt's Lend-Lease program to help Britain and France. At the same time, the United States was about to institute a draft law, which would further reduce the number of orderlies and maintenance workers available to the hospitals.

In the spring of 1940, the hospitals' executive committee recommended closing one floor of the babies' hospital for two months, an economy measure that reflected the unusually high occupancy in all services except pediatrics. Indeed, Robert Bishop reported that "there have been days—even weeks—when every bed on the private service in Lakeside and Maternity has been occupied." By the end of July, patient income for the month totaled over $95,000, an all-time high, and there was actually a small surplus in operating funds.

Nearly half of the paying patients in the hospitals, however, were subscribers to the Cleveland Hospital Service Association insurance plan, and there was a substantial difference between the revenue generated by them and that of the other paying patients. Bishop also pointed out that the paperwork involved in cases of third-party payers was rapidly growing to nightmarish proportions, and that "the detail involved in this connection is voluminous and has increased our expense in the accounting department to a considerable extent."

Potentially more damaging than fiscal or accounting problems, however, was a nascent personnel shortage that threatened to cripple the entire medical center. By midsummer of 1940, with hostilities in Europe intensifying and a growing threat to American neutrality from the aggressive Japanese empire, the Surgeon General's office assigned the designation "Fourth General Hospital of the U.S. Army" to a unit consisting of physicians and nurses from University, City, and St. Vincent's hospitals—in effect, recommissioning "Base Hospital #4," the old "Lakeside Unit" of World War I. The new unit would, in the event of war, drain even further the hospitals' already limited medical staff, because of the eighty-five house officers in the medical center, thirty-six were already members of the Reserve Officers Corps and many would be placed on active duty even before the scheduled call-up in July of 1941.

The Red Cross had also begun to sign up nurses for potential military duty, leaving University Hospitals with fully half of its three hundred graduate nurses subject to an active-duty call-up. Even elaborate plans to train ward aides from applicants from the National Youth Association, a New Deal work-training program, collapsed when it was found that all of the region's NYA members—more than a thousand of them—had already been recruited into local industries.

Despite the continuing headaches presented during 1940, the year ended with University Hospitals showing signs of health in at least one area. For the first time in a decade the hospitals closed out a twelve-month period with a substantial surplus—in excess of $60,000. Of course, the combined deficit for the decade totaled more than $100,000, but Robert Bishop called the debt "infinitesimal compared with that suffered by most of the leading teaching hospitals in the country," many of which counted their deficits in the millions of dollars.

During the first three months of the new year, the medical center's financial health did in fact continue to improve, and by the end of the first quarter of 1941, income exceeded expenses by some $25,000. Staffing problems were, however, an ongoing concern, especially as the pool of available qualified nurses continued to shrink. With a crisis in the offing, the hospitals decided to earmark $10,000 to fund a three-year basic course in nursing for high school graduates, the course to be administered within the university's graduate school of nursing. And not long after, pay raises were at last given to the woefully underpaid nurses already on staff, a move that, as Robert Bishop noted, "resulted in a definite improvement in morale."

Flush with funds for the first time in ten years, the trustees appointed a committee to study the feasibility of starting a Department of Psychiatry, an addition for which Bishop had been arguing for some time. Unfortunately, the feasibility study found that a minimum capital outlay of $500,000 was required to create the department, and the committee admitted that it did not see "any possibility, except by some large gift, of this money being available for a long time to come...."

While the hospitals prospered—at least relative to their preceding ten years—the School of Medicine of Western Reserve University faced its most dismal year ever. With enrollment down in all of the university's schools, and with the severe shrinkage of the university's endowment, Western Reserve had itself been fending off fiscal crises throughout the decade. By 1941, the situation had become so critical that the university was unable to provide its usual annual support to the medical school.

With nowhere else to turn, the medical school approached University Hospitals with hat in hand to ask for monetary assistance. The hospitals' trustees, realizing that the viability of the academic medical center they had worked so hard to create now depended more on the health of the school than on that of the hospital group, immediately took the only step they could to avert disaster. In past years the university's reimbursement payments had helped to keep the hospitals afloat; now University Hospitals would return the favor, granting $20,000 to the medical school to ensure its survival. And the hospitals' board indicated that further grants could also be forthcoming in the future, "provided a similar need should then exist."

With all elements of the academic medical center stabilized and functioning at levels at least close to normal, the mood in the hospitals was more relaxed than at any time in the preceding twelve years. In Cleveland, as across the country, the economy boomed and spirits were lifting. Indeed, by the end of November, planning had already begun for a Christmas party in the wards of the Babies' and Children's Hospital, an annual rite that this year promised to be a particularly cheerful affair. Then, on Sunday, December 7th, a series of news bulletins interrupted regular radio broadcasts to report that Japanese forces had bombed American ships and military installations at Pearl Harbor, Hawaii, in a devastating sneak attack. The following day the United States declared war on Japan; three days later, both Germany and Italy declared war on the United States. The two-year-old conflict in Europe had suddenly escalated to the level of a world war.

Just as it had nearly a quarter of a century before, Cleveland's medical community began to mobilize immediately. The "University Hospitals Fourth General Hospital, U.S. Army"—the new designation of the old "Lakeside Unit" of World War I fame—was offered the opportunity to again become the first American medical unit in the war. The unit's physicians, surgeons, and nurses departed from Cleveland on January 10, 1942; by the end of February they found themselves in Australia, where for the next two years they would treat the Pacific war's wounded and injured in the newly built Royal Melbourne Hospital.

In January of 1941, at the annual meeting of the University Hospitals board, most of the assembled trustees and officers had expressed relief that the medical center had weathered the worst of the Depression's storms and was still afloat, albeit under somewhat reduced sail. That the hospitals had survived intact through the worst prolonged financial cataclysm in American history was a miracle of sorts, but the fact that they had managed in great part to stay the course that had been charted for them so many years before was a truly remarkable accomplishment. Now, looking back at that annual meeting from the perspective of 1942, the members of the board must have found deep irony in one comment made by their administrative director, Robert Bishop. In concluding his assessment of the upcoming twelve months, Bishop had commented hopefully to the trustees that he and the other administrators of the hospitals could "approach the new year with confidence." And, he had added, they would enter 1941 with "the determination to win through— come what may."

CHAPTER EIGHT

Little Joe

America's entry into the Second World War marked the end of the Great Depression that had so ravaged the country over the preceding decade. After the bust of the 1930s, the boom of the early 1940s invigorated virtually all of the nation's businesses and industries, among them the country's hospitals, which together comprised the major portion of what was already coming to be known as the health-care "industry."

For University Hospitals of Cleveland, the relative prosperity of the war years alleviated for a time the desperate economic situation that had brought the institution to its knees during the depths of the Depression. As early as 1941, in fact, the hospitals were already seeing a major improvement in their fiscal health, with an annual operating income that year of some $1.17 million, the highest ever. Indeed, if the value of the hospitals' property, assets, endowment funds, and income from trusts and estates were added together at the time, the result would have shown that the medical center was in effect a $30 million institution—far larger than all but a handful of Cleveland-area companies.

But the war years also proved to be among the most difficult in the hospitals' history. No longer forced to close wards, floors, and entire buildings due to ever-diminishing revenues, the medical center nevertheless faced the same prospect, but for a new reason: a sudden shortage of personnel.

Of the fifty-three Cleveland physicians, surgeons, pathologists, X-ray specialists, and dentists serving in Australia in the Army's Fourth General Hospital, for example, thirty-four came from University Hospitals. Fifteen of the sixty nurses going overseas were also from the medical center, and although the number and proportion in the latter group were smaller, it was in the nursing corps that the hospitals encountered their most pressing problems.

The perennial second-class citizens of medicine, nurses had suddenly become a commodity as precious as gold to health-care providers. So many women were leaving stateside hospitals either to serve overseas in the military or to take higher-paying jobs in domestic industry that health-care institutions around the country had to scramble to fill the growing vacancies on their staffs.

In 1941, for example, University Hospitals started the year with two hundred and fifty general-duty nurses, each working a forty-hour week. By April of 1942, the hospitals had only one hundred and twelve full-time nurses—each working a forty-eight-hour week—with eighty part-time nurses and some four hundred volunteers from the community helping out wherever they could. Another eighty-eight students were enrolled in the nursing course for high school graduates that had been started the year before, but these trainees would not be available for duty until 1944.

By the summer of 1942, the number of full-time general-duty nurses employed in the hospitals was down to just eighty-five. The nursing shortage had become so dire that dozens of beds were pulled out of service, and a limit was placed on the number of new admissions. Adding to the problem was a turnover rate of more than seventy percent for hospital service personnel, some of whom were leaving to serve in the armed forces while others were snatching up high-paying jobs in industry. Lay volunteers continued to provide help throughout the medical center, but government-imposed gasoline rationing limited their availability. By the end of 1942, therefore, virtually every department in the hospitals had instituted labor-saving schemes to maintain a modicum of service. In the kitchens, for example, the dearth of workers willing to wash dishes resulted in a new policy that saw meals for ward patients served on paper plates.

At the hospitals' annual meeting in April 1943, administrative director Robert Bishop reported to the trustees that, despite the fact that all of the nation's health-care institutions had been designated as "essential industries," few could compete with hotels, laundries, and the like for semi-skilled or even unskilled service workers. University Hospitals itself, Bishop reported, was now so desperate for such employees that he had been reduced to hiring laundresses who were only sixteen years old.

Nurses, of course, were still at a premium—so much so, in fact, that Bishop planned to establish an employees' day nursery within Babies and

Childrens Hospital.* His hope was that older, married nurses would be willing to return to the hospital work force on at least a part-time basis if they knew that day care was available for their children. A different strategy was tried at Rainbow Hospital, where free room and board were offered to selected students from a nearby women's college in return for morning and evening work in the hospital.

Bishop's main point in his report to the trustees, however, centered on what he called the "trend in hospital earnings." The director explained that extensive enrollment growth in the Cleveland Hospital Service Association insurance plan in 1942 had resulted in an increase in hospital earnings from that source of about $150,000 over figures for 1940. The CHSA boasted of some 500,000 subscribers, an enormous group that accounted for nearly sixty-five percent of all paid care in the medical center's hospitals.

This increase was accompanied, however, by a drop of some $50,000 in earnings from full-paying, uninsured private patients. And because CHSA reimbursement covered only the actual costs of care provided, the hospital could not recover the approximately $2-a-day profit it normally derived from the full-pay patients, a margin that was used to subsidize the cost of providing unreimbursed care to staff cases.

In the end, the medical center actually incurred a $5,000 net loss from its CHSA admissions in 1942. And if the number of CHSA patients continued to increase—as Bishop was certain it would—there would be not only further losses but also less room in the hospital for directly billable private patients. The inevitable result, he said, was that, over time, "our earnings are bound to decrease."

Beginning in May of 1943, Bishop reported, CHSA would add an "item of depreciation in buildings and equipment" into its per capita reimbursement payments. But this additional sum would be relatively small, and Bishop could not foresee a time when the association might be in a position to increase it. The reality, according to Bishop, was that, "only those hospitals that have endowment funds…will be able to carry on any free work."

The director called the problem of reimbursement the most important that the hospitals faced, not because of its immediate financial consequences but because it was, in effect, a ticking time bomb. The growing

---

*Apostrophes were dropped from the hospital's official name by the time of the war.

crisis in health-care insurance would one day reach an acute stage, he believed, and then the situation would "undoubtedly result in a compulsory indemnity plan under Social Security, with government supervision and regulation." The very thought of any government control of the processes of health-care delivery was frightening to most in medicine, but the prospect of mandated payment limits that Bishop foresaw was an eventuality that shook the hospitals' trustees to the core.

As the year wore on, the medical center's existing problems only grew worse. Even as the number of admissions continued to increase, the hospitals remained woefully understaffed, particularly within the nursing corps. The ongoing problem of net losses from CHSA cases also deepened through the year, but by October a new worry had arisen. Reports out of California revealed that nurses there had organized a union and had already secured a wage package of up to $170 a month. At the time the highest monthly salary for a nurse in a Cleveland hospital was still only $155, and the medical center itself was only paying $120 a month. The news from the West Coast sent the hospitals' trustees into a fit of hand-wringing. On top of the mounting losses from CHSA cases, plus the $10 monthly raises that had been instituted to retain defecting service workers, the prospect of having to increase nurses' salaries by as much as forty percent raised the gloomy specter of Depression-era-sized deficits again.

By the end of 1943 the hospitals were indeed running a deficit of nearly $25,000, but the economics of the moment were actually of less immediate import than the ongoing personnel shortages. Director Bishop told the board that virtually every department was being hobbled by the lack of quality service workers. Even more disturbing was the situation in nursing. Indeed, so desperate were the hospitals for trained personnel that at one point they actually hired a nurse of Japanese descent, a remarkable decision in light of the widespread hatred and suspicion of all Japanese—even those born and raised in the United States—which had engulfed the country in the wake of Pearl Harbor.

Characteristically, however, Bishop used the opportunity of the year's annual meeting to dwell less on problems than on possibilities. With the war still raging in Europe and in the Pacific, and with the medical center itself plagued by a growing number of seemingly insoluble dilemmas, Bishop nonetheless presented to the trustees an agenda of strategic moves for which he felt the hospitals should begin planning immediately. At a time when even the medical center's annual report could not be published due to the rationing of paper and ink, Bishop was already thinking ahead to a postwar world and to the hospitals' position in it.

Bishop's proposals included two longstanding ideas, both of which had been relegated to the status of low-priority issues during the lean years of the Depression: an addition to be built onto MacDonald House for the gynecology department (the longtime desire of obstetrics chairman Arthur Bill), and the establishment of a full-fledged Department of Psychiatry. Bishop also proposed the creation of an educational program, to help returning veterans pick up their residencies where they had been interrupted by the war.

The most radical idea that Bishop presented, however, was the establishment—in its own new building—of a separate Outpatient Department for paying patients. Once again displaying his unique understanding of the changing nature of health-care delivery, Bishop argued for "a pay clinic service which would attract a different type of patient than is now attracted by and permitted to come to our Outpatient Department." He pointed out that the University of Chicago had already instituted a similar service, and although it had not met with "the whole-hearted approval of the Chicago Academy of Medicine" (who zealously guarded the interests of the city's private practitioners), it was a development "along a line that I believe is bound to come." Local physicians in private practice who abhorred the Chicago-style plan would come to accept the idea in Cleveland, Bishop insisted, "when, if and as we have [outpatient] medical-care plans comparable to hospital-service plans such as we have at the present time. [And] that day is rapidly approaching...."

Bishop could already foresee the time when insurance carriers would begin to write policies that covered not only hospital stays but also outpatient care, and he knew that University Hospitals would have to be prepared to take advantage of the new development when it came, if the medical center were to compete successfully for private patients. Just a few blocks away, George Crile's Cleveland Clinic was already siphoning away a percentage of the paying patients who might otherwise have patronized the medical center, and that trend, Bishop feared, could only continue. Ultimately, without a sufficient base of private patients to help offset the cost of providing free care to the needy, University Hospitals could one day find itself unable to fulfill one of the fundamental tasks of its historic mission.

Bishop's proposals, raised at a time when there was still no end to the war in sight, may have seemed to some of the trustees as nothing more than a purely hypothetical wish list. But the hospitals' director had concluded that after the war the federal government would in all likelihood make available funds for expansion of what would inevitably become an overburdened national hospital system. And by then, he urged, "our plans should [already] be matured to secure such benefits...."

Bishop's presentation proved so persuasive that the board appointed a committee to evaluate several possible improvements that might be implemented once the war was at last over. By the winter of 1945, however, Bishop was back before the board with another new idea—this one not just visionary but downright daring. In typical fashion, Bishop felt no compunction whatever about raising his radical proposal to the trustees, despite the fact that, if implemented, his plan would be of more immediate benefit to the medical school of Western Reserve University than to the hospitals themselves, and that, ultimately, the cost to the medical center could total roughly half a million dollars.

Bishop rightly saw that the continuing viability of University Hospitals depended in large measure on the health of its affiliated medical school, and at the time, the medical school was in serious trouble. Western Reserve itself had still not recovered fully from the Depression, and the university's ability to sustain its graduate program in medicine—which had weathered the 1930s only with the financial assistance of the hospitals—was seriously in question. The medical school had seen a drastic drop in enrollment, due in part, of course, to the exigencies of the war. But the school was also crippled internally by a lack of leadership and by the petty jealousies of its faculty members.

The spirit of cooperation that had so impressed Abraham Flexner during his visit to the school nearly forty years before had long since evaporated, and in its place was a divisive system of de facto principalities and battling factions. Professors vied with each other for prestige and power, one measurement of which was how thoroughly they could intimidate and overwork their students. Indeed, the faculty's seeming utter disregard for the welfare of their own students had turned medical education at Western Reserve into a war of attrition, as more and more class members dropped out and fewer and fewer new students enrolled. The reputation of the school that Flexner had once called one of the three best in the country was in danger of sinking to a point below the horizon.

Like virtually all of his predecessors, Torald Sollmann, dean of the medical school since 1928, had grown conservative to the point of ossification over the years, and it was on his watch that the school had begun its precipitous slide toward mediocrity. In June of 1944, Sollmann finally retired at the age of seventy, but no new dean was named to replace him. For eight months the school did not have even Sollmann's shaky hand on the tiller, until Robert Bishop at last raised his concerns in a letter to University Hospitals board president Henry S. Curtiss.

"We are at the crossroads in medical education," Bishop wrote to Curtiss early in 1945. "The financial difficulties of the university are presenting severe handicaps from the standpoint of growth and development of the medical school, and it is only a matter of time...before [the situation] will be reflected within the hospitals themselves."

Bishop proposed that two steps be taken at once, not just to stabilize the medical school but to safeguard the future of the hospitals as well. First, he urged the trustees of both the hospitals and the university to "take the initiative in insisting that a new dean be appointed at once," someone who could "provide the...leadership so badly needed...." Second, Bishop proposed that, "in their own protection," the trustees of the hospitals "should be willing to underwrite this new dean and his new program over a period of five years at an annual outlay of $100,000."

The situation was so critical, Bishop explained, that "unless prompt action is taken the medical school and hospitals will have suffered irreparable damage." After the war, he wrote, medical education was "bound to undergo a radical reorganization. Several of the leading medical schools in this country are already planning such a reorganization and will unquestionably assume leadership in the field." At Western Reserve, however, it was Bishop's contention that "we are not even marking time; we are slipping daily.... Certainly it seems to me that our board of trustees should have the faith of our predecessors and be willing to take the initiative and leadership that is so badly needed."

Bishop already had a candidate in mind to fill the vacancy at the top of the medical school, a man who was, in his words, "available within our ranks." He was referring to the hospitals' chief of medicine, Joseph T. Wearn. Bishop had been a Wearn partisan since 1929, when the younger man had first arrived in Cleveland and made the audacious demand that the configuration of the new Lakeside building—then in the midst of construction—be changed to accommodate more laboratory space. Understanding the importance of Wearn's ideas to the future of the hospital, Bishop had thrown the full weight of his influence behind him at the time. Now he was about to do so again, and for exactly the same reason.

Joe Wearn had already proved himself as a physician, researcher, and leader, first at Harvard—where he worked on important studies of the heart and kidney—and later at University Hospitals. But he was also an urbane and witty man, widely read, and with a multitude of varied interests. A born diplomat, he was a commanding presence who led not through intimidation but with charm and genuine enthusiasm. Nearsighted, balding, and so diminutive as to be almost elfin in stature, he was known to many of his associates by the affectionate nickname "Little Joe."

Wearn and his wife were friends of the Bishops; the two couples lived near each other and were comfortable in the same social circles. But it was more than Bishop's personal affection for Wearn that prompted the hospitals' director to recommend that his friend be named dean of the medical school. If Wearn were allowed to bring in new department heads throughout the school and implement new programs of teaching and research, Bishop was convinced that the institution could be not only saved but pushed to new heights.

Like Bishop, Wearn saw that the future of the medical center was largely dependent on the stability of its affiliated medical school. Wearn also had radical notions about the direction of medical education, and he possessed the powers of persuasion necessary to get his new ideas implemented. Indeed, at the time Joe Wearn may well have been the only man in the country capable of both preserving the integrity of the hospitals and resuscitating the moribund medical school. He was also eager to try.

In April 1945, after two months of internal discussion, the University Hospitals board approved Robert Bishop's plan to underwrite the medical school with subsidies of $100,000 in each of the following five years, the money to come from the accumulated income of one of the hospital's larger endowment funds. Less than a month later, Joseph Treloar Wearn's nomination as dean of Western Reserve's medical school was also approved. Although the members of the hospitals' board did not realize it at the time, they had put in place all of the elements necessary for a full-scale revolution.

§

Independent of the higher machinations going on within the medical center's board room, however, the daily business of the hospitals managed to continue, despite the devastating effects of the war. The logistics of the vast health-care complex were especially hard hit, particularly within some of the more mundane areas of the institution. Because of the worker shortage among laundry, housekeeping, and maintenance personnel, for example, the need for volunteer help increased dramatically, so much so that from 1942 through the end of 1944 more than 1,600 individuals contributed a total of 220,000 hours of service—and this despite gasoline rationing, which severely curtailed the mobility of many of the would-be volunteers. The few remaining social workers in the hospitals' Social Service Department were also stretched to the limit, overwhelmed by the huge number of children who had been left in the "care" of irresponsible relatives while the children's mothers either worked in defense plants or followed their husbands to stateside military camps.

Nowhere were wartime constraints felt more profoundly, however, than in the hospitals' nursing corps; at one point, for example, only fifty-three full-time general-duty nurses were at work in the entire complex. Staffing levels eventually reached so low a level that the medical center finally took the bold step of breaking with longstanding citywide precedent by accepting "colored student nurses" and hiring "colored dietitian aides," as well as employing one black and two more Japanese-American general-duty nurses in 1945. Robert Bishop told the board of trustees that these moves not only improved the level of staffing within the hospitals, they also represented "a further contribution to the betterment of interracial relationships."

Even the collapse of Germany and the end of hostilities in Europe in May of 1945 brought no immediate relief for the beleaguered hospitals; the war in the Pacific continued, and with scant hope that the Japanese would surrender anytime soon, no stateside institutions could hope for a timely return to normal prewar operations. Meanwhile, Joe Wearn, the medical school's newly named dean, faced the daunting task of replacing nine department heads, all of whom were either scheduled to retire or planning to leave for other reasons. Happily for Wearn, the opportunity to remake the school by filling it with a faculty that shared his progressive views coincided with the need to fill the vacancies.

Of particular urgency was the Department of Pediatrics, which had been the fiefdom of Henry J. Gerstenberger for more than three decades. Gerstenberger, who was already sixty-four, had for years been running the Babies and Childrens Hospital as if he considered it his private clinic, denying access not only to certain doctors but even to the parents of some patients. Then, in the summer of 1944, three junior members of the

pediatric staff reported to Robert Bishop that Gerstenberger was conducting uncontrolled experiments on hospitalized children. As had happened during a similar incident in 1918, an internal investigation sub-
stantiated the charges against Gerstenberger. Instead of the mild reprimand he had received after the earlier incident, however, Gerstenberger
was asked to take a "leave of absence" until his official retirement at the
end of the 1944-45 academic year.

The search for a new departmental chief had been ongoing for some
months by the time Joe Wearn was named dean of the medical school in
May of 1945. And although Wearn had little input in the selection
process, in June he joined in the unanimous faculty vote approving the
nomination of Charles F. McKhann as head of pediatrics. McKhann came
to Cleveland with a solid research background, first at Harvard and then
at the University of Michigan, where he had investigated, among other
subjects, the poliomyelitis virus. His most recent position, however, had
been as assistant to the president of Parke, Davis, a pharmaceutical company, which made him one of a growing number of physicians whose research efforts were funded, either directly or indirectly, by drug makers.

With McKhann in place, Wearn turned his attention to the larger task
of remaking the medical school and, by extension, the hospitals themselves. One of his first initiatives was a move that prepared the way for
the fulfillment of one of the medical center's longstanding goals: the
creation of the hospitals' first full-fledged psychiatry department. In 1937,
Wearn had created a division of psychiatry within the Department of
Medicine by appointing Edward O. Harper and Neil McDermott, two
young psychiatrists from eastern schools, as instructors in medicine. Because he had an abiding interest in the mind's effect on the body, Wearn
routinely invited Harper and McDermott to lecture to his own classes, as
well as to accompany his staff on ward rounds, thereby creating, in effect,
one of the country's first integrated programs of psychiatric and medical
education. It was not surprising, then, that in August of 1945—the same
month as Japan's final surrender and the end of World War II, and just
three months after being named dean—Wearn recruited a former psychiatric consultant to the Surgeon General of the Army Air Corps, Douglas
D. Bond.

A Freudian psychoanalyst, Bond was a graduate of Harvard and had
earned his medical degree from the University of Pennsylvania. He was
a personal friend of Anna Freud, daughter of the founder of psychoanaly-
sis, and he had formed numerous other important professional friend-

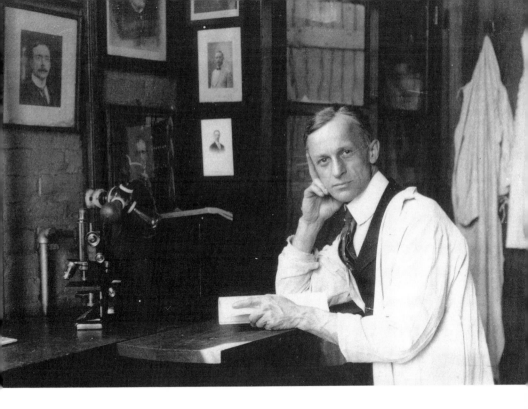

ABOVE: Harvey Cushing, who changed Lakeside without ever leaving Baltimore. (Alan Mason Chesney Medical Archives of The Johns Hopkins Medical Institutions) BELOW: Maternity Hospital supervisor Calvina MacDonald. (UHC)

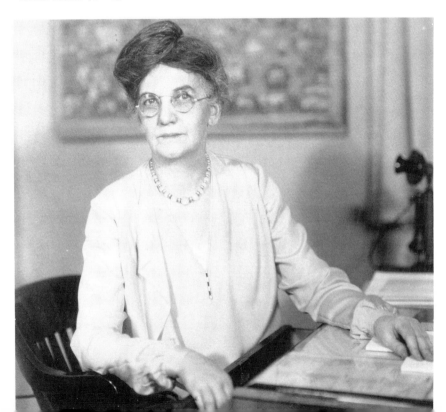

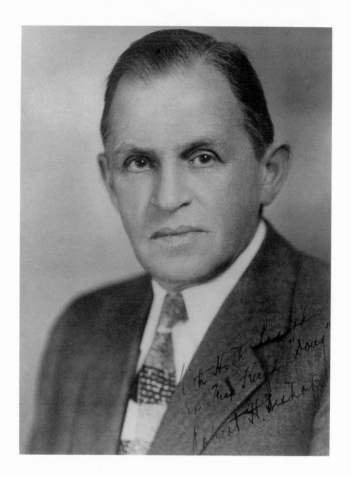

ABOVE: Robert Bishop, charged with leading the new University Hospitals through the difficult years of the Depression. BELOW: The new medical campus as seen from the north in 1925, with Maternity and Babies' and Childrens' Hospitals nearing completion. (UHC)

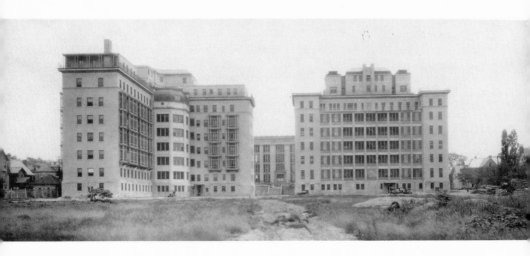

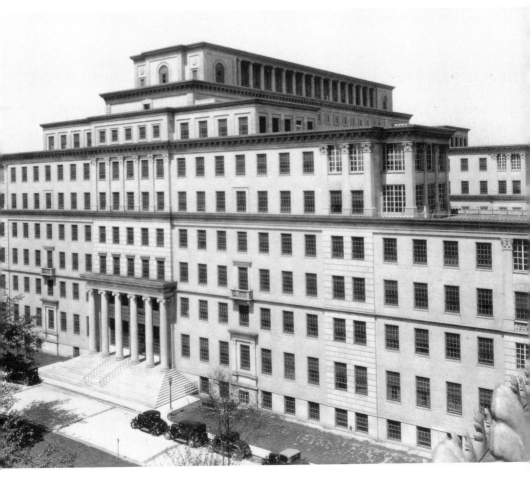

The main entrance of Lakeside Hospital, circa 1932, cornerstone of the medical center complex in University Circle. (UHC)

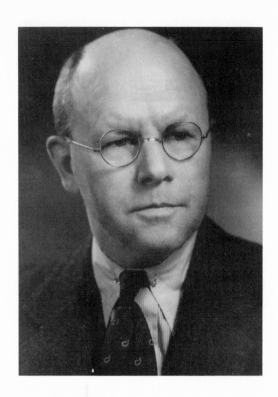

ABOVE: Joseph T. Wearn, driving force behind the 1952 "new curriculum" and the expansion of the hospitals. BELOW: Innovative cardiac surgeon Claude Beck. (UHC)

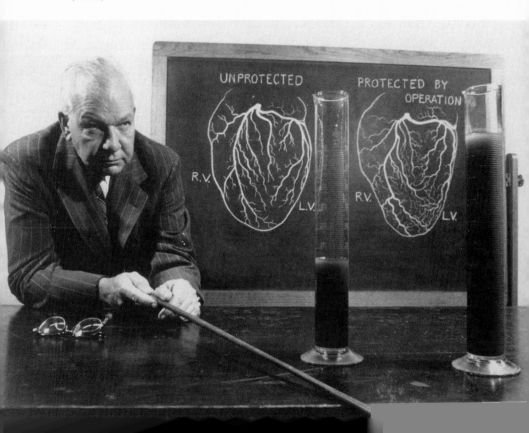

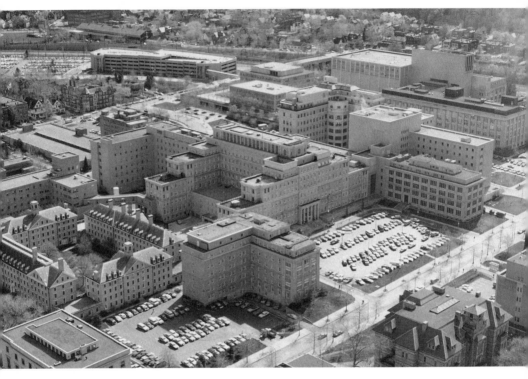

The medical campus of University Hospitals of Cleveland in the 1970s. (UHC)

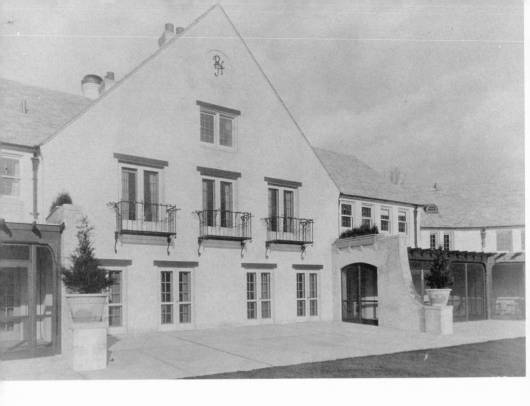

ABOVE: The old Rainbow Hospital in suburban South Euclid (Cleveland Press Collection/Cleveland State University Archives) BELOW: University Suburban Health Center, located on Rainbow's former site. (University Suburban Health Center)

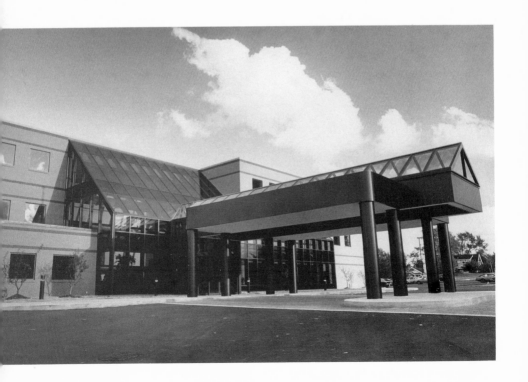

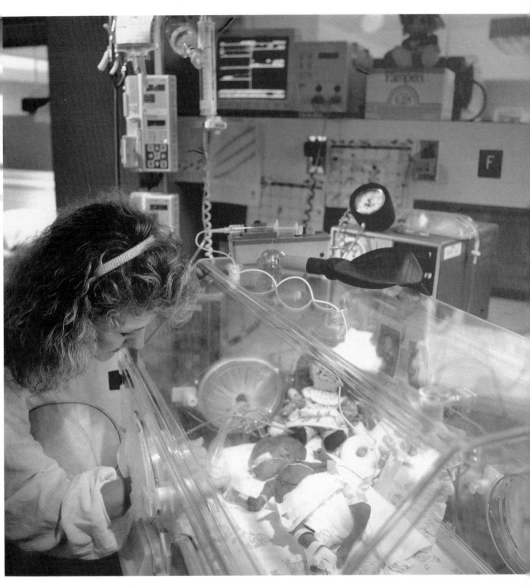

A premature infant receiving care in the new Neonatal Intensive Care Unit.
(Rainbow Babies and Childrens Hospital)

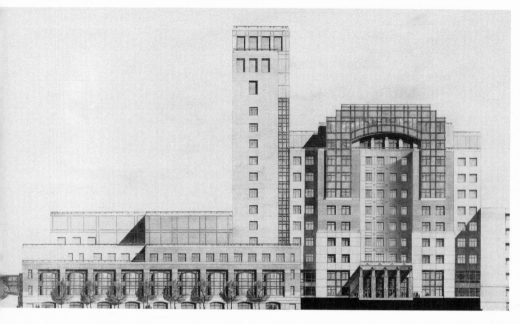

The proposed Bed Tower complex, major component of the medical center's master plan for the future. (UHC)

ships around the world. Indeed, Bond was so widely known and respected that not long after his arrival in Cleveland he was able to convince Maurits and Anny Katan, two internationally renowned European psychoanalysts, to join his staff at the medical center. Both came to work in Bond's division despite the substantial financial sacrifice the move entailed.

Wearn's next coup, in April of 1946, was to persuade John Dingle to come to Cleveland with the four-man team he had led under the Army's wartime Epidemiological Board. As director of the Commission on Acute Respiratory Diseases, Dingle had been able to use large and stable control groups of subjects for his studies on the effects and spread of respiratory disease, and he hoped to continue the work in a peacetime setting. His appointment as head of the medical school's new Department of Preventive Medicine would, in the words of one representative of the Rockefeller Foundation, "immediately put Western Reserve medical school in the lead in such work in the country." Ironically, the preventive medicine department was created at a time when many of the endowment funds of both the hospitals and the medical school were invested in, among other things, the stocks of liquor and tobacco companies.*

While Joe Wearn was busy on his shopping spree for talent, however, the hospitals themselves remained in a state of turmoil. The year 1945 had seen an unprecedented number of admissions to University Hospitals, at a time when the medical center was ill equipped to handle the load. The jump in attendance was both a blessing and curse, because although income from all sources grew substantially, the strain on the depleted ranks of workers within the hospitals grew apace. The hundreds of volunteers upon whom the medical center had relied so heavily during the war—almost 300,000 hours of work were donated by them through 1945—had for the most part stopped coming after V-J Day. And the nursing corps, whose diminished size had been one of the motivating factors behind the volunteer efforts, did not return to its prewar strength even after the end of hostilities. Two-thirds of all nurses serving in the war

---

*Yale University had also been trying to entice Dingle and his group (a physician, a pediatrician, a biostatistician, and a bacteriologist), but the eastern school had been unable to raise the money needed to underwrite the team. Wearn, however, had two advantages in that regard: not only the hospitals' $100,000 annual grant to the medical school, but also a large gift from the Elisabeth Severance Prentiss Foundation, a fund created by the widow of Lakeside's former chief surgeon, Dudley P. Allen.

had come from hospitals, but upon discharge many were either starting families, seeking higher education with the benefits they derived under the G.I. Bill of Rights, or entering more remunerative areas of nursing.

Operating income for the hospitals was, nevertheless, up substantially, even more than operating expenses, which were fueled by a rapidly increasing rate of inflation. Yet Robert Bishop expressed his concern about fiscal matters at the April 1946 hospital annual meeting, worrying openly about the medical center's "questionable ability to continue to increase our earnings in the same proportion that our expenses increase." Primary among his fears were salary levels within the hospitals; although they had risen by nearly twenty-two percent since 1940, most were still lower —and in some cases, *far* lower—than those offered in private industry. A new minimum wage of sixty-five cents an hour was also being considered by Congress at the time, and if such a national standard were to be established, Bishop knew that the hospitals would "have to be prepared to go a long way toward meeting that rate even though it comes to a question of curtailment of activities."

Bishop also warned the hospitals' board of another looming crisis: the outpatient clinics, once the most crowded and highly used areas of the medical center, had been seeing fewer patients of late, and the prognosis was for even further reductions in demand. Indeed, clinic visits had dropped in half since 1941, going from 148,000 to 73,000 annually, which, as Bishop noted, raised the question of the hospitals' "continuing ability to secure sufficient teaching material from the indigent group of patients."

The problems at the outpatient clinics were attributed to two basic factors: the general prosperity of the country, which enabled many more individuals to seek care from private doctors rather than from free clinics; and the remarkably high percentage of Clevelanders covered by health insurance. Realizing that a change of approach was inevitable, therefore, Bishop again strongly recommended the establishment of a "pay clinic," similar to the one already functioning at the University of Chicago. The new clinic could be not only "a new source of teaching material," Bishop explained, but it would also generate additional funds to help support the still-struggling medical school.

As the year wore on, however, it became apparent that the school was not the only element of the medical center that was suffering financially. Postwar inflation continued to force up the prices of food and other commodities, so much so that the hospitals had to raise the rates on private rooms by twenty percent just to catch up. Another request for an increase in reimbursement rates from the Cleveland Hospital Service Association also helped to defray rising expenses, but the long-range outlook was not encouraging.

Ironically, by the summer of 1946 the hospitals had begun to show signs of overcrowding, particularly at MacDonald House, which simply could not keep up with demand. The phenomenon that would come to be known as the postwar "baby boom" was taxing the facilities of maternity hospitals all over the country, but at the medical center the problem was exacerbated by the ongoing nursing shortage, which had forced the closure of entire wards throughout the hospitals. Robert Bishop called the outlook "alarming," noting that not only was the school of nursing having difficulty filling its classes, but the nurses then at work in the hospitals were grumbling about their low pay and forty-eight-hour work weeks. To avert an open revolt, the hospitals instituted pay raises for general-duty nurses, bringing their salaries up to a maximum of $200 a month. The operating deficit that inevitably resulted from this and other increased expenses would be met by the only means available: another upward adjustment of room rates, the increase to be effective as of January 1, 1947.

Finally convinced of the need to develop additional sources of revenue for the medical center, the trustees at last moved on what was by then Robert Bishop's three-year-old proposal. Early in the new year the board approved the creation of an outpatient clinic for paying patients, although not in Lakeside, the most obvious location. The new clinic was to be a part of the Babies and Childrens Hospital, where chief of pediatrics Charles McKhann believed the facility "would make available to pediatricians services not now available in this section of the country." McKhann's comment mirrored the sentiments of the trustees, who, in approving the new clinic, had concluded that all of the hospitals within the medical center would eventually have to "rely on serving the doctors of the community rather than the people directly."

The board's apparently abrupt change of course for the hospitals—from serving "the people directly" to serving "the doctors of the community"—was in fact a decision based on the most logical of deductions. As Robert Bishop had been the first to recognize, the medical center was beset by external pressures to which its constituent hospitals would simply have to yield if they were to survive. And since the onset of the Depression, those pressures had been exerted less by changes in the practice or delivery of health care than by the changing ways in which the hospitals' income was derived.

All of the University Hospitals member institutions had begun life as the eleemosynary undertakings of the most prominent citizens of the region. Each had already undergone the metamorphosis from being an individual general hospital to being one element of an academic medical center, with the personnel, equipment, and cooperative expertise that allowed them all to provide a level of care superior to that available in their previous incarnations. But with the advent of subsidies from local government for care of the poor, followed by the rise of private insurers, the "indigent class"—which each of the hospitals had originally been founded to serve and from which the academic medical center procured most of its teaching material—was, in effect, disappearing.

Over the years the purview of the hospitals had grown to encompass both the class that had created them and the burgeoning middle class, the latter a group that had sprung up precisely because of the presence of the businesses and industries forged by the former. The middle class, with the relatively inexpensive insurance available through the Cleveland Hospital Service Association and other providers, could now afford to take advantage of the health-care services formerly provided only to the very poor or the very rich. In that respect, therefore, the hospitals had indirectly created a new market for their services, and they had then been forced to adjust their goals to meet the new demands.

The steady decline in both the number of the hospitals' private benefactors and the ability of those remaining to provide the type of blank-check support associated with a Samuel Mather, for example, was another element in the complex set of factors forcing change upon the medical center. Increasingly, local, state, and federal governments had taken the place of the hospitals' original saints as major sources of funding, especially as the research component of the academic medical center came to the fore. Seemingly overnight, various arms of government, as well as pharmaceutical companies and philanthropic foundations, were supplying the bulk of funds needed to underwrite care for the poor, laboratory research, and medical education.

Indeed, at the same time that the University Hospitals board was debating the direction of the institution, the Cleveland Foundation was offering the medical center a $70,000 grant to support the new Department of Preventive Medicine. In Washington, Congress was considering the Hill-Burton Act, a bill that would provide federal funds to match state funds for the construction of hospitals in underserved areas around the country. The Senate was also debating a bill introduced by Ohioan Robert Taft that called for federal funds to match state aid for the indigent. And the Taft proposal was nothing more than an attempt to block passage of the Wagner-Murray-Dingle bill, which, if it were to pass, would mandate compulsory federal health insurance for all citizens.

Years before, when the sole concern of a hospital such as Lakeside had been to provide health care for as great a number of the city's poor as could be managed, questions about room rates, insurance reimbursement, government stipends, and other forms of income had not even been raised. The hospital relied for its financial lifeblood on such individuals as Samuel Mather, who was both willing and able to play the role of the kindly and benevolent Uncle Sam. Now, the new realities of health-care delivery saw hospitals not only vying with each other for paying patients, but also coming to depend on subsidies from such entities as the federal government—a less generous and far less sympathetic Uncle Sam.

Ironically, it was Sam Mather's own son-in-law, Robert Bishop, who had first recognized the necessity for change. As early as 1931, as the Depression began to tighten its grip on the country, Bishop had explained to the hospitals' trustees that it would no longer be possible to "render an unlimited amount of free service" to the community. Those days were gone, Bishop had made clear at the time, because in future the hospitals could only continue to function if they kept in mind the new reality: "Medical care is something which should be paid for...."

§

Operating expenses for the entire hospital group exceeded $3 million for the first time at the end of 1946, leaving a frighteningly large deficit of approximately $200,000. Of course, University Hospitals was not the only academic medical center trapped amidst the spiraling costs of supplies, commodities, and wages, not to mention the ongoing personnel shortages which resulted in expensive overtime payments for those actually working. At the April 1947 annual meeting, Robert Bishop reported that hospitals around the country were experiencing their largest operating deficits in history, even worse than during the Depression years. The medical center board could at least derive some solace from the fact that teaching hospitals in the East were facing deficits of up to half a million dollars.

Nevertheless, the per-day cost of patient care was rising steadily, and the momentum was alarming and seemingly unstoppable. "Hospital costs under our present system cannot continue to mount year after year without endangering the future of our institution," Bishop told the board, "and yet, frankly, I see nothing to stop them for a very considerable time ahead...." Bishop reiterated his concern about the level of philanthropic donations to the medical center, saying that the ability of individuals to help finance such institutions was "rapidly diminishing."

While costs continued to rise, however, so, too, did demand. The flood of obstetrical patients at MacDonald House, for example, forced the imposition of an eight-day limit on hospitalization, at a time when the standard stay for maternity cases was roughly two weeks. And all of the hospitals in the group faced critical shortages of nurses, anesthetists, dieticians, technicians, stenographers, typists, ward maids, and other housekeeping positions—almost all of which were jobs traditionally filled by women.

With all of its many problems, the medical center was at least no longer the most expensive hospital in the city; its per capita operating expenses had been squeezed to the point that it was by then only the fourth highest in Cleveland. This small victory was largely the work of Robert Bishop, who had spent much of his career as director of administration attempting to keep the hospitals on an even fiscal keel. Indeed, it was Bishop who had led the medical center through the perilous years of the Depression and the war, and it was Bishop whose insight and bold new ideas were so often the source of positive change within the institution.

After facing so many crises over so many years, however, Bishop had grown tired, and in the summer of 1947 he decided to move into a decidedly less stressful position. He tendered his resignation from the hospitals to assume the directorship of the newly formed "Joint Committee for the Promotion of Medical Education and Research," a fund-raising consortium of representatives from University Hospitals, the Medical School of Western Reserve University, St. Luke's Hospital, and Mt. Sinai Hospital. William B. Seymour, one of the medical center's former assistant directors of administration—and a former practicing physician in the Department of Medicine—was named to replace Bishop.

With Bishop gone, the responsibility for prodding the medical center toward new directions devolved upon Joe Wearn, who in many ways had already taken up the mantle of leadership. Indeed, in May of 1947, Wearn had to update the hospitals' trustees on the changes he had already effected. He pointed out that, thanks in large measure to the $100,000-a-year grant from the hospitals, the medical school had begun "a complete reversal of the...downward trend" that had so devastated the program during the Depression. New departments had been created, and six new chiefs had already been put in place—Arnold D. Welch in Pharmacology, McKhann in Pediatrics, Hymer Friedell in Radiology, Dingle in Preventive Medicine, Harland G. Wood in Biochemistry, and Douglas Bond in the Division of Psychiatry. "Each of these men is eminent in his particular field," said Wearn, "and several of them so outstandingly so that we have been particularly fortunate in securing their affiliation with our institutions." In the following three years, MacDonald House's Arthur Bill, pathology chief Howard Karsner, and head surgeon Carl Lenhart would also be retiring, and with their departure the entire leadership of the school would have been replaced in just five years.

Wearn also offered the trustees two new ideas for the hospitals, both of which could conceivably act as sources of revenue. He proposed the creation of an ambulatory diagnosis center for private patients in Lakeside and Hanna House, to be established along the lines of a similar clinic at Johns Hopkins. The new center would accept referrals from outside physicians, thus broadening the hospital's patient base, and it would free up otherwise wasted beds by allowing patients who were merely waiting for a diagnosis to use space other than that needed by acutely ill paying patients.

Wearn's second proposal was for the establishment of a pay clinic for the Department of Preventive Medicine. Here again, the clinic could not only generate revenue but also provide a steady stream of "material" for the nascent department. If inaugurated, it would be the first such clinic in the country.

As Wearn's new proposals were considered, plans that had been made previously were beginning to come to fruition. In September, Lakeside's first psychiatric ward was opened, in space borrowed from the medical and surgical departments. The new ward was to be considered only a temporary facility, however, because planning was already underway for a separate home for what would eventually become the Department of Psychiatry. The year before, members of the Hanna family, through hospital trustee Leonard C. Hanna, Jr., had announced that they would contribute a total of $1 million toward construction of an addition to the medical center, to honor the memory of Howard Hanna, who had died early in 1945. When completed, the Howard M. Hanna Memorial Building would make University Hospitals the only private medical institution in the city with separate facilities for psychiatric care.

By the spring of 1948, however, a pall of gloom was again descending on the hospitals. At the April annual meeting, director of administration William Seymour revealed that the medical center had sustained a $150,000 operating loss for the previous year. A number of board members chose to downplay the significance of the deficit, citing much larger losses—more than $1 million at Massachusetts General, and nearly $2 million at Columbia Presbyterian in New York—at other similar institutions. But the reality of the situation, as Seymour expressed it, was that the financial picture was "gruesome." He pointed out that "reimbursement [for indigent care] from governmental agencies, both local and national, falls far below the actual cost of services rendered by the hospitals." Although one million people in Cuyahoga County were then enrolled in the Cleveland Hospital Service Association insurance plan—and University Hospitals derived fully seventy percent of its private-patient income from these individuals—continually spiraling costs were forcing the hospitals to raise room rates to a point dangerously close to the public's "limit of tolerance."

The board seemed intent on minimizing the potentially disastrous consequences of the inflationary trend, however, preferring instead to focus on some of the more positive figures in Seymour's report. Between 1931 and 1947, for example, the number of patients treated annually in the hospitals had risen by more than four hundred percent, while the actual number of days each patient spent in the hospital had been sharply reduced. This apparent paradox was in fact good news for the medical center, because the average cost of one day of patient care had almost doubled since 1940, and the expenses were the same to the hospital whether or not they were covered—in full, in part, or not at all—by the patient or by third-party reimbursement.

Of course, another reason for the shorter stays was the combination of high demand and ongoing personnel shortages. It was imperative that patients be discharged as quickly as possible, simply to free up beds. Perhaps the most compelling explanation for the reduced length of stays, however, was penicillin, which had been discovered in 1928 but only became widely available in the 1940s, when large-scale production techniques were perfected. With the advent of penicillin and such other new antibiotics as streptomycin, medicine could for the first time rely on a broadly effective weapon in the age-old war against what had theretofore been the most pernicious killer of all: infection. With these powerful new drugs, patients who might otherwise have been confined to a hospital for weeks or even months could be treated, cured, and discharged in a matter of days.

Positive developments notwithstanding, the hospitals still found themselves deeply in debt, with a $100,000 deficit for just the first half of the year. And the nursing situation was, in Director Seymour's words, "rapidly deteriorating." It would be necessary to both close more wards throughout the medical center and to raise the pay of nurses. And to offset the effect of the latter move, patient rates would also have to be raised immediately, by from $1 to $2.50 a day.

By the time of the April 1949 annual meeting, the fiscal concerns of a few months before had escalated to the level of crisis. The previous year had ended with an operating deficit of $200,000, which amount could be covered only by tapping income from the endowment funds. The reasons for the huge deficit were readily apparent from the statistics compiled in the hospitals' annual report, which was released in printed form for the first time in nearly two decades. In 1931, for example, University Hospitals had admitted thirty-six percent of all indigent cases entering private voluntary hospitals in the city; by 1948 that figure had risen to fifty percent. In 1931, internal salaries constituted only thirty percent of the medical center's annual costs; in 1948 they constituted seventy percent. Income from endowment funds in 1931 had amounted to forty-four percent of the hospitals' total working capital; in 1948 that figure was down to twenty percent, another example of the effect the great number of Cleveland Hospital Service Association subscribers had on the way the hospitals worked.

At one point during the annual meeting, board chairman Henry S. Curtiss rose to address the subject of primary concern for everyone present. For the first time since the end of the Depression, Curtiss called attention to the medical center's continually rising operating costs, and he offered a word of warning for the future. It would be necessary, he said, to raise substantially the rates paid by Cleveland Hospital Service Association subscribers to meet the rising expenses, but he cautioned that, from then on, the trustees themselves would have to take the initiative in "restricting [operating] costs as much as possible." As the University

Hospitals representative to the CHSA board, Curtiss knew that the insurer could not continue to raise its subscribers' rates indefinitely. Sooner or later, a confrontation was inevitable, and the consequences for the hospitals could be disastrous.

Even with its growing fiscal concerns, however, the medical center continued to plan expansion of its facilities. In May the process of assembling parcels of land for the new Hanna Memorial psychiatric building began. By August, the trustees had approved a $70,000 expenditure to create a "premature infant suite," consisting of a half-dozen six-bed wards on the seventh floor of the Babies and Childrens Hospital. The medical center's first formal infants' intensive-care facility would replace a jury-rigged ward that had been in operation for some time, but which was of inadequate capacity and provided less than ideal protection from infection.

At the same time that the hospitals were preparing to invest in new and remodeled facilities, however, the scenario that Henry Curtiss had warned of just a few months before was already being played out. In early autumn, University Hospitals was informed by the Cleveland Hospital Service Association that "further increases in hospital rates of reimbursement cannot be met with funds available to the association." Believing the postwar inflation to have long-since peaked, the insurer was sending out a warning to all Cleveland hospitals that it would no longer "accept the responsibility to pay higher rates...." While in previous years the medical center had been able to negotiate higher reimbursement rates almost at will, now the service association's board was taking a stand, forcing the hospitals to at last accept the responsibility for cost containment. The insurance system on whose reimbursements the University Hospitals group had relied for sustenance for so many years was suddenly telling the hospitals, "No more."

§

By the beginning of the new decade, there was progress in at least one area of longtime concern: nursing. After instituting pay raises and a forty-hour work week, the hospitals began to attract more nurses back to the fold, and by January of 1950 there were a total of two hundred and sixty graduate staff nurses working in the medical center—more than at any time in the previous eight years. Even more dramatic, however, was the progress being made on a complete overhaul of both the medical curriculum and the manner in which it would be presented to students. As Joe Wearn explained to the hospitals' board, he and the group of young revolutionaries he had assembled—known within the medical school simply as "Joe's Boys"—were busily creating an entirely new method of teaching medicine, a system that streamlined the process, eliminated courses of questionable merit, and brought the student into the hospitals more immediately and more directly, to obtain more first-hand, supervised experience than previous students had ever enjoyed.

The plans also involved what Wearn called "the breaking down of departmental walls," a development that would have been inconceivable under the old system of fiefdoms and jealously guarded power. For Wearn and his "boys," however, cooperation and shared knowledge were the only ways to ensure progress, particularly in reviving those areas of research that had become largely moribund over the years.

Indeed, it was with an eye toward strengthening the level of research at the hospitals that Wearn nominated the replacement for Arthur Bill, who had finally retired in 1948 after a thirty-year association with the MacDonald House maternity hospital. No replacement had been named immediately upon Bill's resignation because Wearn was intent on finding what he considered the right man for the job, a man with a background in the laboratory who would bring his influence to bear on the overwhelmingly practice-oriented Department of Obstetrics. Not until early in 1950, therefore, would the dean appoint Gilbert Vosburgh, a brash, young research-minded obstetrician from Johns Hopkins, to head the department at University Hospitals.

By that time the hospitals themselves were showing signs of renewed vigor, so much so that a small brochure titled "Report to the Community" was published and disseminated throughout the city. Reminiscent of the annual reports of an earlier age, the booklet was designed to serve double duty: it contained both a raft of information about the current state of the hospitals, and a gentle nudge to potential contributors to the endowment funds.

Under the heading "Highlights of 1949," for example, the booklet listed a mind-boggling array of statistics: 27,537 patients received 261,585 days of care during the year; 4,543 babies were born at MacDonald House, while an additional 694 births were supervised in the still-functioning "home delivery" program; 12,580 patients had visited the Emergency Department.

The hospitals' 1,972 employees conducted 14,076 surgical operations; administered 16,957 anesthetic procedures; performed 223,273 laboratory examinations; administered 39,287 X-ray examinations and treatments; conducted 4,294 transfusions from the hospitals' own blood bank; served 1,312,255 "well-balanced and tasty" meals; and washed and processed 3,544,955 pounds of laundry, more than 13 pounds of laundry per patient, per day.

Recalling the nineteenth-century practice of public appeals for funds, the 1950 publication also included a short message from board president Harvey Brown, Jr., who asked the "farsighted friends of University Hospitals" to again help "enlarge our endowment resources" to ensure that the medical center's "humanitarian task" would continue. Despite their overwhelming reliance on income derived from third-party payers, the hospitals were indeed continuing to call on their endowments, to cover the annual deficits that accrued because of the disparity between the rate of reimbursement received for indigent care and the actual cost of that care. In fact, at the time there was a real if only dimly perceived danger that the hospitals could become so dependent on their endowments that the principal of the funds themselves might one day be invaded and so thoroughly depleted that it could never be refunded completely. For this reason, Brown's message to the public ended with a statement not unlike those written by his predecessors more than half a century before: "The hospital trustees will be glad to discuss any gift, large or small, with prospective donors."

As board chairman Henry Curtiss explained at the trustees' annual meeting in April, University Hospitals was already furnishing fifty-one percent of indigent-care services rendered in Cuyahoga County, and the annual reimbursement payments from the Community Fund were never sufficient to cover the actual cost of care delivered. In fact, the total amount of all such unreimbursed expenses was "more than the deficit incurred in operations for the year 1949."

Director of administration William Seymour pointed out that staff patients could be either referrals from the county relief office, for whom the hospitals were reimbursed at a rate of only $10.50 a day; Welfare Federation-referred patients, whose care was billed at approximately $10.50 per day, although the hospitals never actually received full payment; or other poor patients, who paid in accordance with their ability. Large annual losses were, therefore, inevitable, because "the only possibility we have of controlling income [that is, *increasing* it] is in the class of private patients...which amounts to only thirteen percent of our income."

Nonetheless, Seymour reported to the trustees that the medical center had actually achieved a semblance of order for the first time since the onset of the Depression. Despite a sixty-eight percent increase in the cost of living over the decade just ended, when Seymour compared the institution to other university hospitals in the eastern United States he found Cleveland's situation to be more balanced and secure. "Our costs have risen, but appear to be stabilizing," Seymour explained. "Our financial position, although susceptible of improvement, is definitely not precarious; and we have no personnel shortage."

Just two months later, however, the question of personnel shortages again came to the fore, as the United States entered the military conflict in Korea. For the second time in less than a decade, trained medical personnel were called to active duty, again raising the possibility of severe cutbacks of service within University Hospitals. To preempt the onset of another nursing crisis, the hospitals soon raised the monthly wages of general-duty nurses. At the same time, however, food and commodity prices began to rise more swiftly, and by November, across-the-board pay raises of roughly five percent were instituted to ensure a steady supply of maintenance and housekeeping employees. Then, in December, hospital employees voted overwhelmingly to subscribe to Social Security pension benefits under the Federal Insurance Contributions Act. By the end of the year, the hospitals' share of the FICA contributions, combined with the costs engendered by the pay raises, had created an additional annual expense of some $175,000.

As if the pressures of the war were not sufficient to induce worry among the board, the advent of 1951 also saw the sudden departure of pediatrics chief Charles McKhann. Along with W.D. Belnap, a fellow in pediatrics, and associate surgeon Claude Beck, McKhann had been conducting a series of experimental surgical treatments on some one hundred and twenty-five patients, including ninety-three children of whom the youngest was just nine months of age. The operation they performed had been devised on the theory that by increasing the flow of blood to the cerebral cortex, the effects of everything from epilepsy and cerebral palsy to mental retardation could be reversed. The surgery itself created a connection between the carotid artery and the jugular vein, in effect force-feeding the brain with a higher volume of arterial blood. The procedure became known as the "buzz operation," because patients reported "hearing" a buzzing sound in their heads after the surgery was performed.

The experimenters claimed "improvement" in roughly half of their patients, but these results were based primarily on subjective appraisals and were questioned from the start by other staff physicians. Indeed, the suspicion soon arose that even the marginally positive results reported by the team may have been overstatements, and some staffers voiced the opinion that figures had been deliberately manipulated. If even the lowest numbers were inflated, then the procedure had been an unmitigated disaster from the start and should have been stopped early on. This suspicion was given credence when even before a Medical Council investigating committee had the opportunity to advise the board of trustees of its findings, McKhann voluntarily submitted his resignation. And as had happened so often before in similar circumstances, the board then decided that "no further action seemed to be indicated, and that further discussion and publicity would not be beneficial and should be avoided."

The most surprising aspect of the McKhann affair may well have been the participation of Claude Beck, one of the most prominent surgeons on the University Hospitals staff. Associate surgeon under Carl Lenhart and chief of the neurosurgery division, Beck was a brilliant innovator who had already devised a number of techniques to attack the problem of lowered blood supply to the heart. In 1935 he performed the first widely successful surgical treatment of coronary artery disease—the "Beck I" operation, in which he scuffed the heart of a patient with an abrasive to foster the growth of new capillaries. In 1948 he devised the "Beck II" operation, in which revascularization of the heart was accomplished by grafting a segment of vein from the aorta to the coronary sinus. (The Beck II operation preceded by twenty years the advent of coronary bypass surgery, which used a vein graft from the aorta to a point beyond the occlusion of a blocked coronary artery.) And in 1947 Beck became the first surgeon to successfully use electric shock to return a fibrillating heart to normal rhythm during surgery.

In the 1920s, with Elliott Cutler, Beck performed the first operations on the heart's mitral valve, conducting open-heart surgery on a working, beating heart, decades before the invention of the heart-lung machine. Indeed, Beck himself in the 1940s would postulate the creation of just such a device, as well as the possibility that one day heart transplants and the use of artificial organs would become fairly routine matters.

A large, heavy-set, almost elephantine man of serious mien (incongruously, he also bore a striking facial resemblance to the comic actor W.C. Fields), Beck was nonetheless a delicate and meticulous surgeon. His broad hands and thick fingers belied the dexterity and skill he brought to every operation. He was so well known for the slow and steady pace he set in the operating theater that a colleague once remarked on the superfluousness of the clock on the wall of his surgical suite. When Beck was operating, it was said, the appropriate means of marking the passage of time was not a clock but a calendar.

As head of neurosurgery Beck was the logical man to be asked to participate in the clinical end of the McKhann experiments. Why he *did* participate in so questionable an enterprise, however, and why he did not monitor the results more carefully, is problematic. The experimentors may well have fallen into the trap of "finding" the results that they wanted to find. It would not, of course, have been the first time in the annals of Cleveland medicine that bias might have influenced the results of an investigation.*

Beck's involvement in the McKhann experiments may also have been one of the reasons he had not been chosen to replace the retiring Carl Lenhart earlier in the year. Although Joe Wearn did not go outside the medical center to find a new chief of surgery, he bypassed Beck and settled on William D. Holden, one of five assistant surgeons who had worked under Lenhart and Beck. Holden was only thirty-seven years old at the time, but he was already a committed teacher and he made plain to Wearn that he would consider his approval as director to be a mandate to fill the surgery department with a full-time staff of like-minded individuals. This was, of course, precisely what Wearn wanted to hear.

While Joe Wearn concentrated on rebuilding the medical school's internal structure, however, the daily operations of the hospitals themselves were again becoming mired in trouble. The Korean conflict, for example, was sapping the strength of the institution, much like the two world wars had done in previous years. Wearn himself noted to the trustees that

---

*In one such episode in the nineteenth century, a famous local surgeon was presented with a patient afflicted with a huge growth in one testicle. After performing a careful examination of the patient the surgeon asked his practice partner for his opinion of the case. The second doctor correctly pronounced the patient's problem to be a large tumor. "No," said the surgeon excitedly. "It is a baby. I could feel its knees and neck." Convinced he had stumbled upon the ultimate medical anomaly, the surgeon proceeded to operate. Only after a tumor, not a child, had been removed from the patient did an unrepentant Horace Ackley grudgingly admit that his diagnosis may have been in error.

several members of the house staff had been called to active duty in the service, and that because of the shortage of physicians the normal two-year internship had been cut to just one year.

William Seymour added further bad news when he told the board that the hospitals were again logging large operating deficits that were consuming all of the available income from the hospitals' general endowment funds. As for the personnel question, unemployment levels nationwide had been low even before the war in Korea, but now competition for general unskilled or semiskilled workers was intense. "In the 1942 crisis a great many people—workers and volunteers alike—worked in hospitals out of a sense of patriotic duty," Seymour explained, "but this sense is notably lacking at the present time, and our help situation is suffering accordingly." There was no immediate crisis, he continued, but it was clear that "any sudden development which would aggravate the international situation would...put us in a position where operation of the hospital would have to be restricted...."

In June, room rates were again increased in an attempt to slow the rising tide of red ink. The general forty-hour work week, instituted "in cooperation with all other hospitals in the area," also added to expenses. At the same time, the cost of supplies continued to rise, and the hospitals were forced to spend enormous amounts of money just to maintain basic services. An oral thermometer, for example, cost less than fifty cents, but using almost three thousand of them a year brought the total annual bill to more than $1,400. The cost of syringes exceeded $15,000, rubber gloves amounted to nearly $3,000, and even cotton balls raised the tally by more than $7,200. These and other increased expenses only added to a growing deficit that by the end of July exceeded $150,000.

Despite a looming financial crisis, the medical center proceeded with plans to build what was still being called the "premature suite" in Babies and Childrens Hospital, thanks to a $100,000 gift from Mrs. John H. Hord. The promised Hanna Memorial psychiatry building was also at last about to be started, after land on Abington Road was acquired through a complicated land swap involving the hospitals, the university, and one of the university's fraternities.

At the start of 1952, however, Director Seymour sounded a more urgent warning to the board about the desperate need for more working capital. The hospitals were already "far behind in the payment of current accounts," and the situation was affecting their credit rating with suppliers. In addition, the previous year's outstanding cash operating deficit, plus recent expenditures for equipment and other capital items, totaled nearly $300,000. Seymour's recommendation was to begin taking "cash advances" from general endowments—actually using the principal of certain funds, and leaving an IOU to be repaid later.

The hospitals' fiscal woes were aggravated by the advent of another nursing shortage, which was a result of wartime demand. From a high of two hundred and sixty-five graduate nurses at work in the medical center only a few years before—which was itself a number below the optimum level of staffing—the ranks had been thinned to just one hundred and eighty-two. The shortage was felt most acutely in obstetrics, which was already overburdened due to the huge volume of admissions resulting from the baby boom. With an entire private floor closed for lack of nurses, MacDonald House was forced to discharge new mothers far earlier than normal, simply to free up beds for new patients. And since the vast majority of MacDonald admissions were private patients, the closing of an entire floor constituted a serious loss of potentially valuable billable days. "If [even] twelve more nurses were available for that service," Seymour explained, "we would be able to pick up an additional six thousand patient days with [annual] revenue of approximately $120,000."

Seymour had already met with the heads of all the clinical departments to try to come up with a plan for recruiting more nurses, especially those who would be willing to work the hated 11 p.m.-to-7 a.m. shift. (Even bonus pay for the night shift was proving an inadequate incentive.) The department chiefs had rejected the ideas of closing staff beds, of using volunteer help or senior medical students, or even of reopening the old employees' day nursery, to lure back nurses who had left the profession to raise families. The only possible expedient was to institute a "radically increased pay schedule," but this most obvious possibility was roundly rejected by the board of trustees; even with better pay there was "no assurance" that more nurses would be forthcoming, and if they were not, the hospitals would be stuck paying higher wages to their existing corps of nurses. In the end, the board merely appointed another committee to consider the matter.

The medical center's old standards of service seemed in imminent danger of retrenchment. The hospitals were treating more than double the number of patients they had seen in 1933, with a staff that was roughly the same size as that of nearly two decades before and a nursing corps that was actually smaller. In fact, by the spring of 1952 the nursing problem had become so acute that in some divisions only one nurse was on duty at any given time—a level of staffing that William Seymour, with some understatement, called an "irreducible minimum."

At the board's annual meeting that year, Seymour outlined most of the hospitals' problem areas, but he minimized their potential consequences. "We should not feel too apologetic about...minor deficiencies of service in some areas," he said, "[because] the overall quantitative and qualitative medical results are continuously better." The apparent complacency of both Seymour and the board, however, was precisely the wrong attitude to adopt at the time. The leaders of the medical center seemed oblivious to a growing attitude among the public: that medical care alone, no matter how skillful or effective, was only one element of hospitalization.

Patients were coming to expect more of physicians and hospitals— more personal attention, more prompt service, and more comfortable accommodations. In an era of full employment, with the hardships of the Depression and the war years behind them and with a vast segment of the population covered by all-inclusive health insurance, more people were beginning to consider not just the kind of treatment they could receive at a hospital but also the types of amenities that the hospital could provide. And as competition for patients began to grow more serious among the city's health-care institutions, the "secondary" aspects that Seymour and the board seemed to dismiss as unimportant were actually becoming primary reasons for patients to choose one hospital over another.

As if to reinforce the notion that the medical center was immune from a possible defection of public patronage, Seymour told the trustees that "this institution is a vital and necessary unit of our community." He added that "no individual or individuals are as important as the whole," and concluded by saying that "we cannot let distractions in any particular area affect our judgment or belief in the overwhelming force for good which we possess...."

Seymour's impassioned speech actually served two purposes. In one sense it was a rallying cry for the faithful, but on another level it was a very personal act of self-defense. Seymour was, in effect, asking for the board's support of his position in a messy little affair then ongoing in MacDonald House, a situation that had started as a mere dispute but that had blossomed into a full-fledged confrontation.

In addition to the obvious problems engendered by the nursing shortage, MacDonald House had been rocked for months by internal dissension, an uprising of sorts led by the members of the hospital's visiting staff of private practitioners. The turmoil derived from the hospital's fundamental problem: throughout its existence the institution had been the virtually autonomous domain of its first director, Arthur Bill.

One of the hallmarks of the maternity hospital during Bill's tenure was the large number of outside obstetricians who constituted the visiting staff. Indeed, of all the component hospitals of the medical center, only at MacDonald House had the preponderance of admissions over the years been the paying patients of nonstaff, private physicians—the so-called "part-timers," as opposed to the full-time teaching and research-oriented staffs of other departments. And the visiting staff at MacDonald House consisted almost entirely of obstetricians whose large and lucrative private practices left them only limited time to devote to either teaching or research—both of which, ostensibly, were requirements for physicians seeking admitting privileges at the medical center.

In 1950, after Bill's retirement, Joe Wearn chose Gilbert Vosburgh from Johns Hopkins as the new head of MacDonald House, precisely because Vosburgh was a well-known researcher and educator—a classic academic-medical man. Indeed, one of Vosburgh's first tasks at the hospital was to assemble his own loyal staff of full-time physicians for MacDonald House, a staff both willing and able to engage in the type of teaching and research work that was being carried out in all of the medical center's other departments. And with his new physicians in place, Vosburgh had begun to commandeer for staff patients some of the beds that had previously been allocated for use by private cases.

At the time, MacDonald House was admitting four times the number of patients it had seen in 1927, even though it had fewer nurses than had been available that same year. Most of the cases admitted were private, because, as an investigation by the Medical Council would later conclude, "there has been no control whatever placed on the admission of the private patients of the visiting staff." And because the one floor of the hospital already closed due to the nursing shortage had been a private floor, Vosburgh's new initiatives only further reduced the number of beds available for the paying patients of the outside obstetricians.

Not a particularly gifted manager or administrator, Vosburgh failed to explain his program adequately to the members of the visiting staff, which left them feeling besieged. Bitter at what they perceived as a sudden and inexplicable constriction of their "rights," members of the visiting staff began to air their grievances by 1950. Instead of talking directly to Vosburgh, or to the hospitals' Medical Council, the director of administration, or even the board of trustees, however, the obstetricians chose to publicize their concerns in another quarter. Before long, hospital trustees were receiving letters, petitions, and personal inquiries from MacDonald House *patients*, all of whom had been told by their physicians that the ongoing cutback of private beds was only the first step in what would inevitably be the complete elimination of private cases from the hospital.

Alarmed at the rumors—which were, in fact, false—spread by some members of the MacDonald visiting staff, and themselves feeling besieged, the trustees appointed a board committee to investigate. They then asked the hospitals' Medical Council to look into the affair as well. Before the council could conclude its investigation, however, the visiting staff finally communicated directly with new board president John C. Virden (chairman of the Federal Reserve Bank of Cleveland), Seymour, and Vosburgh. In a February 1952 letter, the members of the visiting staff accused the hospitals of maintaining a "policy of attrition" against them. As a result of the increase in the number of staff patients at MacDonald, they said, the hospital's waiting room "often resembles a flophouse," and they quoted "many" unnamed private patients who, they claimed, had "heatedly stated they will not return to the disorganized confusion and tenement-like rooming that they have experienced recently."

The visiting staff went so far as to send a copy of its letter to the local newspapers, all of which weighed in immediately with articles about the turmoil in the hospitals. (The *Plain Dealer* even ran an anti-Vosburgh editorial under the headline "Tragic Failure.") Not long after, however, the Medical Council investigating committee, chaired by Douglas Bond, submitted a blistering report to the board, a report that few trustees wanted to see. Blame for the hysteria at MacDonald House was allocated in proportion to the parties responsible: Vosburgh, for his lack of leadership and communication skills; Seymour and the trustees, for not providing "outstanding help"; and most of all the visiting staff, who, the committee commented, did not give Vosburgh even the hint of their "full and loyal cooperation."

"The visiting staff of MacDonald House, with a few exceptions, has demonstrated little insight into the objectives of a teaching hospital," said the report. Although most members of the visiting staff were "able practitioners" who took justifiable pride "in the quality of practice in MacDonald House," still most were "not willing or not able to accept the kind of teaching responsibility, research activity or administrative duties expected of comparable staff members in other clinical departments of University Hospitals."

The hospitals' administrators and trustees were also culpable because they had never made plain to former head obstetrician Arthur Bill or to the visiting staff "a clear understanding of the objectives of University Hospitals." For many years, therefore, there had been "a much greater emphasis" placed on the admission of private patients than on the maintenance of teaching and research programs. (In one pre-Vosburgh year, for example, fully seventy-five percent of MacDonald House admissions had been of private patients.) When Vosburgh brought in his new full-time staff members, the move had been "interpreted by some of the visiting staff as a threat to their private practice."

The Medical Council report supported Vosburgh and insisted that he be given "a reasonable chance to develop his programs," even if that resulted in "the withdrawal of some of the members of the visiting staff who are not in sympathy with his objectives...." A limit on the number of private admissions was recommended, as well as a limit on the number of obstetricians who would be "given the privilege of practice in MacDonald House." Finally, the report boldly questioned the hospitals' board itself, asking "whether some of [the trustees] fully comprehend their obligations to the hospitals and the public, whose representatives they are in guiding this institution."

The report was discussed at the April 1952 annual meeting, but no action was taken at the time. A little more than a week later, however, William Seymour submitted a lengthy memo to the board detailing suggested changes which might alleviate "general problems concerning the entire operation of the hospitals." Among his recommendations, Seymour proposed that the easiest way to restore order in MacDonald House was to fire Gilbert Vosburgh.

Opposition to this idea arose immediately from most of the medical center's department heads, and particularly from chief of medicine Joe Wearn, who had, in his capacity as dean, recruited Vosburgh in the first place. Two days later, under attack from the full-time staff and having won no support from the board of trustees, Seymour submitted his own resignation to board president John C. Virden. Without attempting to change Seymour's mind, Virden counseled him to hold his resignation until the MacDonald House controversy could be settled.

Seymour agreed to wait, and no mention of his pending resignation was made publicly or even, for that matter, in meetings of the board.

Unfortunately, an improbable comedy of errors involving the wounded egos of three different local newspaper reporters shortly resulted in the publication of a biting article in the Cleveland *Press* on the MacDonald House turmoil and Seymour's resignation. Three days later, an article in the Cleveland *News*—a piece printed even after Seymour had asked the *News'* publisher not to do so—quoted him as saying that he was indeed resigning, because he could no longer be "head of a hospital I am not running." In the same *News* article, Joe Wearn was quoted as saying that some members of the MacDonald House visiting staff had been "plotting to 'get Vosburgh.'"

Wearn and Seymour later attempted to limit the damage done by the articles by releasing a joint statement for publication in the *News*. They claimed that "statements had been made and attributed to them which had been confusing and misinterpreted." Neither man flatly denied the implication of the articles, however, and neither claimed to have been misquoted.

Three months later, Seymour did in fact officially resign as director of the hospitals, after which he reentered the Department of Medicine as an assistant clinical professor. The MacDonald House affair, however, had already tarnished the carefully polished image of University Hospitals. It was a remarkable development in the nearly century-long relationship between the hospitals and the city's newspapers, which, as recently as twenty-five years before, had served as the principal boosters of the citywide campaigns to raise funds to build the new medical center. Negative press had been a rarity in the era of Samuel Mather and the rest of the original saints, but that time was over. Suddenly, the hospitals' oldest allies were growing cold and distant, and no amount of persuasion could keep them from casting a critical eye on the inner workings of the institution.

The deeper meaning of the MacDonald House affair, however, had less to do with newspaper headlines than with the future of the hospitals themselves. It was, in its way, a milestone, because it marked the ultimate triumph of the ideal of academic medicine. Founded as havens for the poor and indigent, the hospitals had in time grown increasingly accommodating to more and more private patients, and had also begun to rely upon the revenues derived from them to help maintain operations. The attractive public image of the medical center as the city's preeminent health-care institution had brought first the upper class and then—as health insurance became ubiquitous—the middle class to its doors, and in the rush to make room for the new patients, a substantial portion of the hospitals' other missions had slowly been eroded.

Nowhere had the influx of paying patients been more dramatic than at MacDonald House, which had attained a certain cachet as *the* maternity hospital in the city. And when Joe Wearn began to reverse the process of "privatization" by filling departmental vacancies with research- and education-oriented physicians, uproar ensued. The basic functions of an academic medical center—all of which relied either directly or indirectly on a steady supply not of private but of staff patients—were again being brought to the fore. And because those functions were being emphasized so strongly within the hospitals, many private patients began to feel that insufficient attention was being paid to their needs—that their interests were being sacrificed on the altar of academic medicine.

A patient who could not be seen by his attending physician because that doctor was either leading a group of interns on rounds, teaching a class, or engaging in a time-consuming laboratory project might easily feel that he or she was being neglected. And a patient who could not even be admitted to the hospital because the number of private beds had been reduced to make room for more staff cases would, of course, turn elsewhere for care. It was the fundamental problem of all academic medical centers: how to balance the needs of all of the hospital's many constituents without alienating that segment of the population whose patronage provided a substantial portion of the hospital's operating funds each year.

At University Hospitals, the pendulum that had in recent years swung more toward the interests of private patients was now swinging back toward the ideal of academic medicine. And while the shift of direction again set the hospitals on the path toward many of its long-established goals, it also inevitably produced a multitude of new problems that would, eventually, have to be confronted.

§

As if to sweep away the memory of the unpleasant episodes at Mac-Donald House and the resignation of William Seymour, the search for a new director of administration for the medical center was conducted in record time. At the end of July 1952, the trustees offered the post to

Stanley A. Ferguson, who came highly recommended from similar positions at Cleveland's City Hospital and, before that, the University of Chicago. Seymour stayed on the job until October, however, and in the interim he faced a number of immediate crises.

Foremost among these was the deepening nursing shortage, and early in August the hospitals were forced to take a radical step. Desperate for qualified personnel, the board authorized the expenditure of roughly $45,000 a year to institute a scholarship program for nursing students. The program provided a full scholarship to the Bolton School of Nursing to any student who contracted to work in University Hospitals for one year upon graduation. Other inducements included free rooms in the nurses' dormitories for graduate nurses who wished to enroll in the school's "Advanced Professional" program, as well as free tuition to nurses enrolling in *any* courses—whether or not they were related to medicine—offered at Western Reserve.

At the same time, there was a sudden increase in the number of poliomyelitis cases reported in the city. The epidemic raised the possibility that City Hospital's pediatrics department—where most of Cleveland's acute polio cases were sent—would be swamped with patients and unable to carry the full load. If that were to occur, Babies and Childrens Hospital would be called upon to take in the overflow, and in that eventuality it would become necessary to halt the admission of virtually all elective cases. Thus, the children's hospital would be put in the position of limiting private admissions, the same stricture that had precipitated the still-unresolved MacDonald House uproar.

To make matters worse, the medical center's operating deficit for only the first seven months of the year had already reached the $300,000 level. Without the likes of a Sam Mather, who could and did routinely chip in whatever was necessary to balance the books at the end of the year, the board of trustees was forced to tap the principal of hospital discretionary endowment funds to cover deficits. But industrialist R. Livingston Ireland, chairman of the board's finance committee, expressed his growing horror at the apparently cavalier attitude adopted by the rest of the board toward these encroachments on the endowments. Ireland wrote to board president John Virden to warn that the trustees were "endangering the base upon which operation of the hospitals must stand."

Ireland pointed out, for example, that of the more than $1.8 million in discretionary funds contributed to the hospitals since 1940, all but $179,000 had been spent to cover operating deficits or to provide working capital. "In order to keep the institution solvent," Ireland told the full board, "it is necessary either to contract its present facilities and services to a level that can be supported with current endowment income, or additional endowment must be provided to support the present level of expenditures."

Just two months after this ominous warning, however, the hospitals again dipped into endowment principal in the amount of $400,000, bringing to $1.2 million the amount "advanced" from the endowment portfolio since 1948. Ireland again called attention to the consensus among members of the finance committee that some "quick action" should be taken to put the operations of the hospitals upon a balanced-budget basis. Each encroachment on the endowments, Ireland warned, constituted yet another step toward "the liquidation of the capital funds of the institution."

Calling the financial picture "shocking," Ireland chastised the board for not having taken steps to "effect such economies of operation as would stop further liquidation of the resources which generous benefactors have provided...." He concluded by saying that all members of the committee agreed that "it is imperative...that there be a full appreciation of the seriousness of what is going on, before it is too late."

Meanwhile, the MacDonald House controversy continued unabated. At one point the trustees even received a petition bearing the signatures of more than one hundred and fifty individuals—most of them private patients from MacDonald—which demanded a written clarification of the hospital's policy on private patients. "From what we have learned by the experience of ourselves and others it would be easy to conclude that the management no longer wishes to serve private patients," the petitioners wrote. "If you have come to that decision, then why not make a formal declaration, and we shall take our support elsewhere."

No amount of persuasion could change the minds of the private patients, whose anger had been stoked by the rumors spread by the visiting staff. And those same physicians had continued to treat Gilbert Vosburgh as a pariah, until the young head of obstetrics actually grew ill under the strain. Finally, in November, the visiting staff officially requested of Joe Wearn that Vosburgh be "relieved of his present position." Wearn refused, but by the penultimate day of 1952 Vosburgh himself had had enough. He tendered his resignation and announced that he would return to the department as only an associate obstetrician. In a statement released to the press, he indicated that his resignation was "the product of the unwillingness of part of the visiting staff to countenance" the "purpose for which a true university hospital exists"; namely, to "further knowledge by teaching and pursuing research."

Vosburgh's abdication of leadership in the department was both a relief to the visiting staff at MacDonald House and a blow to Joe Wearn and his handpicked group of department heads. But the primacy of academic medicine's place in the hospitals had already been firmly established in principle, and even Vosburgh's resignation could not change that. Wearn's vision of a renewed and revitalized academic medical center was becoming a reality. Patient care—particularly the care of private patients—would, of course, remain one of the three pillars of the hospitals' traditional mission. But no longer would private concerns subsume the overriding importance of the research and education programs that Little Joe was putting in place.

CHAPTER NINE

Sea Change

The first class of medical students to participate in Western Reserve's "New Curriculum" discovered a program of instruction far different from any that had come before. In the past, individual disciplines had always seemed to be separated by impregnable departmental walls, which severely limited cooperation and interaction between faculty members. But Joe Wearn tore down the walls of division using an ingenious stratagem: he took control of the curriculum away from individual department heads and put it into the hands of a committee consisting of the three hundred members of the general faculty.

Matriculating under the old curriculum had been a bit like being served a large bowl of stew but then being told to eat each ingredient in its entirety before consuming any of the others. No individual ingredient could complement or enhance any other, and the final effect was less of having eaten a satisfying meal than of having been force-fed representative elements of the basic food groups. The new curriculum, however, was integrated into a more logical and understandable sequence, so that related subjects could be taught together instead of being presented individually. The student was exposed to all aspects of medicine more quickly than before, and could see more clearly the relationships between what had formerly been presented as virtually discrete areas of knowledge.

Established practice had always dictated, for example, that the first year of study was devoted exclusively to the laboratory sciences and anatomy, the latter of which included dissection of cadavers. Under the new program, students were immediately introduced to the clinical side of medicine as well, each student being assigned to follow the progress of a pregnant mother, her baby, and the rest of her family over a four-year period. Students gained a greater appreciation for the wide range of medical problems encountered within a typical family and for the preventive aspects of health care. And students started their study of medicine by looking at life, rather than at death.

To accomplish these changes, Wearn created the Committee of the General Faculty on Medical Education and then recruited three dedicated men—Jack Caughey, T. Hale Ham, and Harland Wood—to push the process along. Caughey, from New York's Columbia Presbyterian Medical Center; Ham, from Harvard; and Wood, from the University of Minnesota, were of diverse backgrounds and temperaments, but each shared with Wearn (and with Douglas Bond, another important member of the team) a singular trait: they subscribed to the revolutionary notion that, in medical education, the welfare of the student should come first.

The curriculum experiment was funded in large part by grants from the Commonwealth Fund, a New York-based philanthropy created by Mrs. Stephen V. Harkness, an old friend of both the medical school and the original Lakeside Hospital. With such solid financial backing, Wearn was able to bring together all the talent he needed to revolutionize the educational program of the medical school. He did not, however, enjoy the same luxury when it came to filling vacant posts in the clinical departments of the hospitals. For those positions, he could call on only those resources that were normally available.

Nevertheless, by the beginning of 1953 he was able to secure two badly needed department chiefs for the medical center. Allan C. Barnes came from the Ohio State University College of Medicine to become the new director of obstetrics and gynecology, and Frank E. Nulsen left the University of Pennsylvania Medical School to assume the post of chief neurosurgeon. Both men were valuable additions to the staff, particularly Nulsen, who brought with him highly specialized expertise in his field. His 1949 innovation of the hydrocephalus shunt—a method by which to drain excess cerebrospinal fluid from around the brain—had become the first effective treatment of what was commonly known as "water on the brain," a condition in newborns that, previously, had been nearly always fatal. His arrival in Cleveland both expanded the capabilities and furthered the reputation of the Babies and Childrens Hospital.

Wearn's usual method of filling vacant posts on the faculty was to act as a one-man search committee, but in the appointments of both Barnes and Nulsen he did not work alone. After the near-mutiny that had arisen in the wake of Wearn's choice of Gilbert Vosburgh as head of MacDonald House, the boards of both University Hospitals and Western Reserve University decided to create an advisory committee to oversee just such decisions, with the hope that similar fiascos could be avoided in future.

A "Joint Executive Agency," consisting of the presidents of both the hospitals and the university (John C. Virden and John S. Millis, respectively), as well as the dean of the medical school (Wearn himself) and the hospitals' director of administration (Stanley Ferguson, who had already replaced the departing William Seymour), was created in December of 1952 to "facilitate decision making" when problems arose concerning "operation, personnel, expenditures and programs" within the hospitals and the university's schools of medicine, dentistry, and nursing. Thus, before appointments were offered to either Barnes or Nulsen, the JEA made a point of becoming, in Virden's words, "intimately involved" in the process.

The oversight committee's purview included making recommendations to the boards of trustees when "a change in basic policy in either or both [of the] institutions" was indicated. The agency was also designed to serve as a forum for airing internal grievances and as an arbiter of those grievances, to solve problems before they could spill out into the light of public scrutiny. And to preclude the sort of mix-up that had actually precipitated the biting newspaper articles about Seymour, Wearn, and Vosburgh in the spring of 1952 (a snafu in which two reporters were inadvertently promised exclusivity on the same otherwise innocuous story), the JEA even created a "voluntary code through which all three Cleveland newspapers would be treated equally in the release of publicity." Indeed, by that time Stanley Ferguson himself had already entered into "discussions...with representatives of the local newspapers to assure orderly and efficient methods of publicity."

By the April 1953 annual meeting of the hospitals' board, therefore, President Virden could cheerfully report to the rest of the trustees that the atmosphere within the institution seemed to be returning to normal and that, in the opinion of respected professionals from other cities, the medical center was "growing steadily in prestige and reputation...." Internally, however, Wearn and some other members of the senior staff still harbored doubts about the board itself, which had been the object of stern criticism from the Medical Council committee that had investigated the Vosburgh affair. The report had asked whether all of the trustees "fully comprehend their obligations to the hospitals," citing evidence that the board seemed to neither understand nor support the notion that, in an academic medical center such as theirs, the educational and research com-

ponents of its mission had to be maintained even at the price of occasionally inconveniencing private patients.

Virden used the annual meeting to acknowledge the criticisms of the
board and to offer assurances that in future the trustees would indeed be
more mindful of their responsibilities. He told his colleagues that they
had "come to a crossroads," and that each trustee should forget "the past
and any unpleasantness which may have occurred." They should, he said,
express their "full sympathy with the program and objectives" of the
medical center, and all "must give strong support to the development of
our hospital as an institution devoted to furnishing the best of medical
care, which can be accomplished only through medical education and research."

Virden's statement was a clear and strong endorsement of the ideal of
academic medicine, as well as a reversal of previous attitudes held by
many of the trustees. By saying that "the best of medical care" could be
furnished "*only* [italics added] through medical education and research,"
he was, in effect, bestowing formal recognition on the primacy of
academic medicine over private concerns. And he was also rallying his
colleagues on the board to embrace that position. By extension, Virden's
remarks were also an endorsement of Joe Wearn and the programs he
had initiated; indeed, the statement placed so much emphasis on the importance of education and research that an observer could be forgiven the
suspicion that Virden's remarks had been heavily influenced—if not actually scripted—by Wearn and his "boys." And if further proof were needed of Wearn's influence on the operations of the hospitals it would come
in the very next item on the agenda of the annual meeting: the report of
a Special Joint Committee of seven trustees from both the hospitals and
the university.

The committee had been formed to investigate the causes of the medical center's recurring deficits and to suggest ways to "restore the hospitals' operations to solvency." Its report cited many of the economic
hardships entailed in maintaining an academic medical center, revealing
that "medically indigent" staff patients, for example, cost the hospitals $9
a day over and above the reimbursement received for them from Cuyahoga County and the Welfare Federation; that the largely charitable Outpatient Department was itself losing about $200,000 each year; and that
Cleveland Hospital Service Association payments did not cover that part
of patients' bills attributed to the cost of teaching and research, which
amounted to some $75,000 annually. "On the basis of these facts," the

report concluded, "it would appear at first blush that the budget could be balanced by the simple device of reducing the number of days of patient care for staff patients and increasing the number of days of patient care for private patients...."

But such an expedient would not work, according to the committee report, because "the further reduction of staff facilities would so seriously handicap the teaching, clinical and research activities of the hospitals that the danger of losing members of the faculty of the medical school to other institutions would become more than a mere possibility. At the same time, such further reduction of staff facilities would imperil the standing of the hospitals for teaching interns, residents, nurses and medical students."

The hospitals had already seen a de facto reduction in staff beds that was due primarily to ongoing nursing shortages, with a drop of more than twenty-five percent since 1931. As a result, by the end of 1952 only half of the medical center's total number of beds were available for staff patients, a percentage that, as the committee report noted, placed University Hospitals "lower than any other comparable teaching institution" in the country—so low, in fact, as to be at "a rock-bottom level."

Rather than limiting the number of staff cases to reduce spending, the committee suggested, other remedies should be applied. Unfortunately, all but one of the committee's recommendations were either unreasonable in the extreme or virtually impossible to implement. Director of administration Ferguson, for example, was expected to "reduce the cost of operations" while either reducing the expenses or increasing the revenue of the Outpatient Department. (Just how Ferguson was to manage this bit of legerdemain was left unspecified.) Ferguson was also expected to "produce an enlarged supply of nursing personnel," as if he could single-handedly persuade more individuals to enter the profession. The board itself would try to negotiate a more favorable rate of reimbursement from Cuyahoga County, the Welfare Federation, and the CHSA, each of which had proved growingly recalcitrant in the recent past over precisely that subject.

Only one of the committee's recommendations was actually practicable, but it constituted a radical departure from the hospitals' previous standards. It was based on the committee's belief that "the advancement of medical education...and medical knowledge," not "care of the sick and injured," had become the medical center's principal function, and that the trustees themselves would "violate the trust placed in them by the many benefactors who have generously provided [the hospitals'] facilities and other resources unless its policies are designed to continue these lofty purposes." To that end, the committee recommended that "a careful study should be made of the feasibility, at least in certain categories, of utilizing private patients for teaching purposes."

Although the concept of using private patients as "teaching material" was not new (such programs were already in effect in a handful of medical centers in other cities), at University Hospitals it represented the most tangible manifestation of the new acceptance of the academic ideal. As the committee report emphasized, each of the medical center's individual hospitals may well have been established to achieve "charitable, scientific and educational" ends, but over time those priorities had been reordered. Now the hospitals' most important functions were educational and scientific, with actual clinical care of the poor or indigent as only the third of the three historic missions. And to further facilitate implementation of the teaching component, even private patients should be enlisted as teaching material.

While the trustees pondered the committee's suggestions, they also faced growing financial difficulties within the medical center. Expenses for the year 1952 had reached $6.5 million—$1 million more than in 1951 —much of which was due to the higher wages the hospitals were forced to pay unskilled personnel, to compete with private industry. The rate of inflation was also spiraling upward, as reflected in continuing increases in the costs of commodities and supplies.

As the 1952 year-end figures showed, the hospitals incurred an operating deficit of more than $400,000, fully four times that of the previous year. Nearly three-quarters of the deficit actually derived from the loss of potential revenue due to the closing of beds in various areas of the hospitals. And the bed closings were themselves a result of the shortage of nurses and other key personnel, many of whom had been called to active military duty in Korea. As in the past, the deficits could be covered only by invading the principal of four discretionary endowment funds.

The Babies and Childrens Hospital was one of the most crowded of the medical center's facilities during the year, due to a summer-long polio epidemic that saw more than two hundred and fifty patients admitted. (Another two hundred and thirty polio patients went to Rainbow Hospital as well.) Other areas of the medical center also experienced increased patient populations, but none was more overcrowded than MacDonald House. Although one floor of the maternity hospital was still closed due to the nursing shortage, nearly five thousand babies were delivered during 1952. To accommodate the flood of patients, postnatal maternal stays had in some cases been reduced to just three days, a recuperative period which at the time was considered barely adequate.

The shortage of general-duty nurses that precipitated the closing of beds throughout the medical center was not quite as extreme as in the previous year, with one hundred and eighty nurses on staff compared with less than one hundred and fifty in 1951. And sixty candidates were to enter the Bolton School of Nursing during 1953, fifty of them doing so with the aid of the scholarships offered by the hospitals in return for work upon graduation. Of course, the student nurses would not be available for duty until the completion of their schooling three years hence, which still left a considerable gap between the number of open nursing positions and the number of nurses on staff.

Another means of adding to the pool of available nurses was advanced in the spring of 1953, however, when it was proposed to discontinue the old in-house School of Nurse-Anesthesia, started more than thirty years before by Agatha Hodgins, George Crile's anesthetist. For some years the trend in medicine had seen doctors supplanting nurses as anesthetists and making the field their exclusive domain, much as physicians had virtually eliminated the midwifery movement at the turn of the century. At University Hospitals, a new Department of Physician-Anesthesia was already in the works, with a new director, Robert A. Hingson (developer of a needleless jet-inoculator), about to be named. The development of the new department would have the dual effect of consolidating physician dominance of the field and—theoretically, at least—freeing nurses for the general-duty work for which they were so desperately needed.

Ironically, just a few months after the termination of the nurse-anesthesia program the Korean conflict came to an end, and nurses on active duty in the military began to return to work in civilian hospitals. The nursing shortage continued to be a problem at University Hospitals, however, because the medical center was, quite simply, in the process of growing. The motivating factor for that growth was, of course, Joe Wearn, who in broadening the scope of the medical school and expanding its purview was, in effect, forcing the hospitals to enlarge their corresponding clinical facilities. As Stanley Ferguson noted to the trustees, the medical center was "now generally faced with the problem of expanding our services to keep up with the expansion of the medical school."

In the spring of 1954, for example, ground was broken for the Hanna

Memorial Building, which would be the home of the future Department of Psychiatry, itself a Wearn initiative, when it came into being. Indeed, the new building was considered so important that construction plans were being finalized even before the necessary funding had been confirmed. The Hanna family had already pledged $1.4 million for the project, and the United States Public Health Service was committed to contributing $260,000. But some $500,000 in federal funds that were supposed to be provided under the provisions of the Hill-Burton Act had been held back by the government, and there was some question as to whether they would ever be released. The possible loss of the federal monies, combined with the nearly $1 million in funds that the hospitals had already committed to obtain on its own, made the task of fund-raising doubly difficult.

That the medical center could be so heavily reliant on government-supplied funds was indicative of the ongoing changes in the hospitals' sources of income. Not only were they dependent on public and private insurers to cover much of the cost of operations, but now they had to rely on public monies for many capital expenses as well. Throughout the year 1953, in fact, the medical center received very few individual donations, and most of these were fairly small in size. The preponderance of money received was in the form of institutional grants for specific research projects, from such sources as the Department of the Navy (for a study on an artificial kidney) and the U.S. Public Health Service, as well as from such charitable entities as the Cleveland Area Heart Society and the Society for Crippled Children. Another major portion of incoming funds was provided by Baxter Laboratories, Upjohn Company, Pfizer Labs, and Wyeth Laboratories—all pharmaceutical concerns, and all underwriting clinical trials of new drugs.

Funds earmarked for specific uses, however, did nothing to alleviate the medical center's ongoing fiscal woes, which included not only annual operating deficits but also a seemingly insuperable problem of cash flow. In the spring of 1954, therefore, the hospitals again drew down large sums from the endowment principal, to cover a $110,000 deficit and to provide $130,000 of working capital. As was his custom, Finance Committee chairman R.L. Ireland took the opportunity to give his standard warning about the practice of tapping the endowments, this time calling the situation "perilous."

Despite the obvious danger inherent in the continuing raids on the hospitals' endowments, board president Virden painted an optimistic picture of the medical center's current status in his report to the trustees at the 1954 annual meeting. He made special mention of the fact that the long-running turmoil at MacDonald House had all but disappeared since Allan Barnes replaced Gilbert Vosburgh as chief of obstetrics, and that he himself had been "deluged with praise for the situation there, and particularly from those who were most severely critical on past conditions." There was, he said, a "completely new spirit" at MacDonald, especially among the visiting staff, whose complaints had essentially ended when the one closed floor of the facility was reopened and a quota of two hundred and thirty private-patient beds and one hundred and twenty staff beds was instituted.

Virden also pointed out that the demand for services in all of the medical center's facilities had "increased to an extent that is almost unbelievable." Indeed, despite the fact that all of the hospitals' beds that had been pulled out of service over the preceding few years were at last available again, many departments—and particularly the Department of Surgery—were reporting intense overcrowding.

Occupancy rates continued to rise unabated through the summer, thanks in large measure to the slowly growing strength of the nursing corps, which was gradually recovering from the privations of the Korean War years. The summer months also brought another citywide polio epidemic, and the spillover of indigent cases that could not be accommodated at City Hospital were sent to the Babies and Childrens Hospital. The treatment of more than forty of these patients was overseen by Dr. Hilda Case, director of physical medicine and rehabilitation, who was herself but one example of another revolution in the medical center, one that had been ongoing for decades, but most particularly since World War II.

Formerly an exclusively male preserve, the medical staffs of all hospitals had for some time been accepting more female physicians. Although still somewhat rare, female physicians were much more visible than in the earliest days of American medicine, when most medical schools barred women and when a female doctor was considered less an anomaly than a freak of nature. Beginning in the 1920s, in the wake of World War I, and growing throughout the subsequent decades, the progress of women in medicine had been slow but steady. At University Hospitals, for example, there were a dozen female physicians on staff by the early 1950s, a seemingly small number but large in relation to the number of female medical school graduates available at the time. The medical center had yet to appoint its first female surgeon, however, and, remarkably, there were no women physicians in the Department of Obstetrics and Gynecology.

Of course, University Hospitals owed its very existence in large measure to the efforts of Cleveland women. Rainbow Hospital had been founded by a group of women, and women had played key roles in the founding of the Maternity Hospital (which had been a barely viable facility until it was reorganized by another woman—Calvina MacDonald). Women had played important roles in the founding of the Babies and Childrens Hospital and all of its precursor institutions. And of course the Home for the Friendless, the immediate predecessor of Lakeside, was a facility founded and maintained almost exclusively by women.

Over the years Cleveland women had donated substantial sums to the hospitals, most notably the munificent gifts of Mary Severance and her granddaughter, Elisabeth Severance Prentiss. Flora Stone Mather had been a constant friend of Lakeside Hospital and its in-house nursing school, and Western Reserve University's School of Nursing owed its very existence to benefactress Frances Payne Bolton. Even into the second half of the twentieth century the tradition of personal involvement in the day-to-day operations and affairs of the hospitals was kept alive by many Cleveland women. The Friends of University Hospitals, for example, operated a Hospitality Shop and Snack Bar inside Lakeside, and the proceeds of their work—combined with that of the Baby Photo Service they initiated in MacDonald House—amounted each year to some $20,000 worth of donations to the medical center, in the form of equipment, furniture, and scholarships to nursing candidates. The Woman's Committee, descendant of Lakeside's old Board of Lady Managers, continued to raise funds for furnishings, equipment, landscaping, and holiday parties in the children's wards. And even the longstanding women's sewing groups, which in a previous era had made surgical dressings and bandages, were still functioning, although now they produced hand puppets, one of which was given to each child admitted to the hospitals.

§

The rising demand for hospital services in the mid-1950s was by no means a phenomenon limited to University Hospitals of Cleveland.

Across the country similar increases were seen at other academic medical centers, as well as at private and public hospitals of all sizes. Concurrent with the growth in demand, however, was the related phenomenon of rising costs. By the beginning of 1955 the cost of health care was a growing concern nationwide, and a national commission chaired by the president of the University of North Carolina was named to investigate the situation. But the commission's final report effectively ignored the most obvious influences on hospital costs: widespread new construction (with a subsequent rise in overhead costs), and the beginning of a nation-wide buying spree of newly developed equipment that was the product of rapid technological advances. Instead, the report cited only the general rate of inflation as the motivating factor behind escalating costs.

In light of the seemingly uncontrolled rate of growth in hospital costs, the medical center's $3,500 year-end deficit for 1954 was remarkably low. Director of administration Stanley Ferguson attributed the modest figure to the tidal wave of new patients—most of them private—that had broken over the hospitals during the year, producing a substantial rise in income. But "much of the service now being given is of a kind [that] was neither available nor possible a few years ago," Ferguson went on, warning that "illnesses of a more complex nature" were now being diagnosed and treated at the hospitals. Because treatment of more complex medical problems required more in the way of facilities, equipment, and personnel, future higher costs for all parties involved were, he believed, virtually inevitable.

One prominent example of the correlation between medical progress and higher costs could be found in the treatment of cancer, which had progressed phenomenally in just the preceding ten years. In the medical center's Institute of Pathology, requests for examinations of cells to identify malignancies had grown to such proportions that department chief Alan Moritz and his staff were performing some ten thousand tumor diagnoses each year. Paradoxically, it was medicine's own great triumphs over many previously uncontrollable diseases that had helped to prolong the lives of individuals, thus allowing them to reach the advanced age at which point many cancers began to occur. And many of the tumors that were revealed through biopsy could by that time be effectively treated, primarily with radiation therapy. Indeed, the demand for such treatment was so great that in 1954 the medical center installed a two-million-volt Van de Graeff generator, a four-ton radiation-therapy device costing some $80,000. Because of its great size and weight, the generator could only be housed in an underground structure, a room adjoining Lakeside that was built at substantial cost to the hospitals.

The new radiation machine was one of the weapons in the arsenal of the Department of Radiology, whose director, Hymer Friedell, had arrived at the medical center in 1946 after a stint with the Manhattan Project, which had developed the atomic bombs that were dropped on Hiroshima and Nagasaki to end the war in the Pacific. In fact, Friedell had been one of the first scientists to enter Hiroshima after the bombing, to study the effects of radiation on the surviving population of the city. In Cleveland, however, he used his expertise to oversee a more beneficial use of the atom. Friedell also advanced the use of radioisotope therapy; the first practical Strontium 90 applicator was designed and constructed at University Hospitals under his direction, and it quickly became the prototype of beta-ray applicators not only in the United States but in many parts of the world.*

The changing nature of health care was precisely the subject of an inquiry by the medical center's new Committee on Plans and Development, which was chaired by John Dingle. The committee attempted to chart the nature of the changes in medicine that had taken place over the preceding few years and to predict those future changes that would logically follow. Based on these studies, the committee's report, issued at the very end of 1954, delineated a rudimentary blueprint for physical change at the medical center, to accommodate the vastly expanded agenda of programs and objectives it recommended for both the hospitals and the medical school.

By the spring of 1955 the hospitals' board of trustees had not only accepted the conclusions of the report but had actually retained the architectural firm of Garfield, Harris, Robinson and Schafer—the same firm that had designed the Babies and Childrens Hospital and Mac-Donald House three decades before—to develop a preliminary master plan for eventual fulfillment of all the newly identified needs. Extensive remodeling of existing structures on the medical campus would have to be undertaken, and a host of new buildings would have to be constructed to house new services, if the report's recommendations were to be implemented. At the time, almost all of the hospitals' departments were

---

*Although the Van de Graeff generator was Friedell's responsibility, the machine was most often operated by the department's chief therapy technician, a woman with the unusually appropriate name of Elnora Glow.

already operating in cramped quarters, and some were dangerously over-loaded. As board president Virden later noted, the hospitals had been designed and built more than a quarter century before to provide service to a limited number of patients, yet they were now being called upon "to handle a much greater volume than they were ever expected to handle."

The Dingle committee's ambitious plans—which were, in effect, a guide for growth over the ensuing twenty-five years—were a response to the needs generated by the expanding medical school. But such growth would not come cheaply; as Virden noted, financing the implementation of the Dingle committee recommendations would require an enormous fund-raising effort, a campaign to rival the hugely successful ones of the 1920s that had built the medical center itself. By that time, the long-delayed $500,000 grant of Hill-Burton monies had finally been received, which eliminated for the moment any concern about completing the funding of the new psychiatry building. But as Virden acknowledged, "In an institution of this kind, the need for funds is always with us."

Even as the hospital trustees considered the recommendations of the Dingle committee, Joe Wearn continued to appoint new faculty members. The midsummer start of the academic year of 1955, for example, saw the addition of a new associate physician in the Division of Psychiatry. Benjamin Spock, author of *The Common Sense Book of Baby and Child Care*, became the most famous pediatrician never to practice in the Department of Pediatrics. Spock, whose 1946 book was the child-rearing bible for the new parents of the "baby boom" generation, worked on a revised version of *Baby and Child Care* while at the medical center. He also hosted a nationally broadcast television show about parenting that featured Cleveland families as guest subjects.

By the end of the year 1955, Joe Wearn, who was approaching age sixty-three, lightened his workload somewhat by stepping down as director of the Department of Medicine. Replaced by Robert Ebert of the University of Chicago, Wearn nevertheless retained his appointment as dean of the medical school, devoting most of his energies to teaching and to overseeing the progress of the school's new curriculum. The first class of students to experience all four years of the new curriculum were about to receive their degrees, and although some changes and fine-tuning of the program were ongoing, the overall response to the experiment was more than gratifying. The same school that only a few years before had been hard pressed to fill its class quotas was now turning away hundreds of applicants. And the success of the school produced a spillover effect for the hospitals: for the thirty-eight internships that were available in 1955, for example, the medical center received nearly four hundred and fifty applications.

The hospitals' finances received a welcome boost early in 1956 when the Cleveland Hospital Service Association raised the rate of reimbursement it paid for the care of private patients. At about the same time, Cuyahoga County increased its daily payment for indigent cases to $22.06 a day, more than double the rate of the preceding year. The large increases in reimbursement payments were a consequence of the rising national rate of inflation, which was fueled even further on March 1st by the federal government's newly mandated minimum wage of $1 an hour. Although the hospitals were not affected directly by changes in the minimum wage—health-care institutions and other nonprofit organizations were exempt from the rule at the time—they would still have to match the wages offered by private industry, to keep their service personnel from taking similar jobs elsewhere. Indeed, shortages of clerical staff and male attendants were an ongoing problem.

Other internal costs were growing as well. The annual nursing scholarship subsidies provided by the hospitals, for example, had to be raised by almost sixty percent to match the increase in tuition instituted at the school of nursing. (The trustees were only too happy to approve this extra expenditure, however, because of "the great benefit received by the hospitals from this subsidy plan.") In addition, the medical center's half of its employees' Social Security contributions, plus the hospitals' own pension plan for retirees, constituted a $160,000 annual expenditure that could only grow larger in future. And to forestall potential defections from the nursing corps, the starting salary of staff nurses was being raised from $250 to $270 a month.

Yet despite the forces of spiraling inflation, the hospitals actually ended the year 1955 with a small surplus. The April 1956 annual report showed that the medical center had averaged six hundred and twelve inpatients per day—another record—with nearly 115,000 visits to the Outpatient Department and more than 18,000 cases treated in the Emergency Room. With such a large and steady patient population providing the bulk of the hospitals' income, the medical center found itself in a situation that was virtually the reverse of the one that had obtained in its earliest years. Previously, almost all income had come from the gifts of individuals and from the fledgling endowment funds; now, only fifteen percent of annual income was being derived from the interest on endowments.

Unfortunately, cash flow was still so great a problem that the hospitals continued to invade endowment principal to obtain working capital, which was used not only to pay the bills of suppliers but also—in light of the Dingle committee recommendations for expansion—to purchase properties in the immediate vicinity of the medical center as they became available on the market. Thus, despite a five-year bull market that had run up substantially the value of those endowment funds invested in securities, Finance Committee chairman R. Livingston Ireland used the committee's annual report to deliver what by then had become his traditional yearly warning about "the situation under which the endowment funds are being constantly depleted...."

The rest of the board did not share Ireland's urgency about the state of the endowments, however, and even a change of officers at the end of the year did not alter attitudes. When John Virden resigned as president in December, his replacement, Charles B. Lansing—who was also chairman of the board of Western Reserve University—expressed neither concern over the endowments nor any plans to discontinue the policy that had begun during Virden's tenure. Of course, at the time there simply were no alternatives.

The tactical use of endowment principal as working capital was a source of potential trouble for the medical center, but other initiatives inspired by Virden had already proved invaluable. He had personally attempted to help rebuild morale throughout the medical center at the time of the Vosburgh flap, and he had tried to rebuild the deteriorating bond between the hospitals and the community. His success on both fronts was apparent when the hospitals went looking for private donors to contribute toward the renovation and remodeling of MacDonald House and the construction of the new psychiatry building, the Hanna Pavilion, which finally opened in April of 1956.

Indeed, the public relations aspect of Virden's presidency was one of his more meaningful contributions. The hospitals had been stung badly by the negative newspaper coverage of the MacDonald House affair, which they had felt much more keenly than another institution might have because they had been coddled for so many years by the local newspapers. During Virden's tenure the medical center created and staffed its own permanent office of public relations, which for the first time in the hospitals' history allowed the institution to disseminate news and information through a single official voice. Before long the public relations office was conducting open-house programs during which press representatives were led on guided tours through various functioning departments of the hospitals, a practice that produced a number of glowing newspaper articles about University Hospitals. To further polish their image in the community, the hospitals even produced a short informational film about the institution—*A Place for Healing*—which was made available to schools and civic groups.

Of course, some of the best publicity the medical center garnered came about as a direct result of the work going on there. The Babies and Childrens Hospital was a particular favorite of the press, especially after the creation of the new Cystic Fibrosis Center in 1957. The local branch of the Cystic Fibrosis Foundation presented the hospital with a $100,000 grant to create a treatment program for CF patients, who suffered from an uncontrollable buildup of thick mucus in the lungs and the digestive system that usually resulted in death by age four. Department chief William Wallace assigned a young pediatrician named Leroy Matthews to the center, and Matthews devised a new treatment protocol that included mist tents to ease patients' breathing and postural drainage, a therapy of thumping the back and chest to loosen heavy mucus. Matthews' techniques dramatically lowered the death rate of patients and made the Cystic Fibrosis Center one of the best-known clinics in the country. In fact, Matthews' program was so highly regarded that the first national Cystic Fibrosis Research and Teaching Center Conference ever assembled was held in Cleveland.

The Cystic Fibrosis Center was just one of the programs that were changing the public's perception of the Babies and Childrens Hospital. As Stanley Ferguson noted at the 1957 annual meeting, the childrens' hospital was the first of the medical center's component institutions to be recognized and used as a tertiary-care facility, with a large percentage of patients coming for specialized care either through the referrals of outside physicians or as transfers from other hospitals. (Of some two hundred infants admitted to the hospital's premature suite in 1956, for example, forty-eight were transfers from primary-care facilities.) And a similar trend was beginning to be seen at the other hospitals within the group, all of which constituted a form of dividend from the massive investment the medical center had made in the ideal of academic medicine.

Ironically, the medical center's heady reputation had a deleterious effect on the teaching component of the institution's mission. As director of surgery William Holden noted, the vast majority of referral cases coming to the hospitals were patients whose hospitalization costs were covered by private insurance. And as more private patients entered the hospital, the ward services—what Holden called "the very heart of physician education"—were being threatened as never before. Holden told the board of trustees that "efforts...of a vigorous and visionary nature" would be required if the hospitals were to assure the necessary number of staff cases needed to maintain uninterrupted clinical training of young physicians.

The Pediatrics Department had, on its own, already addressed the problem of "teaching material," albeit in a quiet and seemingly innocent way. Director William Wallace had simply reorganized the floor assignments of the Babies and Childrens Hospital, which had previously been the means of segregating private from staff patients. Under the new program, all patients, no matter what their economic status, were segregated by age: school-age and early adolescent patients on the third floor, children up to the age of two years on the fourth floor, and preschoolers on the fifth floor. The new system made nursing and recreational programs more efficient, but it also meant that the typical medical student or intern had, in Wallace's words, "increasing contact with children from all socio-economic levels and, therefore, a broader view of his coming responsibilities." In effect, Wallace had turned all of the children in the hospital into teaching material.

One residual effect of the realignment of Babies and Childrens was a noticeable improvement in the efficiency of the hospital, an important byproduct since demand for bed space continued to grow. At the same time, however, the city's other health-care provider for children—Rainbow Hospital—found itself with a rapidly *decreasing* patient population. The problem at Rainbow was the same as that which some years before had made anachronisms of the area's old tuberculosis sanitariums and "fresh air" camps: quite simply, medicine itself had made most of the hospital's functions irrelevant.

A joint committee of members of the medical school faculty and the hospitals' Medical Council had already investigated the situation at Rainbow, and by the summer of 1957 the committee's report was made available. The study found that the emergence of "preventive and specific therapies of many childhood diseases formerly requiring long-term convalescence" had effectively eliminated the bulk of Rainbow's potential patient base. Rickets, osteomyelitis, rheumatic heart disease, and tuberculosis could all be either prevented or treated with relative ease, and these were the types of cases for which Rainbow had been designed. Even polio, which in the preceding few years had raged across the country with particular vehemence, was now on the verge of being controlled, thanks to the newly available "killed-virus" vaccine developed by Jonas Salk.

At the same time, the general prosperity of the region had improved the home environments of the socioeconomic groups whose children were most affected by disease, effectively eliminating the need for a separate facility that provided extended convalescence away from home. Modern nutritional concepts, antibiotics, potent immunizations, anesthesia, blood transfusion, and improved surgical techniques—all had combined to sharply reduce the number of children requiring the type of care that Rainbow had traditionally provided. "As a consequence of these changes," the report noted, "the utilization of Rainbow's facilities has diminished despite growth of the local population."

The most recent patient census at Rainbow had revealed that the hospital was filling on average only about forty of its one hundred beds each day. Most cases were now orthopedic problems, and the majority of these patients were under the "management" of private orthopedic surgeons. The medical center's interns, residents, and house physicians, therefore, oversaw the care of only a handful of staff cases, which, as the committee report noted, left "teaching and research at a low ebb" and "no uniform program of patient care."

There was, nonetheless, a very real need for short-term treatment for crippling conditions such as congenital orthopedic deformities, cerebral palsy, and osteochondrosis of the spine and the hip, as well as for disabilities resulting from accident or injury. And for some complex problems requiring the attention of specially trained physicians, nurses, and physiotherapists, long-term hospitalization was still the best means of providing treatment. "It is only within the confines of a medical center," the report concluded, "that the great majority of these patients can be safely treated and cared for."

The committee report acknowledged that there was indeed a place for Rainbow Hospital among the member institutions of University Hospitals, but that to survive, Rainbow would have to integrate services "for both inpatients and outpatients." Ambulatory cases that could convalesce at home or receive rehabilitation treatment on an outpatient basis should become substantial elements in Rainbow's patient population, because advances in medical science had rendered the hospital's old program untenable.

But to change that program while the hospital remained at its old location would require construction of expensive new facilities and the addition of new professional staff, the report noted. If, however, the old hospital buildings on Green Road were to be closed and the property sold off, a new building—erected adjacent to Babies and Childrens Hospital—could provide complete care for all patients at substantially less cost, care that could include all the services offered in the existing facilities of the medical center.

The committee's recommendation to build a new Rainbow in the middle of the medical center's campus was both logical and economical, but such a drastic move required ample study before it could be implemented. The Rainbow trustees in particular had to consider whether they wanted to cede control of the institution to the University Hospitals board. Meanwhile, however, other capital improvements at the medical center were already in progress. The renovation of MacDonald House was completed during the year, which allowed the maternity hospital to increase the size of its monthly quotas of private and staff patients. The new guidelines allowed for two hundred and fifty private cases and one hundred and thirty staff patients, which, director of obstetrics Allan Barnes observed, came close to balancing supply with demand.

Actually, the hiring of additional nurses in MacDonald House had been just as important as the building's renovation in expanding the monthly quotas. Even with the subsidies and scholarships the hospitals provided to ensure a steady supply of registered nurses, the medical center faced constant shortages of trained personnel. Indeed, an entire division within Lakeside had been closed for some time due to the lack of available nursing personnel. The division was reopened only after being staffed with Licensed Practical Nurses, in what the hospital administration called "an experiment" for patients requiring only "minor care."

Because registered nurses were in such high demand across the country, the medical center was forced to continually reappraise its salary rates to remain competitive with other hospitals. Starting salaries for general-duty nurses were raised from $270 to $295 per month in 1957, for example, yet by early 1958 it was apparent to Stanley Ferguson that another increase would soon be necessary, "to meet national competition." The pay of maintenance and service personnel would also have to be increased by an average of more than $4 a week, because high demand by private industry was draining the labor pool.

Despite continually increasing expenses, however, the medical center was able to record a $100,000 surplus for the year 1957, a phenomenal turnaround from earlier in the decade. The main reason for the surprising excess was that room rates had again been raised, and a corresponding increase in payments had been won from the Cleveland Hospital Service Association, which a few months before had merged with the Akron Hospital Association to broaden its subscriber base under the new organizational name "Blue Cross of Northeastern Ohio."

The hospitals' own solid financial foundation did nothing, however, to alleviate what seemed to have become the chronic problem of cash flow. The annual cost of operating the medical center had by then reached $9 million, but the amount of cash on hand at any given moment was pitifully small. The resulting cash squeeze left many of the hospitals' suppliers holding unpaid bills for as long as five months. It was still necessary, therefore, to draw cash advances from the principal of the endowment funds, although the hospitals had begun to charge themselves interest on these "loans." At the time, however, a total of more than $800,000 had been drained from the funds for operations, plus another $350,000 for building and equipment replacement. And in the upcoming fiscal year, Ferguson projected the need of at least $85,000 more.

Even that figure soon proved optimistic, however, because by the end of 1958 a nationwide recession had significantly raised the number of unemployed in Cleveland. During the year a large number of patients found themselves unable to pay their hospital bills, and many more had become true medical indigents after losing their jobs and, consequently, their insurance. The only positive aspect of the economic slowdown for the medical center was the sudden availability of a large pool of workers. For the first time in almost two decades, Stanley Ferguson could report to the board that almost all of the hospitals' service and maintenance positions were filled. Additional registered nurses had also become available, so that by the end of the year the medical center had a higher number of full-time nurses on staff than at any time since before the start of World War II.

Despite the economic downturn, all of the medical center's component hospitals found that their biggest problem was overcrowding. Director of surgery William Holden begged for an additional surgical suite because the existing facilities simply could not keep up with demand, especially since open-heart surgery had become a regularly scheduled procedure. And Robert Ebert's Department of Medicine was desperate for more private beds, because the department was dangerously close to losing many of the outside physicians—the "part-timers"—who taught in the medical school in return for admitting privileges to the hospitals. Without open beds for their patients, the part-timers found that admitting privileges were, in fact, pointless. And if the part-timers left, then the staff physicians would have to pick up the outsiders' share of teaching responsibilities in addition to their own, which would leave them no time to actually see patients.

The most heavily crowded of the medical center's clinical services was the Department of Pediatrics, which continued to set new admissions records every year. By 1959, however, director William Wallace was openly expressing his frustration at working in a building that was "constructed at a time when the chief resource of the physician was to remove the sick child from the view of the community and observe the natural history of his disease." New and effective methods of intervention —such as the types of operations performed by Robert J. Izant, who in 1958 had returned to his alma mater from Boston's Childrens Medical Center to become the first practitioner in northern Ohio to specialize in pediatric surgery—might seem "miraculous" to the physician of even twenty years before, said Wallace. But it was growing increasingly difficult to utilize such methods "in a building as archaic as Babies and Childrens."

The only department in the entire medical group not recording excessive overcrowding was obstetrics, which for the first time since the end of the war saw a slight decline in the number of births at MacDonald House. Director Allan Barnes insisted, however, that the maternity hospital could not stand pat but would also require expanded facilities. Another baby boom was coming, he said, an explosion of births engendered by the original boomers who would, he was certain, start having children of their own at the same rate as their parents, beginning in the late 1960s.

By the end of 1959, formal plans for expansion of the medical center were well underway. All of the new additions, as well as the changes to be made within existing structures, were responses to the recommendations contained in the 1954 Dingle Committee report, which had delineated the full degree to which growth of the medical center's facilities had failed to match the growth of its clinical services over the preceding twenty years. Many of the trustees had been surprised to learn, for example, that even some of the hospitals' most basic elements had for some time been woefully inadequate. As the committee had noted, there was far too little space for the efficient storage of medical records; many receiving docks were too small to handle deliveries from modern trucks; and even the capacity of the lines supplying water to the hospitals was inadequate. Before the first new building could be started, therefore, it would be necessary to spend some $9 million just on internal improvements.

To get a firm idea of exactly how much money would be needed for the entire building program, a committee of trustees from University Hospitals and Western Reserve recommended the creation of a Joint Committee for Development. The new committee was charged with determining the monetary needs of the medical center for both new construction and additions to the endowment funds. A second entity, the University Medical Center Development Committee, whose honorary chairman was George Humphrey, took the place of Robert Bishop's old Joint Committee for the Advancement of Medical Education and Research, to bring the fund-raising case to the public.

Early in 1960, the Joint Committee for Development concluded its study by projecting a cost of $28 million for the entire expansion program. By that time, however, the hospitals already enjoyed a solid foundation upon which to base their capital-funds drive. The Leonard C. Hanna, Jr., Fund had just provided a $10 million gift, $4 million of which was designated for improvements and new buildings, with the remaining $6 million earmarked for use as supporting endowment.*

Among the many new facilities tentatively slated to be built on the medical campus was a $2 million building to be used exclusively for ambulatory patients. So large an expenditure for what amounted to an outpatient department on a grand scale was entirely justified, however, because ambulatory patients had, in fact, become vital to the teaching

---

*Curiously, at the same time as the multimillion dollar gift of the Hanna Fund, the medical center also saw an upswing in the number of in-kind contributions it received from individual donors. In the days of the original Lakeside, such gifts had typically consisted of bandages, bed linens, clothing, and foodstuffs. By the beginning of the 1960s, however, they were more likely to be either magazine subscriptions or television sets for the youngsters in the Babies and Childrens Hospital.

component of the hospitals. Joe Wearn, who had been replaced by Douglas Bond as dean of the medical school the year before and had taken up the job of vice president for medical affairs at the university, explained the situation at the hospitals' April 1960 annual meeting.

As a class, said Wearn, young adults were simply disappearing from the hospitals' inpatient populations. As a result, medical students and interns were now "seldom able to observe many illnesses which were common twenty-five years ago." When younger patients did come to the hospitals, they came, for the most part, as ambulatory cases. (Indeed, the number of ambulatory patients at that point was greater than at any time in the medical center's history.) But the net effect of the changes, said Wearn, was that the hospitals' inpatient populations were aging rapidly. "Twenty-five years ago the average age of ward patients was thirty-seven," he explained. "Five years ago it was fifty-seven, and now it is sixty and going up."

These figures were confirmed by Stanley Ferguson, who had found that the average inpatient in 1959 stayed in hospital two and a half days longer than his counterpart in 1949. "We believe this change is primarily attributable to the increasing age of the patients admitted for care," said Ferguson, who noted that such a trend was national in scope. "As the number of oldsters in our population increases, they will need increasing amounts of hospital service, and their average length of stay will be higher than for younger segments of the population."

The wholesale demographic shift in the medical center's patient population was occurring because of fundamental changes in the effectiveness of medicine itself. Before World War II, the object of medical care had for the most part been to allow an individual to reach the ripe old age of forty without first succumbing to or being completely disabled by disease or injury. After the war, the products of clinical pharmacology (antibiotics, corticosteroids, antihypertensive agents, and even tranquilizers), as well as new and more effective surgical techniques (cardiac catheterization for diagnosis, open- and closed-cardiac surgery), had all become readily available and fairly routine. And at that point, medicine became able to virtually guarantee that an individual could not only achieve age forty, but that such a milestone would constitute merely *middle age*.

Having succeeded in eliminating many of the "old" killers, however, medicine had inadvertently prepared the ground for a crop of such "new" diseases as heart disease and cancer, both of which tend to appear later in life. And because treatments for these "new" ailments were more complex and time-consuming, not only the average age but the average length-of-stay of hospital patients was tending to rise. Most younger individuals with less serious ailments were treated on an outpatient basis, which made it essential that a teaching institution like University Hospitals make room for more ambulatory patients if it were to maintain an adequate educational program.

One other negative side effect of medical progress was also becoming apparent, at least to director of medicine Robert Ebert. As new areas of interest were explored and as narrow areas of expertise developed within the profession, many physicians were beginning to specialize, limiting their practices to specific fields. Now, said Ebert, there was simply too much information for any individual physician to absorb. Thus, the full-time members of his own department, who were traditionally expected to be "equally expert in the areas of teaching, research and patient care," were of late finding that such a goal was "fast becoming an impossible task...."

But clinical considerations would prove to be of secondary importance to the medical center during the year 1960, which was an inauspicious time to be considering a fund-raising effort for a program of expansion. The curse that had plagued the hospitals since the earliest days of the original Lakeside—each announcement of a plan to enlarge facilities had been followed immediately by a nationwide economic downturn— seemed still to be in effect. The stock market plunged precipitously early in the year, and a full-blown recession ensued. It was a particularly disheartening turn of events, because the medical center was beginning to operate regularly at a surplus, and the future looked more stable than it had for years. Even R. Livingston Ireland, the Jeremiah of the Finance Committee, gave an optimistic report at the hospitals' annual meeting in April, venturing the possibility that "within a few years some of the [$1 million-plus thus far] advanced for working capital may be returned for investment."

Ireland's hopeful premise would, however, be revised during the year. In 1958, the Cuyahoga County Board of Commissioners had taken over responsibility for the operations of City Hospital, which was then renamed Metropolitan General. After studying health-care costs around the city, the county found that treatment costs for indigent patients in private hospitals were higher than those at Metro, so in 1960 the Board of Commissioners unilaterally cut a substantial portion of the usual reimbursement payments it had been making to University Hospitals, St.

Vincent's, St. Luke's, and Mt. Sinai. This left the four private institutions seeing the same number of indigent patients as before but being reimbursed for only a fraction of their costs. As their deficits began to mount during the year, the four hospitals filed suit to stop the county's cutbacks and reinstate the former rates of reimbursement. The case dragged on into 1961 without resolution, and in March of that year, St. Vincent's actually began to turn away patients.

The extent of the county's reimbursement cuts was painfully obvious at the medical center, which recorded a year-end operating deficit of $150,000. Director of administration Stanley Ferguson noted in his April 1961 annual report that there had been a daily average of six hundred and seventy-seven patients in the hospitals during the year (another record high), with some 168,000 visits to the medical center's ambulatory clinics. Only Rainbow Hospital showed a decreasing number of patients, but formal action on the idea of integrating a new Rainbow facility into the University Circle medical campus had yet to be taken.

The major issue addressed at the hospitals' annual meeting was the year's huge operating deficit, which was a direct result of the county's cutbacks. Ferguson reminded the trustees that although the hospitals had been founded "for the purpose of giving aid to the sick, friendless and poor, the failure of local government to continue financial responsibility for some of these people" constituted a serious threat to that "basic purpose." The county's actions were doubly harmful, said Ferguson, because not only was the medical center's "ability to give care" affected, but the abdication of local responsibility could "only hasten the development of programs at the federal level to fill these needs."

The old bugaboo of federal involvement in the processes of health care was a notion still abhorrent to most members of the medical center's board. And despite the fact that the hospitals were already heavily dependent on public money in the form of reimbursement payments from county government (so dependent, in fact, that they would go to court to ensure the continued availability of such monies), the fear of federal intrusion was a longstanding and overriding concern.

Within just a few years, however, Ferguson and the rest of the medical center community would find themselves in the awkward position of actually welcoming the advent of federal health-insurance programs. With their heavy unilateral cutbacks in reimbursement payments, the county commissioners managed to accomplish the impossible: they made federal intrusion look good in comparison.

§

Even as the year's operating deficit continued to mount, however, progress was being made on the capital improvements so long under consideration by the medical center. A formal decision was made to follow the Medical Council committee's 1957 recommendation to build a new Rainbow Hospital adjacent to the existing facilities of the Babies and Childrens Hospital. Then, in midsummer, the medical center received a $500,000 gift from the Leonard C. Hanna, Jr., Fund, the money to be put toward the cost of constructing the new Rainbow. The same fund also provided $1 million for the expansion of Hanna House, as well as $500,000 for use by the medical school.

The Hanna gifts were welcome additions to the medical center's fledgling capital fund, which was soon to be tapped for the first project of the building program. A research-laboratory structure to be owned jointly by the hospitals and the medical school was to be erected contiguous to Lakeside along its eastern wall. The research building would cost some $5.2 million, but the medical center already had $1.2 million of the total in the form of a grant from the U.S. Public Health Service, as well as another $40,000 that had come in the form of a gift from Cleveland's Republic Steel Corporation. The new structure would house laboratories for the departments of medicine, surgery, radiology, and preventive medicine, and would be named for the man most responsible for the explosive growth of research at the hospitals over the preceding decade: Joseph Treloar Wearn.

As the hospitals expanded to fill the needs of a new age in medicine, however, they were also forced to meet the demands of a new age engendered by another profession. Previously, the medical center had not needed to carry large and expensive institutional malpractice insurance policies because Ohio law had always provided eleemosynary institutions with immunity from liability for the negligence of their employees. In 1956, however, the Ohio Supreme Court ruled in favor of the plaintiff in a malpractice suit against one of the state's charitable hospitals, a ruling that effectively eliminated the longstanding doctrine of immunity. With no limit on the dollar amount of potential judgments against them, hospitals around the state immediately began to purchase more insurance. The medical center held back for as long as it could, but in 1959, a lawsuit filed by a patient whose plastic-surgery procedure had failed raised the specter of a possible $1 million judgment against University Hospitals. Although the case was eventually settled out of court for a much smaller sum, the hospitals were sufficiently shaken by the episode to increase their malpractice coverage from $600,000 to $5 million.

The fear of potentially disastrous lawsuits was, in fact, one of the subjects that concerned the hospitals' Medical Council as it once again took up the question of the paucity of inpatient "teaching material" in the medical center. The council's Committee on Staff Services, under the chairmanship of Douglas Bond, issued a report in the summer of 1961 that suggested the only way to ensure an adequate number of teaching cases was to rework the definition of the "staff patient." Patients should be accepted to the staff services "if they so choose," said the committee, and an individual's economic situation "would not be used as a criterion for exclusion."

If paying patients were now to be used as teaching material, however, some alterations in the usual operations of the hospitals would have to be initiated. "Changes will be necessary," noted the committee report, "to remove some of the impersonal methods which have resulted from the care of large numbers of patients on a mass basis." The hospitals should upgrade their "emotional and physical atmosphere," and staff physicians would have to be particularly forthcoming in their "relationships with physicians outside University Hospitals." In other words, if some paying patients were to be categorized as staff cases, they would have to be treated with virtually the same consideration then being afforded to private patients.

The committee recommended that the old medical and surgical wards be replaced with "one- and two-bed rooms, with a four-bed unit for intensive care and constant monitoring of acutely ill patients...." And since the new ambulatory-care building would "provide care for both private and staff ambulatory patients," its outpatient clinics should be made more attractive, with decentralized waiting areas and special ancillary services—like X-rays, clinical labs, and physiotherapy—readily available.

Each ambulatory patient would be assigned to a specific member of the senior teaching staff, not unlike the arrangement of attending physicians for inpatients. This would ensure continuity of care and what was called "personalized service," a term more often found in the advertisements of luxury hotels than in descriptions of hospital facilities. And because many of the newly designated "staff patients" would not be true indigents, they would be charged professional fees, just as if the staff doctor attending their case were a private physician. These charges would be accumulated by the hospitals and put into a fund for the support of resident training programs.

At that point, of course, the hospitals were searching rather desperately for any new source of income. By the fall of 1961 it was apparent that the county's severe reimbursement cutbacks were wreaking havoc with the medical center's budget. A projected deficit of more than $175,000 for the year loomed on the horizon, and suppliers' bills once again went unpaid for months at a time. In October the hospitals took another "advance" from the endowments, some $200,000 to use as operating funds. That brought the total of monies advanced over the years to $1.35 million.

Then, early in 1962, the fiscal crisis was exacerbated by the Welfare Federation's announcement that it could no longer continue to increase the amount of its own indigent-care payments to the city's hospitals. Just three years before, payments from the federation and the county had together covered sixty-two percent of the costs of indigent care incurred by the medical center. By the end of 1961, the two entities covered only forty percent of such costs, and that figure now promised to go lower.

It was not surprising, then, that the operating deficit for the year actually exceeded projections, coming in at nearly $200,000. As Stanley Ferguson explained at the April 1962 annual meeting, indigent-patient visits to the ambulatory clinics and the emergency room reached new highs during the year, which had only increased the disparity between the cost of services rendered and the amount of reimbursement received for those services. Within the medical center as a whole there had been a slight drop in the number of days of care provided to paying patients, which also added to the deficit.

One of the reasons for the lower number of inpatients was the slowing local birth rate, which further decreased demand at MacDonald House. "This situation undoubtedly will continue until the predicted rise in birth rate occurs in the late 1960s," said Ferguson, whose comments reflected the belief of not only obstetrics chief Allan Barnes, but most other observers at the hospitals. Ferguson, Barnes and the others all blindly accepted the notion that the generation then coming of age would behave in precisely the same manner as had their parents—marrying at the earliest opportunity and then producing children in record-breaking numbers.*

---

*Just two days before the medical center's annual meeting, an astute observer might have

But the most important business of the 1962 annual meeting was a review of the final report of the University Medical Center Joint Trustee Committee (a slightly expanded successor version of the old Joint Committee for Development). Based on the recommendations for growth first delineated in the by-then eight-year-old Dingle Committee report, the Joint Committee proposed that a $54.8 million fund-raising campaign be undertaken. Of the total to be raised, $10 million would go into endowment funds, while the remainder would pay for the expansion of University Hospitals, Rainbow Hospital, and the Schools of Medicine, Nursing, and Dentistry of Western Reserve University.

Some $4 million would be allocated for new construction at the School of Dentistry. Another $1.5 million would underwrite an additional facility at the Frances Payne Bolton School of Nursing, designed "to eventually accommodate a one hundred percent increase in enrollment." The School of Medicine would receive $14.5 million for new laboratories and a health-science library, as well as for major renovations of the school's main building and the Institute of Pathology.

The rest of the funds—some $24.8 million—would be earmarked for the hospitals. In addition to the planned research and ambulatory buildings and the expansion of Hanna House, Lakeside itself would receive a badly needed $4.5 million renovation and modernization. And the Babies and Childrens Hospital would be remodeled and adapted to incorporate the new facilities for Rainbow, creating, in the committee's words, "a complete child-care center."

The hospitals would attempt to raise a total of $8 million from local and national corporations, $16.5 million from local and national foundations, and $11 million from government grants. The rest was expected to come from individuals, faculty members, alumni, trustees, and a community-wide small-gift appeal, which was to begin immediately and which would continue for more than two years.

The medical center's design for expansion was nothing if not ambitious, but the most important aspect of the program may well have been the planned $10 million addition to the endowment funds. Just two

---

deduced how wrongheaded that belief would prove. Benjamin Spock, whose book on infant care so heavily influenced the child-rearing strategies of the baby boom parents, spent the day leading a "Ban the Bomb" march in downtown Cleveland for the Committee for a Sane Nuclear Policy, of which he was a member. It was only a matter of extrapolation to guess that Spock's "children" might eventually follow the trail he blazed and diverge substantially from the path their parents had followed.

weeks after the announcement of the capital drive, the county commissioners deliberately began to delay making payments of those funds that were still available for reimbursement of indigent care at the hospitals. Coming on top of the county's previous cutbacks, the new delays only heightened the fiscal woes of the medical center, which was projecting a $300,000 operating deficit for the year. Yet another raid on the endowments was, therefore, inevitable, and in May some $200,000 was advanced for working capital.

By then the total amount "advanced" from the endowment funds had reached $1.75 million, a figure so large that R. Livingston Ireland decided to try a new tack in his continuing warnings to the rest of the board of trustees. Ireland pointed out that despite two decades of virtually uninterrupted growth in the value of the stocks in which the medical center's endowments were invested, and despite ongoing additions to the funds over those years, the net amount of money available for "income production" was actually $1.2 million *less* than it had been twenty-two years before. And because of this depletion, the hospitals were annually losing some $50,000 in investment income.

Not long after Ireland's dire warning, the Welfare Federation announced that it was planning to phase out all support for hospitals over the next few years, "on the theory that this activity [is] properly a government responsibility." Those private hospitals in Cleveland that had relied on such support to help defray the costs of indigent care now found themselves in the peculiar position of being told by the Welfare Federation to turn to local government, while at the same time being told by local government to turn elsewhere.

Fortunately, the Blue Cross insurance system continued to provide a major portion of the hospitals' income each year. Yet even that source was faced with growing problems, all of which were directly attributable to the continuously rising cost of health care. Indeed, the merger of the Cleveland and Akron hospital associations that formed the Blue Cross entity in 1957 had itself come about because of higher costs; each group was running dangerously low on reserve funding, and both thought they could strengthen their finances only by pooling resources.

The extent of growth in the cost of hospitalization was, in fact, nothing short of remarkable. In 1934, for example, the then newly created Cleveland Hospital Service Association had been asked to cover the expenses of just seven subscribers who were inpatients at University Hospitals. The average daily payment made to the hospitals then had been just $4.50, and the total for the year had been exactly $486.50. In 1961, there were more than *thirteen thousand* Blue Cross inpatients at the medical center, at a daily cost of $42.68, for a total of nearly $6.25 million in payments. Over the decade of the 1950s, the minimum per diem Blue Cross payment to University Hospitals doubled, while total annual payments during the same period nearly tripled. And since the end of World War II, the rates that Blue Cross charged its subscribers had consequently risen by well over three hundred percent.

As costs continued to rise, however, public reimbursement rates continued to fall. In the spring of 1963 the State of Ohio instituted cutbacks on its own relief funding for indigents, raising the possibility that the medical center would lose an additional $70,000 a year over and above the nearly $300,000 already cut by Cuyahoga County. The hospitals incurred a $367,000 operating deficit in 1962, and all signs pointed toward increasing losses down the road as well. "The trend toward more tests and treatments continues to rise, all of which requires more time of people, more equipment and more supplies," said Stanley Ferguson. "This will mean, in turn, that the cost of care in a hospital such as ours will continue to rise at about the same rate as in the past."

Indeed, even as Ferguson was outlining the problem, work was proceeding on a previously unbudgeted $210,000 Surgical Intensive Care Unit that was being installed on the otherwise vacant sixth floor of the recently opened Wearn Building. And the new building itself, which was originally estimated to cost $4.8 million, had been completed at an actual total cost of more than $5.5 million. It was a small miracle of sorts that in May the medical center required only $250,000 of endowment funds for working capital, but even that relatively modest sum brought to $2 million the total amount advanced from the endowments.

Ultimately, the operating deficit for the year would reach $625,000, and by the time of the April 1964 annual meeting, even the usually unflappable Stanley Ferguson was expressing his consternation at the need to take another large advance. "As a voluntary hospital we [traditionally] provided care to the indigent through the benefaction of individuals of large resources," he said, but over time, "society...somewhat altered this course." For more than thirty years, Ferguson explained, local and state government had been assuming a growing proportion of responsibility for care of the medically indigent, and the hospitals had grown to depend on these subsidies. Of late, however, the medical center was confronted with a situation "in which local and state governments claim they have exhausted their resources." And as a consequence, the hospitals were now cautiously embracing a new idea, one that—in less dire times—would have been considered sheer anathema.

The "new idea" was also the hottest topic at hospitals around the country at the time: the proposal then before Congress to enact a nation-wide system of medical insurance for the aged and the indigent. Part of President Lyndon B. Johnson's "Great Society" package of social benefits, a federally funded medical insurance program was about to become law, just as Robert Bishop had predicted back in 1943. Medicare, which pro-vided coverage for those over age sixty-five, would be administered through the Social Security Administration. Medicaid would reimburse doctors and hospitals for care of the medically indigent, with federal matching funds funneled through the states.

"It appears obvious that the problem of indigent medical care is not going to disappear," said Ferguson, forgetting for the moment that, to the founders of the medical center's individual hospitals, indigent medical care had been not a "problem" but the very motive that had driven them to create the facilities. "If the financing moves to the federal government, it well behooves the voluntary hospital to cautiously explore all the impli-cations that such financing might bring."

In truth, Ferguson was merely bowing to the inevitable, the final stage of a progression that had begun in the middle of the nineteenth century. As the cost of providing health care to the poor had outstripped the abil-ity of "individuals of large resources" to fund it, the burden of such care had shifted from just the wealthiest individual citizens of the community to all members of the community, through citywide charities and city and county taxes. Then, as even these resources began to prove inadequate, the burden shifted again to include all citizens of the state, through tax monies that were provided in amounts that matched each county's local contribution. Now, finally, the burden was again shifting, this time to all citizens of the country through federal taxes. As the costs of health care continued to grow without any control, only the formidable pool of re-sources represented by federal tax revenues could hope to keep up.

In the meantime, however, construction had already begun on the medical center's new $8 million general-service unit—the "Dr. Robert Hamilton Bishop, Jr., Building"—which was to be situated adjacent to Lakeside. The expansion and remodeling of Hanna House and the con-struction of the new "George M. Humphrey Ambulatory Care Center" were also scheduled to begin, despite a projected $500,000 operating deficit for the year. Indeed, the deficit was so great that yet another raid on the endowments had to be made simply to pay the hospitals' usual bills. The additional advance brought the total of money taken from the funds to the alarming figure of $2.5 million.

Even the institution's bleak financial outlook, however, could not dampen the spirits of the hospitals' three thousand employees as they came together in May of 1965 to celebrate the centennial of the founding of the medical center.* The hospitals had, after all, faced more difficult situations over the preceding century, with its seemingly endless series of recessions, depressions, and wars. So it was not surprising that the prevailing atmosphere during the week of centennial events was anything but gloomy. And the mood lasted through the summer, especially when the long-debated Medicare bill was approved by Congress and signed into law at the end of July. Medicare and Medicaid would begin functioning the following year, and although the two federal programs were still regarded with suspicion by many health professionals, some wise observers were beginning to understand their implications for the future.

Indeed, Stanley Ferguson himself made note of the potential effect of the programs, in what may have been the grossest understatement in the century-long history of the medical center. Addressing the subject in an October meeting of the board of trustees, Ferguson said that the new federal insurance system would likely produce "many complications" during its start-up phase. But, he added, "it is believed the plan will be financially advantageous to the hospitals."

---

*The centennial celebration was, of course, one year early, an understandable mistake given the confusing nature of the events surrounding the actual founding of the medical center.

CHAPTER TEN

New Centuries

Douglas Bond believed that the advent of Medicare and Medicaid would result not only in "great improvements for medical care" in the United States, but even, ultimately, the "complete elimination" of medical indigency. He acknowledged that the price of the programs would be high— an estimated $3.5 billion annually once both were in place, beginning in 1967—but the benefits to society as a whole would, he thought, far outstrip their cost. Stanley Ferguson, however, looked closer to home for a more immediate effect from the national health-care initiatives. He foresaw the medical center eventually profiting from Medicare and Medicaid, so much so that he fully expected the programs to "start us on the way to a balanced operating budget."

Of course, the full effect of the federal reimbursement packages would not be felt for some time. As the year 1966 began, therefore, University Hospitals still faced a bleak financial picture, with an operating deficit from the previous year that exceeded $500,000. The bulk of the deficit was traced directly to the ever-increasing number of cases that had been seen in the emergency and ambulatory services during 1965. (Indeed, forty percent of all inpatient admissions that year originated in the Emergency Room, and the number of outpatient visits was actually greater than the number of inpatient days of care.) Only MacDonald House showed a significant decline in admissions of seven percent, an early indication that the expected second baby boom was not, in fact, going to materialize.

There was additional disturbing news at the medical center's April 1966 annual meeting, the first for new board chairman John K. Thompson (former chairman of Cleveland's Union Commerce Bank) and new president Ellery Sedgwick, Jr. (president of Medusa-Portland Cement Company). Yet another shortage of nurses had begun to be felt some months earlier, and by spring the situation was approaching crisis proportions. Some staff beds had already been pulled out of service, and the prospect was for further cutbacks. It was also becoming increasingly difficult to recruit and keep adequate numbers of maintenance and service personnel, because Cleveland was enjoying a period of virtual full employment. And as Stanley Ferguson noted, the individuals that the medical center did manage to hire were not, by and large, "suited to work with people who are ill." (Screening and training new employees had, in fact, become a costly and time-consuming effort.) Replacements also had to be found for departing members of the full-time medical staff. During 1965, for example, both Claude Beck and Alan Moritz had resigned—Beck to retirement and Moritz to return to the general faculty, dropping only his responsibilities as director of the pathology department. At about the same time, Robert Ebert resigned as director of medicine to take up similar duties at Harvard and the Massachusetts General Hospital.

The nursing shortage worsened through the year, and by the end of 1966 an entire wing of beds was closed for a minimum of three months. Earlier, in July, the hospitals had increased nurses' base salary from $435 a month to $450, in an attempt to forestall defections and attract new job applicants. Just a few days later, however, civil disturbances in the nearby Hough neighborhood precipitated two days of rioting that was quelled only after the National Guard was called in to patrol the streets. The question of safety in the University Circle area then became an additional stumbling block to nurse recruitment. Salaries were raised again to $500 a month in January of 1967, but the increase was not enough to counteract the effects of the negative publicity surrounding the riots.

The hospitals ended 1966 with a small net surplus, but it was due primarily to settlement of the longstanding lawsuit against Cuyahoga County to recover nearly $400,000 of unpaid reimbursement for medically indigent cases not paid over the preceding few years. Without the windfall from the county's settlement the medical center would have shown a $360,000 deficit, smaller than the previous year's but still a substantial sum. Ironically, Medicare and Medicaid, far from putting the hospitals "on the way to a balanced operating budget," as Stanley Ferguson had suggested they might, had actually engendered new expenses for the medical center. The need to hire additional personnel to deal with the voluminous and arcane paperwork generated by the programs resulted in an added annual cost to the hospitals of nearly $100,000. In addition, forms were being processed so slowly by the Medicare bureaucracy that the hospitals did not receive their reimbursement payments in anything remotely resembling a timely fashion. Thus, the medical center experienced a cash shortage that necessitated another $250,000 advance from the endowments, which brought to $2.75 million the total "borrowed" from the funds.

Ferguson could report to the 1967 annual meeting, however, that the ongoing capital development campaign was proceeding successfully, with more than $40 million already raised. The former goal of the campaign—$54.8 million—had been adjusted upward to $72 million to include additional renovation work within the complex, but even with the higher goal the campaign was doing well. Ferguson also noted that the University Medical Center Development Committee—the group charged with raising the needed funds—consisted in large part of the children of members of the committees that had raised the funds needed to erect the medical center's original buildings in the 1920s.

Work had already begun on a number of the planned projects on the medical campus. The new Bishop Building, for example, was already partially in use and would soon house not only the radiology department but also the physical therapy division, the medical records department, new kitchens, and a cafeteria. The planned addition to Hanna House was scheduled for completion by autumn, and work on the Rainbow addition to Babies and Childrens Hospital was set to begin at the end of the year. The medical center also planned to purchase the small, independent Benjamin Rose Hospital for the elderly on Abington Road, and assume full responsibility for its patients.

During the remainder of the year the clinical capabilities of the hospitals were further enhanced by the development of full-fledged pulmonary-care and cardiac-care units within Lakeside. Such groupings of personnel and facilities was part of a national trend in medicine, a way to more effectively provide the specialized care becoming available in specific clinical fields. Indeed, specialization was so pervasive within health care that it exceeded the bounds of the merely clinical and spilled over into the administrative side. Stanley Ferguson's title, for example, was changed from "director of administration" to "executive director," and to free him to pursue long-range planning his former operational-oversight responsibilities were relegated to his assistant directors.

A series of delays forestalled progress on the new Rainbow addition for a full year, but by the spring of 1968 all obstacles seemed to have been cleared away. Then, just as work was about to begin, the federal

government instituted a freeze on hospital-construction grants, which
again stopped the project in its tracks. Building costs were rising steadily
at the time, and by September, when new bids were received on the
Rainbow project, the lowest totaled $16 million, $2 million more than the
medical center had originally estimated. Some quick design changes eliminated about $1 million from the budget, but with only $13.3 million
available from donations, another $2 million still had to be raised. The
new building was deemed so important, however, that the board agreed
to make up the difference by tapping the endowments, at least until the
rest of the necessary contributions could be obtained.*

§

As 1969 began, the hospitals moved to implement the recommendations contained in a "Statement of Policy" developed by the Medical
Council. After years of flirting with the idea, the medical center finally
accepted the concept of a "single service," a melding of staff and private
cases into one pool of patients, all of whom would be "available for
teaching and investigation." Other academic medical centers around the
country had already adopted the single-service program, and it was an
inevitable development at University Hospitals after the preceding years'
efforts to derive more teaching material from among the paying patients.

The new single-service program served to further strengthen the educational component of the medical center, but by the end of the year
there was real question as to whether any of the three basic missions of
the hospitals—patient care, teaching, and research—could be sustained
at its usual level. The general rate of inflation was in part to blame, but
another culprit was the outpatient service. Overall the hospitals' operating deficit for 1968 was actually somewhat lower than that of the year
before, but the components of the deficit revealed a disturbing trend. The

---

*At about the same time, the endowments were bolstered by a small but remarkable gift.
Stanley Ferguson informed the trustees that the funds had recently received $520.87 from
the estate of one Irwin H. Milner, who, explained Ferguson, had never forgotten the
"extraordinary fine hospital treatment and service" he received when he had been a patient
in Lakeside some years before. The period of hospitalization that Mr. Milner remembered
so fondly had occurred in 1907.

combined shortfall from the Emergency Room and the outpatient clinics was proportionately greater than that from the inpatient service. Neither Medicaid nor funds from the state's welfare service were available for outpatient care, which was the fastest-growing area in the hospitals.

Basic costs were also rising at heady rates. The minimum wage paid to employees of the medical center, for example, rose by nearly thirteen percent a year between 1967 and 1969. Per diem costs rose almost twenty-two percent during the same period, more than two-and-a-half times the rate at which they had risen in the preceding three years. Even with the bonus of Medicare and Medicaid payments, the medical center saw its gross operating deficits climb at a rate of thirty percent a year. Indeed, the trend was so clear and seemingly so immutable that by the spring of 1970 the hospitals began to consider the possibility of curtailing some patient services in an effort to slow the losses.

The principal villain in the budget story was the cost of ambulatory care, which was not covered by Medicaid and was only partially reimbursed by the county and the state. Nevertheless, some means had to be found to operate an ambulatory service within those constraints. In the autumn of 1970, a special committee chaired by pathology chief Alan Moritz offered the trustees its impressions of outpatient services at other hospitals. Moritz had recently been appointed to the newly created post of chief of staff, a position from which he was to keep the trustees apprised of the conduct of the hospitals, and to act as a liaison between the board and the professional staff as well as among the various professional services. Virtually his first task in the new post was to lead the special committee to investigate ambulatory services in Baltimore and Boston. Like Samuel Mather and his fellow trustees in 1893, the committee looked to Johns Hopkins, Massachusetts General, and other eastern hospitals to find a model after which to pattern their own program.

There was, however, no practical solution to be found to the problem of deficit operations beyond the obvious expedient of trimming budgets. The medical center attempted to cut its own expenses and did manage to trim more than $800,000 from its budget during 1970. But the hospitals amassed a deficit of $260,000 in just the first two months of 1971, so additional cuts—$330,000 from the clinics alone, with additional reductions in service—were proposed. Research and professional-staff functions were also scheduled to be reduced in size, unless each could increase the amount of income it produced.

As if to reinforce the importance of reducing costs, the year-end figures for 1970, presented at the May 1971 annual meeting, showed an astonishing net operating deficit of more than $1 million, even after income from the endowments and special gifts was taken into consideration. This was the highest deficit in the medical center's history, and it was even more worrisome because state and local financing of indigent care was on a perpetual downward slide. In addition, within just a few months all of the nation's hospitals were to become subject to the wage and price controls established by the federal Cost of Living Council, which had been established to try to control the rampaging fires of inflation.

The hospitals stumbled through the remainder of the year with little hope of relief from the burden of their debts. Nevertheless, the medical center could delay no further the long-awaited $7.3-million renovation of Lakeside and MacDonald House. Both buildings had for years required special attention, but little could be done until the other needs of the complex had been met. With a solid capital base from the fund-raising efforts begun in 1965, however, it became possible to schedule the start of work for the end of 1972. The planned five-year overhaul would provide, among other necessities, complete air-conditioning for both buildings. The renovation would also eliminate the last remaining sixteen-bed wards in Lakeside, which were to be turned into one-, two-, and three-bed rooms. In recent years the wards had been virtually unused because most patients simply refused to go into them. Patients had become "consumers" of health care, and they expected certain amenities during hospitalization. They would no longer accept the idea of being "warehoused" in the long, open wards.

Patient attitudes were but one aspect of the rapid and confusing changes that were occurring then in medicine, changes that had been precipitated in part by the advent of Medicare and Medicaid. The high cost of the federal programs greatly exceeded original estimates, and the huge expense—coupled with the cost of the ongoing war in Vietnam—were principal components of inflation. Suddenly, health care—or rather, the *cost* of health care—was a topic of widespread discussion in the country. As Stanley Ferguson noted, "Health care, which...for many years remained well below the surface interests of our general society, suddenly became highly visible on a national scale." Individuals questioned the cost of hospitalization, doctors' fees, insurance—everything associated with the field—yet at the same time demanded more services, more amenities, and more access to care. And so many fantastically effective new procedures had been introduced over the preceding few years that there was also a growing misperception of the omniscience of medicine, a belief that physicians should be able to successfully treat *any* condition. It made for a difficult environment in which to operate a hospital, but most especially an academic medical center.

The degree to which both the practice of medicine and the cost of health care had changed over time was delineated in a report produced in May of 1972 by Walter Pritchard, who succeeded Alan Moritz as chief of staff the year before. In his report, Pritchard painted a picture of the hospitals that would have been unrecognizable to the men and women who had created the institutions a century before. In raw numbers alone the founders would have been stunned to learn that the medical center's staff consisted of more than a hundred and forty full-time physicians, more than four hundred and fifty part-time physicians with admitting privileges, two hundred and sixty residents and interns, more than five hundred registered nurses, and more than three hundred licensed practical nurses. There were a total of thirty-five hundred employees in the medical center, and more than a thousand beds were available for inpatient care.

Sophisticated laboratory equipment and specially trained personnel kept track of the effects of the many drugs newly in use at the time. Groundbreaking investigations, such as Oscar Ratnoff's internationally known work on blood coagulation, continued to spring from the medical center's labs. And new and more complicated surgical procedures had proliferated to an astonishing degree over the preceding decade, particularly in the area of mechanical devices to assist or replace damaged body parts. Total hip replacements had already become fairly routine at the medical center, heart pacemakers were implanted at least once a week, and heart valves were replaced even more often. Cardiologist Herman Hellerstein was even engaged in a program to develop an artificial heart.

Eighty-three patients were admitted to the hospitals every day, while the Emergency Room saw nearly twice that number. Perhaps the most astonishing statistic was the seven hundred and twenty-five daily visits to the outpatient clinics, a figure that also explained in part the growing deficits of the medical center. Of the total $2.73 million gross deficit for 1971, for example, nearly $2 million was directly attributable to the amount of unreimbursed or underreimbursed indigent care provided in the Emergency Room and the ambulatory clinics.

The drain on finances constituted by the ambulatory services was slowed somewhat in September 1972, when the Ohio legislature established a policy of allowing payments for Medicaid patients using the Emergency Room and outpatient clinics. Payments were to be made on the basis of "current reasonable cost," a more realistic factoring of expense by which the hospitals' true costs were for the first time covered completely by reimbursement. Hard lobbying by the medical center and other hospitals in the state had won the provisions, even though the welfare department warned that the new rules might bankrupt the system. Indeed, the state's director of public welfare insisted that there would be restrictions on the length of stay allowed for Medicaid inpatients, which would reduce inpatient income for the hospitals and thereby lessen somewhat the positive effect of the first change.

With a reimbursement procedure that reflected the actual costs of care that it provided, the medical center began to see some hope of eventually achieving a balanced budget. Combined with the windfall of depreciation accruing because of the new construction on the medical campus, the hospitals were actually in a position to begin repaying some of the $3 million that had been borrowed from the endowment funds over the years. The trustees also ordered the start of the renovation of Lakeside, which would be followed by a similar improvement program in Mac-Donald House. Ironically, the maternity hospital was at the time the least-crowded facility on the medical campus, its entire fourth floor closed because of reduced demand. The expected second baby boom had not only not materialized, but there was evidence that the entire country was in the midst of a "baby bust," with no foreseeable prospect of an increase in the number of births.

But if changes in attitude and lifestyle among the younger generation hurt admissions at MacDonald House, it was medicine itself that was producing profound effects elsewhere in the medical center. The new Rainbow Babies and Childrens Hospital, in use by October, was but one example. The many advances of postwar medicine itself had, in effect, killed the old Rainbow Hospital in suburban South Euclid by making most of its services unnecessary. Only a few of the functions of the old hospital—essentially long-term recovery and rehabilitation—were to be incorporated in the new structure on the medical campus, with only the third floor of the expanded children's facility being designated as the "Rainbow floor."

Other changes were also appearing throughout the medical center, but almost all of them resulted in driving up the cost of health care. Indeed, a comparison of the years 1965 and 1972, which encompassed a period of just seven years, revealed how enormous the changes had been. The number of diagnostic radiology procedures performed in the hospitals, for example, rose by more than fifty percent in that time. The number of laboratory tests doubled, as did the use of X-ray therapy. There were dozens of new procedures available as well, including delicate cardio-vascular surgery, an array of new intensive-care procedures, nuclear medicine programs, hip and knee replacements, and renal dialysis. The personnel required to deal with all of the new and expanded programs consequently raised the total number of employees in the medical center by nearly seventy percent.

And all of the hospitals' expenses grew at the same time. Wages were one of the principal sources of increase, but the costs of food, supplies, and simple maintenance also rose. The biggest percentage rise, however, and the one that most accurately reflected the changing nature of health-care delivery, was to be found in the unlikely area of administration. The cost of accounting, billing, collections, and computerization—all related in one way or another to the advent of Medicare and Medicaid and their attendant blizzard of paperwork—rose by an astonishing one hundred and sixty-six percent from 1965.

Indeed, it was the ever-escalating price of health care that was soon prompting cost-containment initiatives from all directions. In the autumn of 1973, for example, the Ohio legislature considered proposals to create "new approaches to the provision of health-care services and control of hospital services and cost." Among the proposals was a "certificate of need" law, which was, in Stanley Ferguson's words, "intended to control the amount and kind of hospital services and facilities [in each region of the state]." Experience with similar laws in other states was, at the time, quite limited, which left Ferguson uneasily contemplating "an additional set of uncertainties" in which to operate, should the law be enacted and implemented.

One longstanding uncertainty was addressed in 1973, however, when Charles C.J. Carpenter was appointed director of the Department of Medicine. The department had been led by a series of interim directors for three years, ever since the untimely death of Austin Weisberger, the first Western Reserve School of Medicine alumnus to be chief of medicine at University Hospitals. The delay in obtaining a permanent replacement for Weisberger was yet another indication of how cutbacks in funding—

in this instance, diminished federal monies—affected the operations of hospitals with large research commitments.

In addition to all of its other concerns, the medical center also had to function within the constraints of a national economy beset by inflation and recession, the former fueled by, and the latter triggered by, the energy crisis created by the embargo of the Organization of Petroleum Exporting Countries that year. Fortunately, at least one initiative of the medical center was paying immediate dividends. The new Rainbow Babies and Childrens Hospital maintained a steady patient census and grew appreciably. In its first year of operations, it was, said Stanley Ferguson, increasingly obvious that Rainbow was becoming "a regional center to which children with a wide range of complicated illness are being referred." The new hospital was doing so well that the board of trustees of the old Rainbow, which had remained intact even after the move to the University Circle location, eventually voted to accept full responsibility for directing all operations of the new hospital, rather than just the "Rainbow floor" as delineated in its original operating agreement with University Hospitals. The Rainbow board also committed to paying one-third of any deficits resulting from operations of the children's facility.

Rainbow's former home on Green Road was demolished, but the movement of city residents to the suburbs that had been ongoing for decades actually produced a new use for the old hospital's site. For years, a group of part-time faculty members had maintained private practices in a medical office building located at the corner of Carnegie Avenue and East 105th Street, just a few blocks from the University Hospitals campus. These physicians, almost all of them internists, were a constant source of referrals to the hospitals until the end of the 1960s, when the urban rioting and social unrest of the decade left many suburban patients fearful of venturing into the city for primary health care. The Carnegie Building physicians soon began to follow their patients to the east, settling in offices scattered throughout the suburbs and referring their patients not to the medical center but to some of the region's outlying community hospitals.

Internist Gerald T. Kent, however, himself a Carnegie Building tenant, came up with the idea of bringing together a number of his colleagues in what he called a "faculty-related practice group." Kent envisioned a single suburban ambulatory-care facility staffed by physicians like himself, who would maintain their teaching ties to the medical center and utilize it as their primary referral center for those patients requiring hospital care. The ambulatory facility could also be a superb educational setting for medical students and residents, allowing them to see and participate in what Kent called "preventive and ongoing care," in addition to the "hospital-based acute and crisis-oriented care" that was so much a part of their training.

After receiving a favorable report from a feasibility study of his idea, in 1969 Kent and his colleagues Hermann Menges, Jr., and Douglas Moore set to work recruiting physicians for the proposed facility and developing its educational program. They looked for an existing building in which to operate, but were persuaded by University Hospitals board members Severance Millikin (son of the late Lakeside ophthalmologist Benjamin Millikin), Stuart Harrison, and Horace Shepard to consider the then empty but still standing Rainbow Hospital. Eventually Millikin convinced the medical center board to buy the Rainbow property, demolish the old hospital, and in its place build a $2 million, forty-thousand-square-foot facility for the group practice. (Millikin, who was chairman of the Elisabeth Severance Prentiss Foundation, also endorsed a $1.25 million grant for the new group, most of which was retained as an endowment to fund the educational program.)

In August of 1973, the University Suburban Health Center opened with a staff of seventeen (fifteen of them internists), along with complete X-ray facilities, a pharmacy and optician's shop, and nutrition and physical therapy services, all available in-house. The new facility not only brought extensive primary-care services to the suburbs, it also immediately became one of the principal sources of private-patient referrals to the tertiary-care hospitals on the medical center's main campus.

Inpatient referrals were vital to the health of the medical center as a balance to the large number of outpatient cases seen in the clinics. The net deficit for 1973, for example, exceeded $1.1 million only because the outpatient department recorded more than 300,000 visits—a record high—during the year. Throughout 1974, however, the hospitals operated free from the recently rescinded federally mandated cost controls that had limited their ability to raise rates. By the end of the year, therefore, the medical center actually showed a small operating surplus. Incredibly, the turnaround occurred despite new limits imposed by the federal government on the maximum amount of reimbursement allowed for certain "routine services," despite wage and salary increases amounting to nearly nine percent, and despite higher energy costs, all of which helped to boost overall medical center expenses by more than twenty-seven percent.

All of the medical center's hospitals enjoyed high rates of occupancy except for MacDonald House, which experienced the twin dilemma of the so-called baby bust and the fact that many suburban families saw no reason to venture into the city for maternity care. But the medical center concentrated on creating new tertiary-care services, and patients soon came to take advantage of the expertise available in such areas as the high-risk pregnancy program created by director of obstetrics Brian Little and his associate Irwin Merkatz. And in the newly expanded neonatology program under pediatricians Avroy Fanaroff and Marshall Klaus, Rainbow Babies and Childrens Hospital admitted more than three hundred newborns in one year, all of them transfers from other local facilities that were not equipped to provide full treatment to gravely ill infants. Early in 1976, Rainbow also opened a twelve-bed Pediatric Intensive Care Unit —the first in the Cleveland area—and converted its third floor for use as an acute orthopedic and surgical unit. Lakeside opened its first Medical Intensive Care Unit, and new subdivisions were created in the rapidly growing fields of oncology, human genetics, and clinical pharmacology.

Changes also took place in the administration of the hospitals, the most notable being the retirement of Stanley Ferguson after twenty-three years at the medical center. Ferguson was replaced at the end of 1976 by Charles B. Womer, who returned to Cleveland after serving for ten years as director of the Yale-New Haven Hospital. Unlike his predecessor, however, Womer would not be executive director of the hospitals. His new title was president and chief executive officer, a change indicative of the ongoing corporatization of health-care delivery. Indeed, the need to run the medical center on a thoroughly businesslike basis was acute, given the operating environment that had grown up around it. As administrator David Clark pointed out at the time, cost reduction had become a "national dilemma," trapping hospitals between an ever-increasing demand for more and better health care and the widespread belief that the cost of that care had somehow to be reduced. A growing national consensus argued that total health-care costs should never be allowed to exceed nine percent of the gross national product, but because the forces of technological progress (combined with the insidious power of inflation) were pushing costs to that limit, "more care for less cost and unit-cost reduction have now emerged as implicit public policy."

Expenses continued to rise uncontrollably, however, and the medical center was forced to raise its room rates by fifteen percent, as well as to increase a variety of service charges. In fact, the inexorable increase in costs actually forced the hospitals to at last proceed with the long-delayed Humphrey ambulatory building. It would, however, be quite a different project than the one that had first been proposed back in 1959.

After a series of delays and seemingly incessant questioning of the viability of the program, formal planning for what was to have been called the Humphrey Ambulatory Referral Center had begun in 1965. Numerous problems continued to appear over the years, however, keeping the project on the drawing board until 1970. By then, the medical center was performing much more primary care in its clinics and Emergency Room than was advisable, seeing nearly double the number of patients of just a decade before. Indeed, the two services had become a steady drain on the finances of the hospitals.

In 1970 the Medical Council recommended the creation of a separate operating division for all of the hospitals' various outpatient services. The board of trustees expressed concern about the plan, pointing out that the medical center could not afford to incur "another deficit operation." The board insisted that before approving the plan it first had to be assured of "the absolute financial integrity" of the proposed division. The trustees also wanted assurances that a new division would service a predefined and limited number of cases, and that the patients themselves would be "representative of all social and economic segments of the community" (that is, not all of them could be medically indigent). They also made plain to the medical council that it was not the medical center's responsibility to "provide open-ended care for the community...." Instead, the hospitals' true role was to establish "exemplary standards of health care and [to] provide a model that can be emulated by other private and public institutions."

At the end of 1970 the Medical Council submitted a revised proposal that included its recommendation for the creation—with other local health-care providers and agencies—of "community-based clinics" for most primary ambulatory care and family health care. Moving a portion of primary care from the medical center to satellite clinics within the community would, it was believed, result in lower costs for all concerned. Such a move would also obviate the necessity for a large new building on the medical campus devoted exclusively to housing all of the medical center's outpatient clinics.

More than four years later, after innumerable studies, discussions, and revisions, a new Medical Council plan proposed construction of a building to house ambulatory surgery facilities, adult emergency services, and admitting offices. The new building would still serve as a referral center for the hospitals, but it would not be the clinic facility that had first been proposed some fifteen years before. Such a building—an ambulatory care center for staff and private outpatients—might, however, be planned for the future.

It was another year before final approval for the project was given, but in January of 1977 the board of trustees at last ordered construction to begin. And the George M. Humphrey Building was scheduled for completion by the autumn of 1978.

§

By the time of the May 1978 annual meeting, the medical center was seeing slight improvements in its ongoing efforts to balance its budget, the first tangible evidence of the accuracy of Stanley Ferguson's 1965 statement that Medicare and Medicaid might indeed prove "financially advantageous" to the hospitals. Both 1976 and 1977 had ended with small net surpluses, despite a national economy that featured continuing high inflation, and despite the costs inherent in the rapid growth of medical-malpractice litigation. The proliferation of malpractice claims represented another fundamental shift in the public's attitude toward medicine and its practitioners, one that had been ongoing for some time. It had been many years since physicians were looked on as demigods of healing, but the widespread use of lawsuits against doctors and hospitals was still something fairly new. Just a decade before, for example, the medical center had required only $5 million of malpractice coverage at a cost of $50,000, and had recorded only about six claims a year. In the growingly litigious atmosphere of the late 1970s, the hospitals faced some thirty claims a year and had to pay $1.3 million annually for $26 million of coverage. It was a far cry from earlier decades, when often the amount the hospitals paid out for insurance premiums was actually greater than the total amount of money paid out in awards to claimants.

One of the reasons for the explosion in malpractice suits was the ongoing development of increasingly complicated medical procedures, the successful application of which could never be guaranteed. Technological advances pushed health care into new realms, particularly at tertiary-care facilities, which were expected not only to keep up with the pace of change but to lead the way. University Hospitals was, for example, one of the first institutions in the country to successfully treat leukemia and aplastic anemia with the experimental technique of bone-marrow transplantation. Yet progress could also produce ways in which to minimize risk. Lakeside's new computerized axial tomography device, or CAT scanner, for example, obviated the necessity for more complicated and potentially hazardous procedures to diagnose brain injuries and disease, and Rainbow's echocardiograph equipment was used for noninvasive ultrasound detection of congenital heart disease in children.

Other advances also gained recognition for their efficacy and worth, notably the infant-bonding concept created by the medical center's John Kennell and Marshall Klaus. The two pediatricians conducted a lengthy study from which they found that, contrary to longstanding belief, the strongest bonds of attachment between women and their newborns were achieved when mothers were encouraged to touch and hold their infants in the first hours and days after birth. As early as the 1960s, Kennell had started to bring parents into the premature nursery to hold their children, who otherwise would be encased in glass-covered incubators and handled only by doctors and nurses. As a result of Kennell's infant-bonding study, which was published in 1971, hospitals around the country adopted a program of encouraging mother-infant interaction. Kennell himself, a latter-day Edward Cushing of modest and unassuming manner, eventually found himself in the unlikely position of appearing on national television to discuss infant bonding.

As the pace of progress within medicine continued to accelerate, so too did the rate of change in the patient population of University Hospitals. A Medical Council study comparing the years 1962 and 1976 found that the number of inpatients from outside Cuyahoga County increased by thirteen percent over the period, with the largest increases coming in the surgical specialties and in pediatrics. It was a clear indication that, in president Charles Womer's words, the medical center was more and more being recognized as a "major referral center for the diagnosis and treatment of conditions which require a high degree of medical specialization, sophisticated instrumentation, and technology and intensive nursing care."

And more areas of specialization were being added all the time. The old division of orthopedics, for example, had grown so large and so well known for its work that it was made a separate department in November of 1978. Neurology, too, was slated to become a department soon. Rainbow Hospital bought its own ambulance to transport critical-care patients —most of them neonatal and pediatric intensive-care cases—from other hospitals and deliver them for treatment to its highly specialized tertiary-care facilities. The annual operating cost of the ambulance was some $30,000, but it was deemed a worthy expense if it helped Rainbow maintain what was called its "leadership position in the treatment of these cases."

Of course, some of the referrals going to the University Circle campus were being generated from the medical center's own outpatient services, particularly from the University Suburban Health Center. Indeed, the Green Road facility was doing so well that there were plans to build an addition to house specialists in ophthalmology, pediatrics, psychiatry, dermatology, and even dentistry. But another reason for the steady number of inpatient cases was the advent of an inhouse program to deal with patients' concerns. New chief of staff Scott R. Inkley, a pulmonary specialist, initiated a program called C.A.R.E. (Concern, Attitude, Responsibility, and Environment), which he described as a "hospital-wide effort to improve relationships with, and attitudes toward, patients and visitors" by developing among hospital staff members an increased awareness of patients' needs and expectations.

Inkley also led a group retreat of department heads and top hospital administrators, at which long-range institutional goals were defined. Out of this meeting came the "Professional Advisory Committee of the Medical Council," which attempted to gather input from staff physicians who were "involved on a day-to-day basis with hospital affairs." Ultimately, the committee made a number of recommendations about the future of the hospital group, primary among which was the need to concentrate more of the medical center's attention on the longtime problem area of ambulatory care.

As the committee noted, outpatient services had to be expanded for a number of reasons, not the least of which was the "increasing pressure" being felt by the entire medical community to decrease the overall number of what were called "hospital bed days." To contain costs, government urged health-care providers to reduce the number of days inpatients stayed in hospital, so that even when the total number of admissions rose (as had been occurring at the medical center), the number of days of care actually fell. The hospitals thus needed more admissions to maintain the same level of patient revenue, and one of the ways to acquire new admissions was through ambulatory referrals.

The committee therefore gave its highest priority to the construction of a new ambulatory-care facility, a building into which all of the hospitals' existing clinics could be moved. This would serve the dual purpose of consolidating the clinics in one new, up-to-date facility and opening up additional room for expansion within each of the hospitals themselves.

By May of 1979, the proposal for the new ambulatory clinic building had been added to the list of needed improvements on the medical campus, a roster of projects that was estimated to require some $42 million to complete. A development campaign to raise funding for the new outpatient building, as well as for additional research laboratories, expanded facilities for the radiology department, added parking, and the modernization of Lakeside, MacDonald House, Hanna Pavilion, the Bishop building, and the Institute of Pathology, was to have been announced publicly shortly thereafter. Unfortunately, the State of Ohio had just initiated a ninety-day moratorium on the issuance of permits to build hospital structures under the new "certificate of need" law, so no action could be taken immediately.

The need for a new clinic building was just one of the problems facing the medical center at the time. Although the hospitals enjoyed a year-end net surplus of nearly $1.5 million at the close of 1978, operating expenses still exceeded operating revenues by more than $2 million. And the shortage of nurses that was affecting hospitals throughout the country was being felt particularly hard in Cleveland. In December of 1978 the city had defaulted on a number of municipal bonds, which not only adversely affected the city's financial status but made Cleveland the butt of jokes from coast to coast. University Hospitals was forced to begin an expanded personnel recruitment effort for nurses, in what Charles Womer called "an effort to offset the negative effects of the national publicity about Cleveland's problems."

Still, the most constant and pressing problem for the medical center was its need to continually cut costs to comply with the seemingly endless flow of edicts and fiats emanating from Washington. Charles Womer went so far as to say that the greatest impediment the hospitals faced at the time was "the increasingly intrusive, stifling, arbitrary, and often contradictory regulation of our affairs by the federal government." And at the hospitals' 1979 annual meeting, Richard H. Stewart, retiring after four years as chairman of the medical center's board, also noted that construction of the new ambulatory-care facilities on the medical campus was, at least in part, a response to the cost-containment demands of government funders on the local, state, and federal levels.

By eliminating many primary- and secondary-care cases from inpatient rolls, however, the hospitals' existing facilities would be grossly underutilized unless even more of an effort to attract what Stewart called "an ever-increasing number of patients from...outlying districts" were made. The medical center had to become known as the region's principal referral center for tertiary care, said Stewart, and to accomplish that goal meant that the hospitals had to offer a "better product" than any of their "competitors" in the area. "To put it bluntly," Stewart explained, "we are no different from any other business. Our product, health care, competes with the same product of other hospitals, just as General Motors [and] Ford compete with their respective products."

Stewart's comparison of health care to automobiles might have seemed out of place to the founders of the individual hospitals within the medical center, but in fact it was an accurate delineation of the environment in which health-care delivery then operated. The cold realism of the marketplace had prevailed for some time and would continue to do so, and the survival of University Hospitals depended in large measure on the ability of its managers to work within that milieu. Indeed, the same realistic viewpoint had been reflected earlier in the year, when a new organizational structure changed the titles and responsibilities of the administrative officers of the medical center and created a very corporate-looking roster of two senior vice presidents, four vice presidents, and three assistant vice presidents.

If Stewart was a pragmatist, however, he was also attuned to the fundamental values that the medical center and its component hospitals had always espoused. He concluded his final remarks to the board by reminding his fellow trustees that the hospitals could not expect to grow unless they maintained the excellence of their teaching and research programs. And most importantly, he added, the care of patients had to be the primary consideration for all medical center employees. "A patient must not become just a number," he said. "He must be given consideration and treated as any one of you would expect to be treated."

Stewart's concern for the treatment of patients was mirrored by that of incoming board chairman Harry J. Bolwell, the chairman and chief executive officer of Cleveland's Midland-Ross Corporation. Bolwell, whose wife was a nurse and whose son was a physician, had an intimate understanding of the needs of patient care, and he believed strongly in maintaining the medical center's historic mission of providing service to the poor. But he also recognized the importance of operating the medical center within the same constraints that any other business would face, and he was determined to balance the needs of patient care and high-quality programs of education and research with a decidedly businesslike approach to management.

As if designed to reinforce Bolwell's point of view, just one month after his election as board chairman the federal government inaugurated new regulations setting limits on the amount of per diem reimbursement available for Medicare and Medicaid inpatients. The new strictures would in all likelihood mean a totally unforeseen $1 million revenue shortfall for the medical center in the coming year. Nevertheless, the hospitals continued to invest heavily in expanding the breadth and depth of patient services. Roughly $7 million was being spent to renovate old facilities and purchase new equipment for the radiology department, whose new director, Ralph Alfidi, had been recruited from the Cleveland Clinic. In addition to establishing a new dermatology department under former Rockefeller University associate physician David Bickers, a chronic-pain clinic within the department of anesthesiology, and a geographic medicine clinic under director Adel A.F. Mahmoud, the hospitals also recruited Jerry Shuck, a trauma and burn-management expert from the University of New Mexico, as the new director of surgery. Groundwork was laid for a more coordinated approach to cancer treatment and research, and a residency program was started in the department of family medicine to further the development of a new generation of general practitioners. GPs were in particularly short supply around the country at the time because the trend in medicine over the preceding three decades had, of course, been toward specialization and subspecialization—a trend, ironically, that had been initiated and led by major academic medical centers such as University Hospitals.

The medical center invested $30,000 for a blood-cell separator required for bone marrow transplants; $16,825 for a sixteen-channel electroencephalograph machine; $20,000 for a single adult echocardiogram machine; $72,000 for a hematology counter; $11,500 for a platelet counter for chemotherapy patients in the oncology center; and $233,772 for a radiographic-fluoroscopic unit. In addition, construction was started on a $3.5 million, three-story building attached to the northern side of Lakeside, which would house receiving docks, offices, and a new Surgical Intensive Care Unit on the top floor. Additional expenses were incurred when, in

an attempt to overcome an acute shortage of qualified nurses that saw
nearly forty of the medical center's beds pulled out of service, salaries
were raised and an aggressive recruitment program initiated.

Although much of the growing expense of operating the medical center was due to the general effects of inflation, the greater part was a
result of the constant need to acquire the new technology of medicine's
latest and most rapidly paced era of change. New equipment, new treatments, and new procedures seemed to pour forth in a torrent throughout
the 1970s, and no tertiary-care center could long survive without incorporating the latest and most effective advances into its programs of
patient care. Since each new addition to the hospitals' arsenal also
required additional trained personnel, the cost of operating the medical
center rose astronomically. In 1949, for example, at the beginning of the
postwar technological explosion, University Hospitals' total annual expenses had amounted to less than $5 million. By 1979, the hospitals' total
annual expenses were close to $100 million.

Nevertheless, in March of 1981, the medical center was prepared to
proceed with its long-delayed ambulatory-care center. The new building
would be erected on Abington Road, along with a new parking structure
and a 10,000-square-foot addition to Rainbow Babies and Childrens
Hospital that would include an expanded Neonatal Intensive Care Unit.
The ambulatory center would have facilities for radiation therapy and a
radiology research center, as well as suites and offices for almost all of
the hospitals' clinical departments. The entire project would cost some
$40 million, to be financed through contributions and tax-exempt revenue
bonds.

Little more than a month later, however, both the federal government
and the State of Ohio—each confounded by the inexorable rise in the cost
of its health-care programs—proposed substantial cutbacks in the levels
of reimbursement to be paid to hospitals through Medicare and Medicaid.
As Charles Womer pointed out to the medical center's trustees, the cutbacks, if they became effective, would "make the present plans for the
new ambulatory care center impracticable." The new building was, consequently, delayed yet again.

Frequently shifting directives from government entities were but one
of the many factors that had to be taken into account whenever the medical center planned either growth or change. And the pace of change had
so accelerated during the 1970s that too often the hospitals could respond
only in piecemeal fashion. Early in 1982 the medical center, with the aid

of an outside consultant, attempted to remedy that situation by developing a realistic view of the market in which it operated and a clearly defined path to follow.

After studying the problem for weeks, vice president William Fissinger reported to the trustees that, because of the unremitting drain on finances represented by the volume of poor and indigent care provided, the only way to maintain that part of the hospitals' historic mission was to balance it with an increase in the number of private referral patients admitted to the hospitals. Wide-ranging interviews in the community had found that the Cleveland Clinic, the only health-care facility in the city recording more days of care than University Hospitals, was perceived as the medical center's only real competitor for referral business. Although local private physicians rated the two institutions as virtually equal in the quality of their technical capabilities and the high caliber of their clinical competence, it was individual patients who were pressuring their primary physicians to send them to the Clinic, because the Clinic was widely perceived as the "final word" on medical subjects. With a broad gap between the reality of the medical center and its perception by the public, there was, said Fissinger, a need to adopt "marketing practices used successfully by industry."

More effectively publicizing the true scope of the hospitals' capabilities and achievements would be a first step. A broad information campaign could also help to keep area doctors more fully aware of the services and expertise available at the medical center. And in an environment that could only grow more competitive over time, it was also important to initiate affiliative joint ventures with other area health-care providers—creating, in effect, a network of local hospitals, with the medical center as the tertiary-care anchor of the system—to ensure a steady flow of referrals.

A written marketing plan was soon in the works, and by May, after Scott Inkley had replaced the departing Charles Womer as president, the medical center was signing a memorandum of agreement with Suburban Community Hospital, in nearby Warrensville Heights. Under the agreement, University Hospitals furnished Suburban with physicians and consultative services for such departments and programs as pulmonary medicine, hematology, and oncology, while Suburban expanded its referral relationship with the medical center. The following month, Heather Hill, a geriatric-care center in Geauga County, also joined the nascent health network when it was officially designated as a "University Hospitals Affiliate."

Even as stronger bonds were formed with outlying hospitals, the medical center's clinical departments continued to expand the range of the services they provided. A Nuclear Magnetic Resonance Imaging machine, which provided safer and more effective diagnostic imaging than standard X-rays, was installed in the Wearn building, making University Hospitals the first facility in the country to possess such state-of-the-art equipment. Both pediatrics and oncology got new chiefs and increased funding, and a proposal for a new cancer center received support and partial funding from the state. The cancer center would be housed in the long-awaited ambulatory-care center, which was finally scheduled to be built, along with additions to MacDonald House, Hanna Pavilion, and the Institute of Pathology, at a total cost of more than $88 million.

The hospitals' financial status was stable as well, despite 1981's year-end gross operating deficit of $1.7 million. Thanks to income from its endowment funds, the medical center actually ended the year with a net surplus of $4 million, which seemed to put the institution on solid footing for its planned future expansions. In December of 1982, however, president Inkley reported to the trustees on the federal government's latest health-care initiative, and suddenly the future did not seem so certain.

Inkley explained that the government was about to initiate a new system by which to reimburse hospitals for the costs of inpatient treatment provided under Medicare and Medicaid. Diagnosis Related Groups, or DRGs, would be put into effect in 1983. Thereafter, hospitals would receive as reimbursement the lesser of the actual cost of a procedure or the group average cost per procedure, the latter a figure to be based on a determination of hospital-specific costs for the year 1982. Illnesses and conditions were grouped into nearly five hundred different categories, and each category was given a code number and assigned a reimbursement value. If a hospital's true cost for a procedure actually exceeded the set value for its category, the hospital had to absorb the difference. If the reverse were true, the hospital profited by the difference. In the end, it was believed, the final tally would balance out. Since government regulators believed that the way to reduce the spiraling cost of health care was to limit the amount of inpatient care delivered, the DRGs did not apply to outpatient treatment; they were, in fact, an incentive to reduce the number of days of care provided within hospital settings.

From 1966 through 1973, Medicare reimbursement had been based on a hospital's actual cost for rendering service. From 1974 through 1982, reimbursement for routine inpatient services had been limited to the lower of actual cost per day or a ceiling cost based on a weighted average for all hospitals of similar bed size. (Ancillaries like X-rays or intensive care were, however, still reimbursed at actual cost.) Now the rules were again being changed, with all procedures coming under the arcane classification system of what Inkley called "the dreaded DRGs."

The imposition of DRGs was the most radical change in health-care delivery since the advent of Medicare and Medicaid themselves. Faced with ever-increasing costs for the hospital health care it reimbursed, government tried to limit that expense by forcing hospitals to promote less expensive outpatient care and by bringing their own expenses in line with fixed amounts that would thereafter be paid for reimbursement. Unfortunately, what the government actually accomplished was to shift a portion of costs to hospitals themselves. But hospitals, unable to lower expenses below an irreducible minimum, still had to pass along those costs to patients eventually. And because the DRGs were actually labor-intensive—new personnel were required to encode patient charts with the DRG codes—hospitals found themselves with even greater expenses than before. The "savings" that the government was trying to effect was actually a shifting of costs; ultimately, someone still had to pay.

§

Despite the prospect of increasingly stringent reimbursement criteria through the medium of DRGs, the medical center continued to expand services. At Rainbow Babies and Childrens Hospital, for example, new programs were initiated to focus on Sudden Infant Death Syndrome, a pernicious killer that was becoming increasingly evident. Eating disorders such as bulimia and anorexia nervosa were also being studied and treated as they began to appear more often in the general population, and the division of otolaryngology was made an independent department. New affiliations with additional suburban hospitals were explored, and an additional suburban outpatient facility was opened. Indeed, so heavy was the emphasis on outpatient care that Lakeside actually closed nineteen underutilized surgical and medical beds. Occupancy rates and total days of care declined at virtually every local hospital, while at University Hospitals, ambulatory surgical procedures amounted to twenty-five percent of all surgical procedures performed.

The cost of health care was becoming an overweening concern for all providers, but most particularly for such tertiary-care facilities as University Hospitals. By the end of 1983, in fact, the medical center was producing reams of computer-generated monthly statistical reports, all designed to provide administrators with a clearer and more precise picture of costs throughout the institution. Charts, graphs, and balance sheets detailed costs and revenues that were broken down by department and even by type of patient.

It was painfully obvious that costs would have to be strictly controlled if University Hospitals were to maintain its historic mission of providing care to what board chairman Harry Bolwell called the institution's "very large indigent patient case load." Bolwell himself not only recognized the need for concern, but for two years he had been working to establish a new management system within the medical center, a system he believed would serve the hospitals well in facing what he described as a "period of fixed resources but unknowable costs."

By May of 1984, Bolwell was ready to announce the creation of a system of six separate management centers within the medical center. Each of the management centers—Medical/Surgical, Pediatric, Obstetrics and Gynecology, Psychiatry, Integrated Health Systems (ambulatory-care programs), and Hospital Services (support services and departments)— would be headed by a single individual who would be responsible for profit and loss within the center. The object was nothing less than to identify and control the costs of patient care throughout the hospitals.

Each center's manager could decide whether to scrap an existing money-losing program or whether to start a proposed new one. "The manager," said Bolwell, "will be responsible for all elements, including the professionals (nurses, physicians, and so on), in his or her area. In other words, the unit will be horizontally and not vertically integrated." Bolwell's plan was quite similar to one that the giant automaker General Motors had recently initiated, but it was the first time such a system had been implemented in the health-care field. Coincidentally, the advent of the new system brought to mind the words of former chairman Richard Stewart, who five years before had urged the board to think of health care as a product, because thenceforth they would have to compete with other area hospitals "just as General Motors" competed with its rivals.

As the new management structure was being put into place, the hospitals themselves continued to expand their tertiary-care capabilities. During 1984, construction proceeded on the new ambulatory referral center, the cancer center (which would be named for former Finance Committee chairman R. Livingston Ireland), a psychiatry pavilion and day hospital for children and adolescents, and additions and improvements to Hanna Pavilion, the Bishop building, Rainbow, and MacDonald House.

Over the next year the medical center obtained a linear accelerator for use in manufacturing radioisotopes for cancer therapy, the state's only Positron Emission Tomography (PET) scanner for tumor identification, and even a helicopter to transfer patients from referring hospitals. New programs were developed in the area of geriatric care, with special emphasis given to the study and treatment of Alzheimer's disease, and a major research program on schizophrenia was initiated. A multimillion-dollar lithotriptor, a new device that accomplished nonsurgical destruction of kidney stones, was obtained through a joint ownership and operating agreement with the Cleveland Clinic—the first major cooperative venture effected by the two institutions.

Meanwhile, inpatient admissions began to rise, particularly in the surgical and medical intensive-care units. At one point, in fact, all thirty-four intensive-care beds were in use, which prompted plans to open an additional eight. Only MacDonald House, which had recently been renamed the MacDonald Hospital for Women, showed an occupancy rate of under eighty percent, and even there new initiatives—such as state-of-the-art birthing and delivery rooms, and a midwifery program—promised to increase the number of admissions.

At the hospitals' annual meeting in the spring of 1986, medical center president Inkley stepped down from his position, and board chairman Bolwell announced his intention to do the same by year's end. Inkley would be replaced by James A. Block, former president of the Rochester New York Area Hospitals Corporation, while the chairmanship would be filled by A. William Reynolds, chief executive officer of the Akron tiremaker GenCorp. In one of his last official acts as president, however, Inkley proposed that the medical center's new ambulatory-care building be named the Harry J. Bolwell Health Center, in recognition of Bolwell's seven years of leadership during what Inkley called a "crucial period" in the history of University Hospitals.

Indeed, one measure of the success of the initiatives undertaken during Bolwell's period at the helm of the institution—the new clinical programs, the added equipment and expertise, and the concerted effort to educate the public about the true value of the medical center—was soon evident, as the hospitals saw a continuing surge of inpatient admissions throughout 1986. Virtually of the medical center's beds were by then in use, and there was particularly heavy demand in the surgery department. Because the types of surgery being performed were much more complex and required so much more time than procedures performed in most community hospitals, operating rooms were usually booked far in advance. To handle the great volume of cases requiring the expertise available only at a tertiary-care center, an additional surgical suite was built and opened early in 1987.

Although full occupancy was no longer a problem for the hospitals, the need to contain costs was nonetheless unremitting. Even as the medical center showed a nearly $11 million net surplus, for example, expenses continued to climb, at one point exceeding budgeted amounts by more than seven percent. A number of insurers, most notably Blue Cross, pressured hospitals to reduce their costs and even sought legislative action to mandate lower charges. Recognizing the new environment in which the medical center operated, both chairman Reynolds and president Block advocated measures that would, it was believed, help to control costs as well as ensure the continued availability of and demand for patient services.

A small number of strategic clinical services would be singled out as "halo" areas, programs whose strengths were already well known but which could be raised to even further heights by concentrating more resources upon them. New marketing programs would also be devised to take advantage of the successes of the halo areas, the reflected glow of which would enhance the reputation of the medical center as a whole. The ultimate goal of the program was for the halo areas to be recognized as "regional leaders in caring for patients" and "national leaders in research and education."

While task forces within the hospitals worked to determine which specific clinical programs would be recommended as halo areas, a consulting team from Boston was brought in to develop a master facilities plan for University Hospitals. In the summer of 1987 the team presented its blueprint for future growth, recommending a "phased renovation and replacement program" to modernize and expand the overcrowded existing facilities and to prepare for future market demands with additional construction.

The first phase of the program called for the construction of a ten-story Bed Tower between Abington and Cornell Roads, which would house two hundred and ten acute-care beds, seventy medical and surgical intensive-care beds, and twenty-one operating rooms. The new facility would also provide space for many of the medical center's ambulatory services, as well as for a host of support services. By locating the new 500,000-square-foot structure directly east of the Wearn Building and north of the Bolwell Health Center, the hospitals would also create a broad courtyard accessible from Euclid Avenue that could serve as the main entrance for the entire medical center. The new entryway would give University Hospitals a Euclid Avenue address for the first time in its history.

Hanna Pavilion and some other buildings would be razed as the elements of the master plan were implemented. More beds would be added in time, along with renovation of many of the older buildings on the medical campus. Additional parking structures were also an important part of the plan, because the continuing growth of not only the hospitals but all of University Circle was already severely straining the infrastructure of the area. Ultimately, the total cost of realizing the ambitious master plan was estimated to be in excess of $300 million, but the huge expense was deemed necessary to ensure the ongoing viability of the medical center and the maintenance of its historic missions.

Even as the hospitals planned their largest and most costly expansion, however, they could not afford to lose sight of the immediate concerns of daily operations. At the same time that more satellite ambulatory facilities and more hospital affiliates were being added to the University Hospitals care network, for example, the medical center still had to compete nationally for nurses in the face of the ongoing shortage of trained personnel. And decreasing rates of reimbursement from both private and public insurers also played havoc not only with hospital finances but even with simple bookkeeping. Medicare and Medicaid had for some time been changing their rates of reimbursement retroactively, as many as four or five times a year. An individual patient's account might therefore continue to be adjusted years after he or she had received treatment, which left the hospitals groping to determine exactly what amount they had or had not received as reimbursement. The system was so bogged down in paperwork that health-care institutions could never determine with precision their true patient income in any given year.

But the momentum for growth within the medical center was undeterred by even the maddening bureaucracy of the federal government. Indeed, by the time of a strategic-planning retreat in September of 1988, a consensus had been achieved to proceed with the enhancement of the chosen halo areas, or "centers of excellence," as they came to be known. Genetics, musculoskeletal medicine, cardiopulmonary medicine, and pediatrics would all be strengthened and expanded. The goal, put simply, was to ensure that University Hospitals would be considered the principal tertiary-care referral center for the entire region of northeastern Ohio.

Of course, to accomplish that goal required substantial expenditures for personnel, facilities, and equipment. With the myriad uncertainties of reimbursement never far from their minds, and with the knowledge that the higher costs of an academic tertiary-care institution were unattractive to many potential patients' employers and insurers, the medical center's management decided to initiate an immediate cost-reduction program, to save $20 million in 1989 "without affecting standards of patient care and other services." Nearly $20 million more of spending reductions were outlined for 1990 and 1991 as well.

By May of 1991, the one hundred and twenty-fifth anniversary of the founding of the medical center, the University Hospitals' network of affiliates had grown to include a total of seven institutions, including two from outside Cuyahoga County—Geauga and Lorain Community hospitals—as well as University MEDNET, one of the largest multispecialty medical group practices in northeastern Ohio, with four locations scattered throughout the region. The University Suburban Health Center, which over the years had expanded three times and added a host of new services and one hundred and forty physicians representing more than thirty specialties, was so successful that it was responsible for a substantial proportion of the commercially insured patients annually referred to the medical center. A preferred provider organization called QualChoice, the area's first hospital-sponsored managed-health-care plan, was also established to contract with area employers to offer more affordable specialty services. At the same time, primary-care units had been created in the hospitals to provide lower-cost care to patients with less serious ailments. New public relations programs were instituted, many of them focusing on the capabilities and achievements of the designated centers of excellence. (The medical center had already been recognized as ranking among the sixty-four best hospitals in the country by a national publication.) Six new directors—Adel Mahmoud in medicine, Victor Goldberg in orthopedics, C. Kent Smith in family medicine, S. Charles Schulz in psychiatry, Robert Ratcheson in neurosurgery, and Wulf Utian in obstetrics and gynecology—had brought their talents and expertise to their respective departments. And work had begun on the massive job of constructing the medical campus's newest asset, the 500,000-square-foot Bed Tower facility.

By 1991, the medical center had evolved into so complex an organization that University Hospitals of Cleveland was but one subsidiary of a larger corporate entity. And the hospitals themselves were so large that their management was delegated to a new position—executive director—which was filled by senior executive vice president Farah Walters, one of a growing number of women in the institution's managerial ranks. At the time, the hospitals maintained nearly a thousand beds and saw some 35,000 inpatients annually. Nearly 400,000 outpatient visits were recorded each year, and the amount of uncompensated care the medical center provided totaled almost $15 million—more than any other private hospital in the state. The Center for Cystic Fibrosis within Rainbow Babies and Childrens Hospital was the largest research and treatment center of its kind in the country, and was credited with having contributed substantially to increasing the life expectancy of CF patients by a factor of seven. The Ireland Cancer Center, one of only seventeen Clinical Cancer Research Centers designated by the National Cancer Institute, provided up-to-date treatments and therapies unavailable at other hospitals. A triple organ transplant—the first in Ohio—was successfully performed by the medical center's transplant team, and MacDonald Womens Hospital recorded the births of some 3,500 babies in its completely modernized and renovated facilities.

Some 1,200 physicians, 1,300 registered nurses, and 4,000 support personnel worked in the medical center, making it one of the city's largest employers. Together, University Hospitals and its affiliated medical school operated more than one hundred laboratories funded by more than $30 million in research grants annually, which made the medical center the largest biomedical research facility in Ohio. The hospitals also boasted the highest occupancy rate of any health-care institution in Cleveland, and patient surveys found a ninety-eight percent rate of satisfaction with the quality of the care provided. The value of the medical center's endowments was at an all-time high, and a substantial portion of the income from the funds was even available for reinvestment—a state of affairs that would no doubt have pleased the late R. Livingston Ireland.

By May of 1991 a well-grounded plan for the future was in place, and the hospitals were poised to enter the new century from a solid and stable foundation. There were, of course, continuing problems with which to contend, and they would have to be dealt with as the hospitals moved forward. Major reductions in Medicare payments of physician fees, for example, were expected in the following year, and the overall cost of health care itself was a national dilemma that affected not just hospitals but virtually everyone in the country. The percentage of the gross national product spent on health care annually had already reached twelve percent—higher by far than the same measure had been just fifteen years before, when the federal government expressed grave fears at the prospect of exceeding even nine percent. And everyone in the health-care industry understood that before a solution could be found, there would inevitably be trying times to endure.

Yet for all the difficulties inherent in the rapidly evolving world of medicine and health-care delivery, the celebratory mood of the medical center's anniversary party in May of 1991 was not diminished. Of all the changes that had occurred since May of 1866, when the first of the medical center's hospitals had been founded in a small frame house on the shore of Lake Erie, none had been so great as to obscure the vision of the men and women who over the years had kept Lakeside, MacDonald, Hanna House, Rainbow Babies and Childrens, Hanna Pavilion, and all the later components of the medical center on the course that had been set so long before.

Social upheavals, financial panics, wars, depressions—some had slowed but none had halted the growth of the medical center. Even the passing of the hospitals' early benefactors had not proved fatal, as new generations of supporters continued the tradition of generosity established by their predecessors. Many things had changed over the hundred-and-twenty-five-year history of the hospitals, including the very pace of change itself, yet somehow the medical center endured. Change had been, after all, merely the impetus for progress.

The anniversary of the hospitals' founding provided an opportunity to look back over the years to 1866, when, in a far different city, far different needs had to be met and far different obstacles had to be overcome. But the medical center was nothing if not a continuum, and the differences between the early and the modern eras were not so great as they may at first glance have appeared. University Hospitals of Cleveland was really the extension of an unbroken line across those years, and if proof were required it could be seen all around the medical campus—in the portrait of Samuel Mather that seemed to watch over patients and visitors as they stepped into Lakeside's main entrance, in a bronze plaque commemorating the life's work of pediatrician Edward Cushing, in the large and imposing building named to honor the memory of Robert Bishop. The facilities, the equipment, the procedures, and the personalities were new and different now, but the legacy was the same.

The founders themselves would have nodded their approval.

Epilogue

On his second day of life, Baby J is introduced to his mother, who has been brought into the Neonatal Intensive Care Unit in a wheelchair from her room in the MacDonald Womens Hospital next door. The NICU's nurses are always advised in advance when a mother is coming to visit her child. If a baby is undergoing a procedure at the time—having its endotracheal tube suctioned clean, for example—its mother will be asked to wait in the unit's reception area.

Warned of an impending maternal visit, the nurses also need to prepare themselves to deal with any eventuality. Some mothers become hysterical when they first enter the NICU and see how tiny and helpless their newborns appear. Others try to leave immediately, or attempt to hide themselves in closets or under the counters that run the length of each nursery. A few have been known to scream at and even strike nurses. Some simply faint, which is why a bottle of smelling salts is always kept close at hand.

Baby J's mother, however, exhibits the most common response seen in the NICU. She sits quietly in her wheelchair, unable to look at her baby. She seems to be studiously examining her own lap, only occasionally glancing up at the attending physician who is trying to fill her in on her baby's condition. Finally, after a few minutes in the unit, she sneaks a look at the tiny creature stretched out on the warming table beside her. She looks away momentarily, but then her gaze returns to the infant.

What she sees is an alarming number of wires and tubes attached to her child. On Baby J's chest are probes for the monitors that give continuous readouts of his heart rate, blood pressure, and rate of respiration. An endotracheal tube, connected to a ventilator that supplies precisely measured quantities of oxygen, protrudes from his mouth. Catheters have been inserted into the vein and one of the two arteries in the stump of his severed umbilical cord. The umbilical venous catheter, or UVC, is used to draw samples for the frequent tests that must be performed to determine the precise concentration levels of oxygen and carbon dioxide in his blood. He also sports an intravenous line running into his left arm, through which he receives nourishment, medications, and "pushes" of normal saline solution. (Pushes are injections, usually of normal saline, administered from needleless syringes that screw onto the plastic stopcocks of IV lines.) When he was first brought into the unit, Baby J received a chin-to-knees X-ray called a "babygram," a precaution to ensure that his UVC, UAC, and endotracheal tube were all positioned correctly. The babygram also gave the NICU doctors their first look at the condition of Baby J's lungs. In this case, the developed X-ray showed what is called a "white out," which meant that his lungs were so immature that he could not possibly survive without the oxygen he received from the ventilator attached to his trache tube.

Despite her qualms, Baby J's mother is encouraged to touch her newborn son, and after a few minutes she is sufficiently comfortable to try. Tentatively, she extends a shaky hand to stroke the child's arm and chest. Then, gradually, she grows more relaxed, even offering a few encouraging words to the tiny infant.

In ensuing weeks she visits often, and on Christmas Day she holds him in her arms for the first time. By then Baby J's warming table is festooned with photographs of family members—his older siblings, for the most part—and a variety of cheerful holiday greeting cards. Almost all of the tables and incubators in the NICU display similar decorations, along with helium balloons, brightly colored stickers, toys, and stuffed animals. They create an almost festive air about the unit, an atmosphere that belies the deadly serious nature of the work that goes on there twenty-four hours a day.

Baby J, for example, had already developed hyperbilirubinemia, a condition in which excessive amounts of bilirubin—an element of bile—are present in the blood. Bilirubin is extremely toxic; when it accumulates in the body it causes jaundice and, if left untreated, can result in death. Since almost all preemies develop what is known in NICU shorthand as "hyperbili," however, the unit was well prepared to deal with another case. The standard treatment of phototherapy from blue fluorescent lights was begun immediately.

Baby J receives nourishment through his IV line. His "feeds" are noted on his chart as "NPN"—neonatal parenteral nutrition, a mixture of vitamins, minerals, proteins, and electrolytes. It will be quite some time before he can accept oral feedings, because for the present he will continue to receive oxygen through his endotracheal tube. As soon as is practicable, however, the unit's doctors and nurses will begin trying to wean him from the vent, bringing him to the point where first he can breathe adequately on a room-air-and-oxygen mix inside a clear plastic hood, and then finally on room air alone. It is imperative that Baby J be weaned from his artificial sources of oxygen because of the dangers they pose. Too much oxygen in the first weeks of life can cause retinopathy, which would leave him blind. Or he could develop bronchopulmonary dysplasia, a stiffening of the lung tissue that makes air exchange difficult and usually leaves a child more prone to colds and pneumonia and more apt to be rehospitalized later.

The NICU staff also has to stay alert for instances of apnea and bradycardia, or "A"s and "B"s, as they are known. Apnea is the complete cessation of breathing for a short period, while bradycardia is a sudden lowering of the heart rate. Both occur frequently to premature infants. One of Baby J's electronic monitors records all of his "A"s and "B"s, and the nurses chart each one carefully. A few are to be expected, but too many are a clear danger signal.

Baby J suffers a relatively low number of "A"s and "B"s in his first few weeks in the NICU, but he is by no means out of danger. Because he is so active he frequently extubates himself by accident, which sets off monitor alarms and keeps his nurses jumping. On New Year's Eve, an attempt to wean him from the vent and into the plastic hood ends when he begins to show signs of cyanosis. He is returned to the vent and given a dose of steroids to promote the growth of his lung tissue. Then, at the age of seven weeks he develops pneumonia, and one lung collapses. He is treated with antibiotics and slowly returns to health. For the next month he shuttles back and forth from the vent to the hood as the NICU staff tries its best to wean him.

Finally, early in February, Baby J makes the leap to room air. Extubated, off the vent, and out of the hood, he will, nonetheless, require some assistance to breathe, so he is fitted with a nasal cannula, a small plastic tube that directs a low concentration of oxygen into his nostrils. Two weeks later he is taken off his warming table and placed in an open crib. Fully dressed now, and alert to his surroundings, he begins to take normal feedings three times a day. He has become a "gainer and grower," and before long he is ready to be transferred to 7-West, the step-down unit for NICU graduates that is on Rainbow Hospital's seventh floor.

Although he still requires some oxygen through the nasal cannula, Baby J progresses well. Some of the NICU nurses, who occasionally go up to 7-West to visit, think he will be discharged on St. Patrick's Day, which would be in keeping with the nickname he has been given. Because most of Baby J's crises and small victories occurred on festive occasions—beginning with his birth on Thanksgiving Day—the nurses have taken to calling him the "holiday baby."

Unfortunately, Baby J must first undergo surgery to repair an inguinal hernia, and his recuperation from that procedure lasts another few weeks. By early April, however, he is sitting up in an infant seat, looking around alertly, and starting to tolerate room air much better than before. Within a few days his parents are called in to receive instructions on how to care for their son when he is discharged. They must learn how to read the apnea monitor that he will continue to wear at home, and they must be shown how to secure the nasal cannula that he will still occasionally require. They also make their first appointments for the follow-up clinic to which they will take their son over the next few months.

Just a few days later Baby J is at last discharged. True to form, the "holiday baby" leaves on Easter weekend. He is one hundred and forty-four days old, and all of his first four months of life have been spent in Rainbow Babies and Childrens Hospital. He weighs a little more than seven pounds now, four times his weight at birth, and he is growing larger and healthier every day. The period of natural gestation that was denied him because of his prematurity had been recreated for him in the artificial womb of the NICU, and now, after four months of care, treatment, and nurturing, he is ready to leave the hospital.

He will see the rest of the world for the first time, and then he will get on with the business of growing up.

Bibliography

Avery, Elroy M., *A History of Cleveland and Its Environs*, Lewis Publishing Co., 1918

Brown, Kent L., ed., *Medicine in Cleveland and Cuyahoga County: 1810-1976*, Academy of Medicine of Cleveland, 1977

Crile, Grace, ed., *George Crile: An Autobiography*, J.B. Lippincott Co., 1947

Flexner, Abraham, *Medical Education in the United States and Canada*, Carnegie Foundation for the Advancement of Teaching, 1909

Fulton, John F., *Harvey Cushing: A Biography*, C.C. Thomas, 1946

Heaton, Margaret E., "The Story of Lakeside Hospital, 1863-1932," Master's thesis, School of Applied Social Sciences, Western Reserve University, 1932

Kent, Gerald T., "History and Development of University Suburban Health Center, 1968—1986," privately published, 1987

Klaus, Marshall, and Fanaroff, Avroy, *Care of the High-Risk Neonate*, W.B. Saunders Co., 1986

Leathers, Shirlee J., *The First 100 Years: A Centennial History of University Hospitals of Cleveland*, University Hospitals of Cleveland, 1965

Ludmerer, Kenneth M., *Learning To Heal: The Development of American Medical Education*, Basic Books, 1985

Marshall, Margaret R., *History of University Hospitals of Cleveland, 1932-1956*, University Hospitals of Cleveland, 1961

Mumford, James G., *A Doctor's Table Talk*, Houghton Mifflin Co., 1912

Orth, Samuel P., *A History of Cleveland, Ohio*, S.J. Clarke Publishing Co., 1910

Rosenberg, Charles E., *The Care of Strangers: The Rise of America's Hospital System*, Basic Books, 1987

Starr, Paul, *The Social Transformation of American Medicine: The Rise of a Sovereign Profession and the Making of a Vast Industry*, Basic Books, 1982

Vogel, Morris J., *The Invention of the Modern Hospital: Boston, 1870-1930*, University of Chicago Press, 1980

Vollstadt, Elizabeth W., *Rainbow Babies and Childrens Hospital: Celebrating 100 Years of Caring*, Rainbow Babies and Childrens Hospital, 1987

Waite, Frederick C., *Western Reserve University Centennial History of the School of Medicine*, Western Reserve University Press, 1946

Weckesser, Elden C., *A Historical Review of the Department of Surgery, Case Western Reserve University*, Case Western Reserve University School of Medicine, Department of Surgery, 1986

Williams, Greer, *Western Reserve's Experiment in Medical Education and Its Outcome*, Oxford University Press, 1980

University Hospitals Archives: minutes of the meetings of the board of trustees, annual reports, administrative and clinical records, official and private papers and correspondence

Case Western Reserve University Archives: minutes of the meetings of the medical school faculty, official and private papers and correspondence

Western Reserve Historical Society Library: Mather and Bishop family collections, George W. Crile collection, Cleveland newspaper collection (*Leader*, *News*, *Press*, and *Plain Dealer*)

Allen Memorial Medical Library: various collections

Cleveland State University: Cleveland *Press* clipping and photograph collection

Cleveland Public Library: various collections

The Johns Hopkins Medical Institutions: publications and reprints

Index

Carved in Memory

Carved in Memory

STORIES BY
WENDELL TROGDON

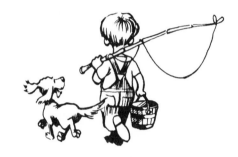

ILLUSTRATED BY GARY VARVEL

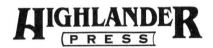

Cover art by Gary Varvel
Cover and book design by Martin Northway
Typography by Students Publishing Co.,
Northwestern University, Evanston
Cover type by Just Your Type, Evanston

A complete list of Highlander Press titles
is available by sending an SASE to:
The Highlander Press
1108 Davis #104
Evanston, IL 60201

Dedication

For Travis, my one-year-old grandson.
May he someday realize that the past
often has an influence on the future.

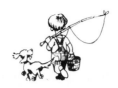

Carved in Memory is the third book compiled by Wendell Trogdon from his nostalgic "Those Were the Days" columns which first appeared in *The Indianapolis News.*

The first book, *Those Were the Days,* was published in 1984, the second, *Those Were the Days: Through the Seasons,* in 1986.

All three are based on life in rural Southern Indiana in the 1930s and 1940s, a time of Depression and war, a time when kerosene lights gave way to electricity, when combines replaced threshing machines, when tractors replaced horses.

It was a time of constant change, but a time when folks held fast to the virtues they had been taught, virtues like honesty, thrift, hard work, and concern for their neighbors.

It was an era worth remembering. This new book is another effort to preserve a bit of history so that readers today and in the future will learn from it.

Contents

Carved in Memory

INTRODUCTION

Memories of Springs Past Endure

It's spring and a man lets his thoughts ripple back through the pages of time. It is an April. Any April around Heltonville, in the 1940s.

Frogs leap from the banks of a farm pond and disappear into the brown murkiness of the splash they create. Youngsters ten to twelve years old disregard their mothers' warnings that the water is still too cold. They disrobe, then flop from the root of a sycamore tree into Back Creek.

A black snake slithers from under a soapstone rock and races through the tall grass toward a hill, there to warm in the sun.

Two boys sit on a creek bank. Straight pins shaped into fishhooks dangle on string from the sassafras bean poles they hold. Beams of sun peak through the trees on the creek bank and reflect off the clear water. The boys pause to appreciate the iridescent beauty of a sunfish darting through the rays.

Off in a pasture, a cow turns to lick her newborn calf, a sign of love that needs no sound. Other cows graze on the tender grass, pausing from time to time to chew their cud.

A colt romps spindle-leggedly through the grass, independent and free, it seems, before returning to the protective custody of its mother.

Out in a field, a dog trots in a furrow, following his master, who sits high atop a tractor. The plow slices through the sod, the moldboard turning over dark soil that smells as new as an unopened book.

A crow drops down, catches a red worm that has wiggled its way out of fresh overturned ground, and soars off to digest its dinner.

A boy is perched on a fender of the Allis-Chalmers, daydreaming of the time when he can plow, disc and cultivate.

In another field, a man seated on a corn planter holds the reins to a team of horses, their hooves deep into the soil that has been worked into a silt. Foamy sweat eases from around the collars on the horses, but they plod on obediently, without protest.

Off in a pig lot, hogs root in search of a supplement to their diet. Sows stretch out, a sign dinner is being served. Their pigs run, squealing, searching for their place at the table.

A woman stooped by years of hard work hoes in her garden, stopping from time to time to view the radishes and onions that are table-ready.

An old man across the road pushes his reel lawnmower, which clips in metallic harmony through the bluegrass. The man stops from time to time to wipe the sweat from the leather lining of the old sun-bleached felt hat he wears.

His wife putters in her flower bed, treating the plants gingerly, the way she does her best china.

They both pause to listen to a locust which has arrived early. It serenades them with an endless tune.

Up the road, another woman hangs the wash on the line, knowing the warm wind will bring new life to petticoats, denim shirts, bib overalls and pillow cases. Tomorrow, she will start her housecleaning, taking furniture out, room by room. She will drape the carpet over a clothes line and order her son to thrash out the accumulated dirt of winter with a rug beater.

In the woods behind her house, mayapple plants cover the ground, their green leaves growing vigorously, getting the most out of their short lives.

In the ford of a creek, the woman's oldest boy washes his 1934 Chevy, his most prized possession, to impress the girl he will take into town for a picture show that night.

When he finishes, he will find a big beech tree, its bark thick and firm. Into it, he will etch with his pocket knife his and the girl's initials inside a heart and carve the date below. It is artwork that will endure generations after their romance fades.

Everywhere it is spring. A time to enjoy. A time to remember.

GETTING BY

Her Breakfasts Were Fit for a King

Zeke called the big breakfast he devoured each day "Millie's morning miracle."

Millie was his wife. Had been for years. Millie and Zeke lived on a farm near Heltonville in the late 1930s with sons Tyke and Tad and their other children. Their home had no electricity, no central heating and no refrigeration.

Refrigeration wasn't needed in the winter. Electricity and central heating would have made things easier for Millie, but she never complained. She was comfortable with the wood range she used to fix meals as well as with the heating stove in the living room.

Breakfast was her specialty. She started thinking after supper about what she would serve the next morning. She prepared the range, putting newspaper in the fire compartment, then adding thin shavings of poplar her sons had sliced from scrap lumber. She laid small pieces of dried wood on top of the kindling.

Millie arose about five each morning and awakened Zeke. He added wood to the few embers left in the pot-bellied stove. Millie set the paper in the range afire and watched it ignite the kindling.

She and Zeke talked softly, careful not to awaken the youngsters in the upstairs bedrooms. In a few minutes, coffee was brewing in the big granite pot. The heat had driven away the chill and Millie went about her work, the queen of her primitive kitchen.

Zeke tugged on his four-buckle overshoes and went out to feed the livestock, knowing a reward awaited his return. The two sons and three daughters who still lived at home were beginning to rouse from their long night's nap. The aroma of baking biscuits, frying tenderloin strips and sizzling sausage crept under the bedroom doors and tempted them to join a new day.

Tyke and Tad dressed and bounded down the stairs, stopping first at the heating stove to soak in the heat, then hurrying to the kitchen to take their seats.

Millie's meal always exceeded their expectations. She served eggs, fresh tenderloin strips, sausage and ham. She passed around a plate loaded with biscuits, followed by thick milk gravy. There was plenty of newly-churned butter, maple syrup, apple butter and an assortment of jams and jellies, canned when the weather was warm and the days were long.

There was little conversation at breakfast. The joy of eating needed no accompaniment.

Neither Zeke nor the boys ever thanked Millie for her efforts. The girls did sometimes, as they helped wash the dishes before leaving for school.

Millie didn't mind, though. She could see her family's approval as they left the table. It was thanks enough to last the entire day, a day when she might heat water in a kettle, wash clothes on a scrub board, press them with irons heated atop the range and spend an hour or two finishing a quilt on the rack in the sitting room.

And she would hear from time to time about how Zeke had bragged to neighbors about the breakfasts she served.

Sharing a Warm Stove and Cold Memories

Tad hunkered down in his mackinaw jacket and fidgeted in the cold leather seat on the school bus, hoping it didn't get stuck again in the snow. He worked his toes inside his shoes to keep his feet warm.

All in all, it had not been one of the most pleasant days in the first-grader's young life, and he was eager to get home and tell his mom and dad all about it.

The temperature had dropped throughout the day and Tad had to wipe off the frost to look out at the snow which was banked as high as the windows in the bus. It was late January, 1936, a winter when the temperature dropped below zero day after day.

A small fan mounted on the dash hummed, keeping ice from forming on the windshield. The driver's breath hung like a cloud as he gripped the steering wheel. A portable kerosene heater near the front provided little warmth toward the back of the bus.

Tad and the other passengers grew colder each mile, their teeth chattering when they tried to talk. The girls huddled together on the seats that ran across the center of the bus. The boys lined the seats along each side.

Tad's ride home from Heltonville covered seven miles and he was happy he didn't have to stay on the bus all the way to the Lawrence-Jackson county line like Walter Owens, who somehow was managing to read a book despite the cold.

Tad stepped off into a snowbank, hurried around the front of the bus and ran for the house, plodding through the snow, stumbling a time or two as his boots crunched a new path. The cattle raised up from drinking from holes they'd stomped in the ice over the creek. They watched him with curious eyes.

Tad hurried to the heating stove where his dad was warming his hands before going to do the chores. "So how were things with Miss Lively today?" he asked.

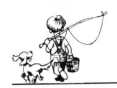
Tad began an unpunctuated, nonstop report about how the school bus had got hung up on the way to school and was pushed by all the students while being pulled out by a team of horses, about some buses being late, about what some of his classmates had worn to keep warm, about everything that he had seen and heard.

He forgot all about what Miss Lively had tried to teach. Then he said, "And Mr. Pierce said we don't have to come to school at all tomorrow 'cause it's too cold to ride on buses and keep the school warm." Mr. Pierce was the principal.

Tad paused long enough to ask his dad: "You ever get off school when it was cold?"

His dad replied, "Never did! But then I only had to walk down one hill and up another to a one-room school that was heated by wood. Everybody else rode a horse."

Tad's mom laughed. "Life was easier back then, Son."

It was then his dad told him he drove a school hack pulled by a team of horses back in 1917. "It was colder that winter than it is now, and there wasn't even a kerosene heater. Talk about being cold.

"I never got hung up, but sometimes I wished the horses had stopped so me and the kids could get off and jump up and down to keep warm," he said.

Tad returned to school a few days later. He didn't mind the cold so much then. But he stored away the memory of a team of horses pulling a school hack through snow when the temperature was below zero. It was the first experience he remembered his dad sharing with him.

Uninvited Guests
Every 17 Years Exactly

Tad hadn't yet turned seven when the cicadas invaded the farm where he lived in 1936. He wasn't old enough to appreciate the sex life of insects, although his dad tried to explain it the best he could without using barnyard language.

His dad called the noisy visitors locusts, but he was a farmer, not an entomologist. Tad would learn later they actually were cicadas.

Tad had seen the shells on trees and bushes. His dad mentioned the locusts had emerged from the ground, found a place to shed their skin and become adults ready to journey into love land.

But the cicadas made little impression on Tad until one afternoon when he and his dad and sisters returned to the eleven-acre tomato field after lunch. A million cicadas, it seemed, had shed their skins at the edge of the field. The shells cracked beneath Tad's bare feet. Some shells were scattered around the hoe Tad had leaned against a tree.

Most of the cicadas had fled to the woods, but a few remained. They were bigger than horseflies with broad heads and had orange-red eyes and wings that seemed never to stop beating.

They buzzed an endless call, high-pitched and shrill, that sounded like "phar-a-oah, phar-a-oah, phar-a-oah."

Tad's dad said the noise was made only by the males, but Tad knew little about birds and bees, locusts or cicadas or mating calls.

"Confounded critters," Tad's father called the locusts. He remembered the locusts from "back in '19," the last time they had appeared in their seventeen-year cycle.

He tried to explain that the locusts came from eggs hatched seventeen years earlier and that the young had dropped into the soil and maintained life by sucking sap from the roots of trees. The wingless nymphs had emerged from the earth to shed their shells and free their wings. The males had wasted no time in beginning their droning call for female companionship.

Once the male and female had mated, the females would perch onto fruit or hardwood trees until their eggs hatched, Tad's father explained. The off-spring would then drop into the ground, there to begin the seventeen-year cycle anew.

It was all too complicated for Tad. He looked confused.

His dad told him not to worry about what he could not yet understand. "Don't fret about it. You can figure it all out in 1953 when the locusts show up again."

Tad laughed. "That's a long time. I'll forget all about locusts by then," he said.

That afternoon Tad and his sisters chopped more weeds than normal. The noise the cicadas made kept them from harping at one another.

The seventeen years passed more quickly than a boy could imagine. Tad did remember that afternoon when the cicadas returned in 1953 ...and again in 1970 ...and once more in 1987.

And life went on. For him and for the cicadas.

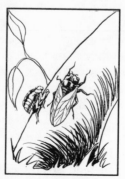

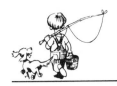

Fresh Warm Milk
Took the Chill Off

News item: Another dairy has made its final home delivery.

* * *

Farm families didn't depend on dairies to deliver their milk, especially during the depressed 1930s and the war-torn 1940s. Jersey, Guernsey and Holstein cows, answering to names like Bossy, Daisy and Spot, did that. The cows provided milk, cream and butter for their owner and some extra change for the cookie jars farm wives kept hidden in corner cupboards.

For youngsters like Tad and Tyke, the cows were a mixed blessing. The boys had to milk, but they were rewarded for their efforts with benefits that outweighed the work involved. And the payoff came quickly.

As soon as the cows were milked, the boys carried the filled, seamless, stainless-steel buckets to the milk house nearby. There, they poured the milk into the open tank atop the separator, a device that, when cranked, created centrifugal force to pull off cream. The skimmed milk came out one spout, the cream the other.

The cream was too rich to drink. And too valuable. Some of it would be saved for use at meals. The remainder would be poured into a cream can to cool in the spring beneath the milk house until Ern Speer came by to take it to a creamery in Seymour.

It was the skimmed milk Tad and Tyke savored. One would crank the separator while the other caught a tin cupful, sipping it slowly, savoring the warmth, a connoisseur by nightly experience.

The milk tasted best in early spring. The grass was lush and green in the pastures, giving the milk a fresh flavor, free from the hint of ragweed that would come later in the summer.

Sundown came early on those spring days, the sun dropping behind the hills to the west, leaving a chill in the air. A cup of warm milk drove off the chill and chased away the pangs of hunger until supper.

The boys' mother churned some of the cream into butter, which was dark yellow from the chlorophyll in the grass. It melted atop fresh, hot biscuits at supper. There would be more butter for breakfast pancakes and thick cream for corn flakes, Wheaties and hot cereal and, later, for strawberries.

Tad and Tyke took the goodness of their home dairy for granted until Jackie, who lived in Heltonville, came to spend the night. Jackie tasted the warm milk from the separator and swallowed approvingly, sticking his cup under the milk spout for another swig.

At supper, he added a thick layer of butter to his biscuits. At breakfast, he applied a coat of butter to his pancakes before adding maple syrup. He had a second bowl of oatmeal just so he could have more cream.

Tad and Tyke told him to eat whatever he wanted.

"The boy looks a bit peaked," their mother whispered to Tyke when he got up from the table.

Tyke replied, "He won't be very long if he keeps eating like he did last night and this morning." His mom smiled.

"I hope you enjoyed your visit," she told Jackie when the boys were ready to leave for school.

Jackie said, "Shore did. Wished we lived on a farm so we could get milk from the cows instead of the store."

From then on, Tad and Tyke had an extra cupful of skimmed milk each night ...with a toast to Jackie's good health.

Improvised Wallpaper
Informed and Entertained

Uppity folks might have laughed and excused themselves as soon as possible. Interior decorators would have scoffed. But neighbors didn't mind when they saw newspapered walls in homes around Heltonville in the 1930s.

The Great Depression had taught people to improvise, to get along with what they had and to make the best of difficult situations. Three or four layers of pages from newspapers and magazines could keep out the cold on long nights. And old newspapers were cheaper and, to youngsters just learning to read, more educational than store-bought wallpaper.

Tad was about eight or nine when a house was built near where he lived and a new family moved in as soon as the roof was on and the partitions were up. He visited them often, became pals with Larry, who was the same age, and watched his parents turn the place into a home.

The walls that divided rooms were made of rough, unplaned green hardwood lumber, direct from the sawmill, with gaps between the boards and blemishes ready to become knotholes. Larry's mother made dishpans full of paste from flour and water warmed on the wood range. She laid out newspapers and used a paint brush to apply the paste, first to the wood and then to the papers. She pasted the pages to the walls, making sure the sheets were hung upright so they could be read.

Larry's mother wasn't content, though, to use only newspapers. From time to time she placed a picture of a Norman Rockwell painting from a *Saturday Evening Post* to break up the type, and she placed comic pages low enough so youngsters could read them. She also cut some color ads and pictures from the magazine and applied them to the news pages as decorations.

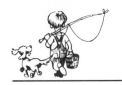

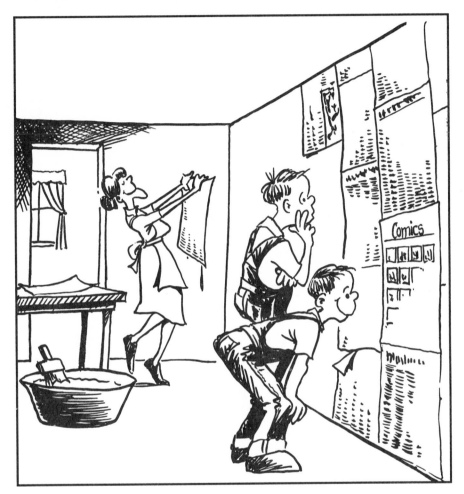

Tad and Larry would wait for each comic page to be mounted on a wall, then read the exploits of Big Chief Wahoo, Mutt and Jeff, "Bringing Up Father," Popeye, Buck Rogers, and Dixie Dugan. The boys, who had sneaked a few smokes of corn silks their second day together, read the brightly colored tobacco ads and wondered how a real cigarette would taste.

Once in a while, Larry's mom would ask them to spread out more newspapers so she could add the paste. She had to wait at times while the boys tried to read the news, most of which was beyond their comprehension. They read about events in Bedford, a place they could relate to, and Indianapolis and Washington, which had no relevancy for them whatsoever.

Tad was still reading and watching when Larry's mom mentioned Tad probably had chores to do at home.

That night after supper, Tad picked up the paper and said, "I reckon I'd better catch up with the news."

It was one of the few times his parents had seen him read anything but the comics, but they didn't question him about it. When he tossed the paper aside, he looked at the painted, planed walls of the sitting room and asked his mom, "Don't you think the room would look better with newspapers on the wall?"

His mom appeared surprised, then replied, "More informative maybe, but I'm not sure any better."

Tad's mother visited Larry's mom the next day and realized where Tad had come up with the idea for newspapered walls. And why he had suddenly become a newspaper reader.

Radio Warned: Backsliders, Beware

America had long ago given up its great experiment. The Eighteenth Amendment to the U.S. Constitution prohibiting the sale of alcoholic beverages had been repealed in 1933.

But that didn't stop Sam Morris. Morris was a radio evangelist who continued to warn the nation it was headed for hell if it didn't once again divorce itself from its love affair with demon rum.

"Backsliders brought back," he said each morning as he roared into the sermon, figuring he could encourage the sinners to change their ways. Morris preached from KERA, "the world's most powerful radio station," which beamed its message across the Rio Grande from Del Rio, Texas, to homes throughout the United States.

The word as preached by Morris came loud and clear into Chig's home about 7:00 each weekday morning. From what Chig could tell, Morris had two missions in life. One was to scare people into salvation by not drinking. The other was to raise money to stay on the air.

Morris had no tolerance for any form of hard drink.

"Whiskey in a pretty bottle with a fancy label and a tax stamp can do just as much harm as a sip from a jug of moonshine," he said.

Morris was usually into his sermon when Chig finished his chores and waited for the bus to rumble down the gravel road en route to school in Heltonville.

Chig would have preferred to listen to WLW out of Cincinnati, but he wasn't about to turn the dial. The program was as important to his mother as Jack Armstrong was to him in the afternoon.

He would, he thought, have been doomed to shoveling coal in the devil's furnace had he not listened. Chig, who was about ten at the time, had no rea-

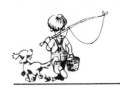

son to doubt what the preacher said. Chig's mom didn't allow liquor in the house. If his dad drank, he never admitted it.

In fact, the only time Chig's dad mentioned the subject was one December morning when Chig's mother said she might send a dollar or two of her egg money to Rev. Morris. "Seems like a nice time of year to do it," she said.

Chig's dad's face turned as red as the stove pipes did sometimes. He stammered a few cuss words and said, "It's your money but givin' money to someone you've never seen to fight for a cause that's done been lost seems kinda foolish to me. If you send that preacher some money, I'm gonna buy myself a pint of liquor just for spite."

Chig's mother looked surprised. She knew better than to say anything just then. Chig kept quiet, too, being smart enough not to take sides in a family argument lest he forfeit a Christmas gift.

His parents didn't say too much to each other for a few days. Chig's mother won the cold war, though. Her husband, caught up in the spirit of Christmas, finally relented and said it would be all right if she wanted to send a check to Sam Morris.

She smiled real big and said, "Praise the Lord. Mr. Morris has brought the backslider back." Then she confessed that she had decided to spend all her money for gifts for the kids.

Her husband was happy. So was Chig. He figured Sam Morris had enough money to remain on the air without help from his mom.

See You in the Funny Papers

Like all ten-year-olds, Tad and Ray argued, but they didn't stay angry long. They lived a half-mile apart and the isolation of their homes meant they'd have to walk a lot further to find other friends. They exchanged visits each Saturday in the late 1930s, spending most of the day together if their fathers didn't have chores for them.

Their greetings were always the same. So were their goodbyes. Tad would stare at Ray when he arrived, act like he'd never seen him before and ask:

"What's your name?"

Ray would reply: "Puddin' Tame! Ask me again and I'll tell you the same."

Ray would hesitate, then ask: "Who are you?"

Tad would respond, "John Brown. Ask me again and I'll knock you down."

Once the introductions were complete, they'd exchange whatever new they'd heard overnight, before talking about the comic strips in the papers their parents took. The comics were avenues to new places and new adventures, giving the boys a view of the world far from their limited environment around Heltonville.

Tad and Ray would talk about "Board and Room" and laugh at the silly cap "The Judge" wore and the antics he tried to pull on his buddy "Emerson." It reminded them of some of the pranks the men at Jerry Jones' elevator in Heltonville pulled on each other.

They talked about "Henry" and the fact he never said anything. All the youngsters Henry's size they knew talked endlessly.

"Dixie Dugan" was young and single, a bit too old to interest either Tad or Ray. They also had trouble identifying with "Mickey Finn," a detective on a big-city police force. But they enjoyed the intrigue of the mysteries Finn solved. "Big Chief Wahoo" was interesting, even though neither boy had ever seen an Indian.

"Popeye," "Olive Oyl" and "Wimpy" made them laugh. They could visualize "Wimpy" eating hamburgers at Al's restaurant on the west side of Courthouse Square in Bedford.

The two boys read the simplistic "Mutt and Jeff" and "Bringing Up Father" and were awed by the imagination of Phil Nowlan and Lt. Dick Calkins, who drew "Buck Rogers, 25th Century, A.D."

But their favorite comic strip was "Joe Palooka." He was an all-American boy, like Jack Armstrong, who proved that good could overcome evil, that modesty was preferable to pride.

"Palooka" won the world championship and kept it for years, fighting foes like "Mister Beagle." Palooka's blond hair dropped over his forehead and always seemed to cover his left eye, but that didn't keep his punches from finding their marks.

The comics kept the boys' thoughts occupied for an hour or so, before they pulled on their jackets, tugged on their sock caps and four-buckle overshoes and set out to run their traps. They didn't mind that the varmints always avoided the traps. The fun was in romping over the hills and through the creeks.

If there was snow on the ground, they'd slide down the hills on sheets of galvanized roofing, before shooting some baskets in the barn loft. From there they would return to the house. The morning paper would have arrived with the mail carrier by then and there would be a new day's comics to read.

They'd comment on the new adventures of their comical friends before Ray would announce it was time for him to head home.

"See you in the funny papers," Tad would say.

Ray would take a couple of steps and reply: "See you in the funny papers upside down."

Neither of them knew the origin of their goodbyes. They were good friends, so it didn't really matter.

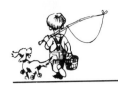

A Special Day Made Tough Men Mellow

C.E. Cummings' general store in Norman was busy as usual that Saturday morning. Some men came and went. Others just came, found a seat near the stove and stayed.

C.E. didn't mind. He liked the men who used his store to spin stories, talk about the weather and complain about how hard times were. And he said nothing when one of them would miss the spit bucket and send a wad of chewing tobacco kerplopping on the oiled wood floor.

They were a hardy group of men, their faces lined with gullies deepened from hours in the wind and cold. Some of them were farmers, some loggers, others so down on their luck they had turned to the WPA for jobs. "WPA" were the initials for the Works Progress Administration, a federal program for men who couldn't find an income elsewhere.

The men wore bib overalls with faded denim jackets and caps with flaps to cover their ears. Their feet were covered with overshoes, most with broken buckles, or gumboots, all caked with red clay.

Valentine's Day was approaching but the men seldom talked about hearts and flowers or love and romance. They were stout and rugged, but easily embarrassed, and kept such topics to themselves.

They were wed to simplicity and gentle women and were aware that the best things in life could be expressed without words. They talked loud, and argued often, but none swore. Profanity was for the barnyards and sawmills, not for places where women might visit.

Tad was at the store that morning in that late 1930s with his dad, who sometimes went to Heltonville, sometimes to Norman, when he needed to buy rivets to fix harness, sugar and salt for the table, or whatever was needed back on the farm.

His dad joined in the conversation, and Tad savored a Three Musketeers candy bar and listened. The men argued for and against Franklin Delano Roosevelt and the New Deal, wondered about "that man Hitler in Germany," discussed the price of corn and laughed at stories told about themselves.

Tad had stood by for maybe thirty minutes before one of the men announced his departure. Trying to be inconspicuous, he eased to the candy jars and whispered for the clerk to scoop out a pound of candy kisses.

One of the other men yelled, "Gettin' some Valentine candy for the old woman, huh?"

The man grinned, but didn't reply. No one else said anything, until an old codger, who looked mean and lean, said, "Worst thing you can do! Buy candy for your wife, she'll either want something every time you come to town or think she has you wrapped around her little finger."

Other men left after buying candy, some orange slices, others caramels, others chocolates or lemon drops, to take home to their wives. Each time, the antagonist had some choice words of ridicule.

After a time, he arose and sauntered toward the back of the store. He whispered softly to the clerk, then waited for her to return with a sack of chocolate-covered peanuts. He eased the sack into his coat pocket and started to walk out, innocently, thinking no one had seen him. He was wrong.

A chorus of comments followed him toward the door. He turned and said, "Didn't say my old woman didn't already have me wrapped around her finger."

The men who remained laughed, then went to the candy jars, one by one, and ordered Valentine candy for their sweethearts.

Cures Were Worse than the Illness

None of the boys in William Wright's class missed many days of school in February 1939. Not even when they had bad colds, sore throats, hacking coughs, fever or chills.

They were afraid the others would call them sissies, which was about the worst thing that could be said about a fourth-grader at Heltonville. And besides, they didn't want to miss the basketball games at noon against E.O. Winklepleck's fifth-grade team.

They often carried to school the odor of home remedies they'd taken for their ailments. The pungent aroma remained with them through the noon hour, permeating the tiny dressing room near the gym. It was an odor that overpowered the mustiness of sweat socks and unwashed uniforms.

Nobody mentioned the smell until Pokey brought it up after one of the games that followed lunch. "Somebody wore a mustard plaster to bed last night," he said, wiping the Vicks salve from his sensitive nose with a big red-patterned handkerchief.

Gordy's face turned red, revealing the "somebody" Pokey had mentioned. "But my cold's a lot better," Gordy said, "and besides, there are a lot worse cures."

That was enough to start a conversation about what their mothers recommended for head colds, chest congestion and sore throats.

Bogey said his favorite cure for a cold and sore throat was his mom's prescription. "A tablespoon or two of peppermint spirits in a glass of water, with sugar added, tastes good," he said.

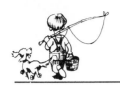

Bob said, "I'm not allowed to take it, but my dad puts whiskey in some warmed lemon juice. Sometimes he comes home from the stone mill so sick he can hardly walk. He'll sip the whiskey and lemon juice and feel fine in the morning."

Bogey wanted to know which he liked best, the whiskey or the lemon juice.

Bob said, "The lemon juice, I guess. He doesn't drink whiskey any other time."

Billy said, "You guys haven't lived until you've been cured of congestion by my ma's solution. She mixes turpentine oil and lard, then rubs it over my chest. Then she takes a towel and pins it inside the tops of my underwear and orders me to bed. I smell that turpentine at night and dream I'm mixin' paint to give the outhouse a new coat."

Pokey reckoned as how turpentine was mild compared to the plaster he wore to bed when he had a cold.

"Mom doesn't use turpentine," he said. "She uses kerosene with lard and rubs that on my chest, and covers it with a warm cloth. If someone happened to strike a match I'd go up in flames."

When the laughter died down, Tad said, "Coal oil on the chest might not be too bad. Wait until you hear what my dad takes for a sore throat."

They all waited, knowing he would tell them.

"He mixes three or four spoons full of kerosene with sugar, and takes that like he would a dose of castor oil," he explained.

The others collectively moaned. "You ever tried that?" Billy asked.

Tad said, "I'd rather have a sore throat. I do let horehound candy, which tastes almost as bad as coal oil, melt in my mouth." It was obvious horehound wasn't his favorite hard candy.

Hubie hadn't said much until then. "My mom feeds us lots of onions and makes us drink onion juice," he explained.

Tad asked him if it cured a cold.

Hubie grinned. "Not always! But it keeps the cold from spreading. Nobody will get close enough to catch my germs."

The bell rang and the boys romped up the steps to the classroom. They'd lost the ball game but learned something about homespun medicine.

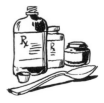

Christmas Required
the Gift of Patience

Tad was a feisty kid, as curious as a calico cat, as snooping as a mongrel pup. And he was as restless as a pig on ice. Especially the week before Christmas.

It was, for him, like waiting for the millennium. The 1939 calendar showed the days were the shortest of the year, but they were the longest for Tad. Endless, they seemed, for a boy of ten, who looked forward to Christmas morning and gifts under the decorated, homegrown Christmas tree.

School at Heltonville was out for the holidays, and Tad had searched every corner of the big farmhouse for presents. He found some boxes, neatly wrapped, but none bore his name. He checked the woodhouse, the milk house, the shed over the cellar. He found nothing there, either.

Each day, he waited for the rural mail carrier, thinking maybe his gifts would come from Montgomery Ward or Sears Roebuck. But the mailman left only Christmas cards, and checks for butter and eggs for Tad's folks.

Tad resigned himself to waiting, plopping down in a chair. He looked as sedentary as the bricks under each leg of the Warm Morning heating stove.

"A watched kettle never boils," his mom said.

"Ain't waitin' for water to boil," Tad replied. "I'm waitin' for Christmas."

His dad finished warming his hands against the stove and said, "If you want the time to pass, the best thing to do is to keep busy. Let's go down to the barn and see what we can find to do."

Tad curried the horses while his dad repaired some harness, then climbed into the loft and shot baskets until light stopped coming through the cracks in the side of the barn. He helped feed the livestock, milked a couple of cows, turned the cream separator and skated a few times down the frozen creek before returning to the house for supper.

Tad had two slices of fresh tenderloin, an oversized helping of mashed potatoes, a couple of biscuits and two pieces of apple pie. He listened to "Lum 'n' Abner" on the battery-powered radio, took the flatiron his mom had warmed and wrapped in the *Bedford Daily Mail,* kicked it down where it could rest against his feet and fell asleep.

The night would pass quickly. Tomorrow, his dad would have to think of something else to keep Tad busy and his mind off Christmas.

Christmas would finally arrive ...and Tad would never learn where his mom had hidden the presents that were under the tree for him.

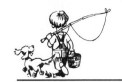

You Could Learn
a Lot in Town

A farm boy could learn a lot in Bedford on a Saturday in December in the late 1930s. All he had to do was listen and watch. It was an educational experience that didn't cost much, which was good because Tad had no money left after Christmas shopping.

Among the things he learned was the fact that men didn't like to shop as much as women did.

As soon as his dad could find a parking place near the Square, he'd stop at the Stone City Bank and write a check for cash. Most of the money went to Tad's mother, who did most of the shopping, except for her own present.

As she walked down I Street to the J.C. Penney store, Tad's dad said: "You buy what you're going to and I'll get Ma's present and we'll meet in the south entrance to the courthouse."

Tad bought his gifts and waited there for his father. Tad was no more than eight or nine, but he was used to being around strangers at the feed mill and grain elevator. He listened to the men exchange stories until his dad arrived.

"Better get you a haircut," his dad said, looking at Tad's shaggy mane which had no part and hung loosely over his forehead. The two walked to Marley's barbershop and waited until one of the Marleys said, "Next," motioning for Tad to climb into the chair.

Tad listened to the men in the shop argue about how good the Bedford Stonecutters were, whether the Monon tracks in front of the shop would ever be relocated around town, the lack of work at the area stone mills and whether Franklin D. Roosevelt was a president or a dictator.

Tad's father didn't care for FDR. "I'm a farmer," he said, "but I don't like the idea of getting money for not doing somethin'. I can make more money for not farmin' than I can farmin'," he said.

Some of the men agreed with him, some didn't. Tad was old enough to know disagreement added spice to the conversation and that some comments were made for the sake of argument.

The barber brushed the loose hair from Tad's shoulder, slapped on some Brilliantine to hold down a cow lick, then dabbed on rose oil for fragrance. His dad paid the barber a quarter and suggested he and Tad have a fish sandwich down the street at Al's cafe.

"Ain't no point in going back to the car. Your mom'll be shopping at least until 2:00 p.m.," he told Tad.

They returned to the courthouse, where all the benches were taken and the wall space filled by men in bib overalls, denim jackets and four-buckle overshoes. Tad listened to the men solve all the problems that existed in the world, and some that didn't.

Tad's pa kept looking at his pocket watch, which he kept in the fob of his bib overalls. He stomped out to the car every fifteen minutes or so, just to see if Tad's mom had returned. His face got redder and redder each time he returned.

About 3:00 p.m. he grabbed Tad by the arm and said, "Let's go to the car. If your ma ain't there, we'll check every store until we find her."

She was waiting at the car. She could tell by the glare on her husband's face it would be wise not to say anything.

They were about halfway home when she turned and asked Tad if he had enjoyed the day.

"Yep!" he said. "Wish we could do this every Saturday."

His dad snorted, sort of like a bull locked in a stall.

It was the only sound he made the rest of the day.

Her Brother
Was a Good Egg

Tad's little sister came storming into the house late one afternoon madder than an old wet hen. She plopped down a bucket and dabbed at a mark on her left hand. The pail was about half-full of eggs, but none of them broke.

She startled Tad so much he forgot he had come into the kitchen to sneak a cookie before supper.

"A darn old hen wouldn't get off her nest so I could get the eggs. Pecked me right there with her beak," the little girl said, angrily eyeing the red welt. "If Dad was here I'd have him wring that old chicken's neck," she added, sniffing back her tears.

Tad was just ten but he knew eggs were a source of income in 1939, not only for his folks, but for other families around Heltonville. Rural families bartered eggs for peanut butter, sugar, salt and assorted staples with the driver of the peddler wagon which came around once each week. The huckster gave the families cash if the eggs were worth more than the items bought.

Tad looked sympathetic, which he rarely did when talking to his sis. "Dad's still out in the field, Marty. But I can take care of that little ol' problem for you."

Marty look skeptical.

"Old hens don't bother me none," he said, remembering to grab a cookie for some quick energy before heading to the chicken house.

He marched to battle, the pail in one hand, his baseball bat in the other.

The nests were compartments built under the roost which stretched along

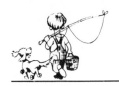

one side of the chicken house. Only one nest was occupied when Tad arrived. The hen that had flogged Marty sat there like a despot, a militant queen ready to wage war with anyone who entered her domain.

Tad tried to push her aside with his left hand and remove the eggs on which she sat with his right. The hen would have none of it. She pecked his hand and raised her wings in combat, stirring up the dust in the nest.

Tad retreated back to the house for a pair of gloves to wear as armor. The hen resumed her defense when Tad returned. This time, he used the bat to raise her off the eggs, then quickly reached in for the two eggs she had attempted to protect.

She flapped out her left wing, banging it against Tad's arm, but he didn't give up. The hen reached out to strike him one last time as he eased out the eggs and placed them gently in the bucket.

His mission had been accomplished. The hen's attempt to raise a brood of chickens had been thwarted.

Tad's mother told him there would be other hens that would try to set before spring turned to summer.

"No problem," Tad said, "now that I've gotten the hang of it." He looked as pleased as a general who had just been honored for a victory.

But his sister looked happier, knowing it would be some time before she had to gather the eggs again.

The Price of Life Was Sometimes Death

Millie's dining-room table was no place for anyone who didn't like fried chicken, especially in June or July in the late '30s and early '40s.

Millie served fried chicken for breakfast, dinner and supper. And it was so good, neither Zeke, her sons and daughters nor her guests ever objected. They would have complained if she hadn't served chicken. It had become a ritual at her house.

Zeke kept the farm profitable, but it was Millie who made sure there was food on the table and some cash in the cookie jar. She did that by keeping a flock of chickens on the farm near Heltonville.

Each March she ordered two to three hundred "straight-run" baby chicks. That meant about half of the chicks were males and about half were females. The females would grow into pullets, then hens, laying enough eggs to feed the family, plus a couple of cases that could be traded to the huckster driver each week.

Males could only grow to be roosters. And roosters who carried on affairs sometimes caused the hens to sit and hatch their own chicks. And a sitting hen provided no income.

That's why the roosters ended up on Millie's table as soon as they became three-pound fryers. As long as the young rooster supply lasted, she'd have sons Tad and Tyke catch at least three of them a day.

It was up to the boys to separate the roosters' heads from their bodies, a chore that didn't bother either boy. They were used to life and death on the farm.

But Bugsy wasn't. He was visiting one day when Tad and Tyke performed the task.

"What happens now?" he asked, looking as if he'd just swallowed a chew of long green tobacco.

Tad, who was ten, the same age as Bugsy, said, "Our job is finished."

That seemed to please Bugsy. Tad added that his mom would pluck the feathers from the fryers, cut them into pieces and soak the pieces in salt water overnight.

"Tomorrow morning, she'll roll each piece in flour that has been sprinkled with salt and pepper," he added. "Then she'll melt some lard in a skillet and put in the legs, thighs, breasts and wings."

Bugsy said he didn't like anything greasy.

"Won't be greasy," Tyke, who was twelve, said in defense of his mom. "Once the chicken is about done, she'll pour off the grease, remove each piece

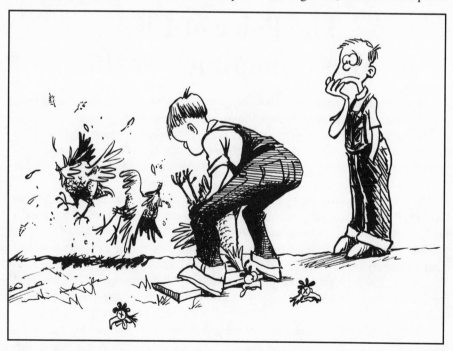

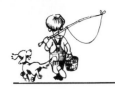

and put it in another skillet that she'll set in the first one. By the time the pieces are brown, all the grease will be gone."

Bugsy forgot his concern overnight. The chicken had been cooked over the wood range when he awoke the next morning. It smelled good and looked crispy and greaseless, as Tyke said it would.

Bugsy had two thighs and a leg before stopping to pour some maple syrup over a hot biscuit. He looked as satisfied as a kitten that had just lapped up a bowl of warm milk.

That afternoon, he helped catch a rooster. And he put its head under a slat of wood, stood on each side of the stick and pulled.

"If you wanta eat, you gotta pay the price," he said, looking both pleased and sad as he watched the headless chicken flop in the grass. It was a lesson every youngster learns, sooner or later, around the farm.

Huckster Truck Was a Store on Wheels

He drove a creaking, rocking huckster truck that brought the city to the country. He was George to his customers, Mr. Hunsucker to their children.

George's truck rumbled through the countryside Monday through Saturday, taking a different route from Louden's store in Bedford each day. George stopped at forty-five to fifty homes on each route, making friends for himself, profits for the Louden boys, Harmon and Pryce. Everything George sold came with a smile and an affordable price.

Folks in the Mundell community east of Heltonville awaited George's visit each Thursday. They could spot his truck in the dry summer months by the dust storm it whipped up as it rumbled over roads built of clay and creek gravel. When March arrived, they could hear the truck laboring through ruts in the roads that had become quagmires after the thaw.

The Chevy didn't always make it through the mud. When it didn't, George would ram the gearshift into reverse, back up, stick the transmission into low and floor-board it through the muck.

Once or twice a week, that didn't work. He remained mired down until a farmer, who was as friendly as George, used a team of horses or mules to yank the truck to a firm footing.

Wes and Edith waited for George to show up, no matter how long it took. They bought big jars of peanut butter, eight loaves of bread, sacks of sugar and assorted groceries from George. When he'd found all the foodstuffs they needed, he'd climb down from the truck, grab a can Wes held and fill it with kerosene. The kerosene was for the lamps in the house and lanterns in the barn.

"Don't forget my mash," Edith would remind George. George pulled down a big bag from the back corner of the truck and set it on the ground. The mash was for Edith's chickens.

George would then figure up the bill, take an order for the following week, and ask, "Anything you want to trade today?"

They usually didn't. A couple of times a year, Edith sold chickens, fryers once they were separated from the pullets, old hens later when the pullets began to lay. That meant George would have to return at night in another truck loaded with coops and help catch the chickens.

It was much the same at the other small farms, except at Jimmy Martin's. George usually had lunch with the Martins. So did his wife, Helen, when she accompanied George on his route.

George passed on news from one house to the other, but he never betrayed a trust. He was once stopped by a youngster who said he wanted to buy a pack of cigarettes for an older friend.

"What's his name?" George asked.

"Don't know," the boy admitted.

George sold him the cigarettes.

"Don't tell my folks," the boy pleaded.

"Just don't tell them I sold them to you," George replied.

A few years later, huckster wagons passed from the scene. Rural families

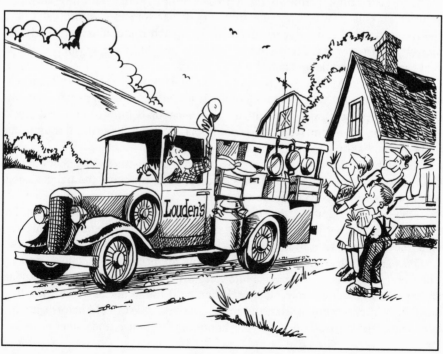

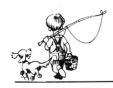

could drive into town to look for the things George had delivered. They found everything they wanted, except the friendship.

* * *

Postscript: George and Helen Hunsucker later moved to Indianapolis, where they still live. George worked as an electrician for Watson-Flagg and Chrysler before retiring.

A Town That Was Endures in Memory

Most of Sherm Umphress' possessions were sold at auction in 1986 at the place where he lived in a spot called Zelma. Some people came to bid on the antique household items and blacksmith tools. Others came to remember the man and the era when he lived and worked.

The antiques cost a pretty penny. The memories were free.

Sherm had been dead almost thirty years. He would have been proud to know the crowd came out as much in tribute to him as they did for the auction.

Sherm and his wife raised seven boys in Zelma from the earnings Sherm made at his blacksmith shop. The sons grew to manhood in the first third of the century when Zelma was a bustling stop on the Chicago, Milwaukee and St. Paul Railroad between Heltonville and Norman Station.

It was a time when farmers drove horses instead of tractors and depended on the village blacksmith to keep plow points sharpened, harness mended and tools repaired. It was a time Elmer, who attended the one-room school in Zelma from 1925 to 1931, recalled.

"The school sat down there," he said, pointing north from Sherm's now abandoned house. "Sherm's blacksmith shop was just beyond the school. The depot was over there," he continued, turning to point toward where Fred Evans lived. Fred is dead now, but his house is still there, abandoned, too.

Passenger trains took riders east to Seymour, west to Bedford. Freight trains took farm produce to market and limestone to Washington for use in government buildings.

Elmer talked about the canning factory Jimmy Cummings once operated across Ind. 58, and about the two stores that were in business when he was in school.

But it was the school that he talked about most. He and Waneta and Thelma, two girls from the neighborhood, entered the first grade together. They learned from Evie Henderson, the teacher, and the students in the other five grades. And they remembered what they had learned.

Elmer remembered strange noises from out of the clouds, when planes began to soar across the sky. "It was an automatic recess when a plane went over. We all went outside to watch as long as we could see it."

And he remembered the time a blimp went over. "That turned out to be an hour recess. It floated slowly from the north to south and we watched until it drifted out of sight."

Elmer recalled when the first train powered by a diesel engine came through Zelma. "I remember an old milk cow Sherm had. The diesel made such a loud and unfamiliar sound, that old milker's legs shook so much she just dropped to her knees trembling."

He wiped the sweat from his brow and talked some more as he looked around at the town as it is today, two mobile homes, one new frame home, two concrete structures and the two abandoned homes.

It was time for Elmer to get back to the sale.

"You didn't mention what you did the other evening," someone reminded him.

What he had done that evening was take Waneta and Thelma to dinner to observe the sixty-first anniversary of their first year in school.

Things that happen a few days ago you forget. You remember things that took place six decades ago.

They Learned To Lean on a "Common Man"

Leston Jones was a common man in an uncommon business. That's one of the reasons families of the dead chose the Jones Funeral Home in Heltonville to arrange services.

Over 59 years, they'd done that 1,464 times--for parents, for sons, for daughters, for aunts and uncles, for the young and the old, for those with money and those without.

They knew the funerals would be handled with dignity and simplicity. With concern, without pretense.

Leston would have been uncomfortable with formality. And so would the relatives of the deceased and those who came from places like Skinridge, Goat Run, Bartlettsville, Meadows, Norman, Zelma, Pleasant Run and Coveyville to pay their respects.

Leston grew up working at the grain elevator his father operated as "J.W. Jones & Son, flour mill and feed store." Leston switched occupations in 1928, when he was twenty-five, buying an existing funeral business. It was a sharp contrast to the grain business and the noise of the mill and the sometimes rau-

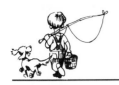

cous manner of the farmers who came to have wheat made into flour and grain ground into feed.

But Leston made the transition successfully. It was a time of economic depression, but he and his wife, Irene, stayed in business, even when a second funeral home opened in town in 1939.

They stayed in business by following the wishes of survivors. Some wanted the caskets and the remains taken to their homes until the funerals. Others preferred calling hours at the funeral parlor. Some wanted services in churches, others at the funeral home.

It was Leston whom the parents of young men killed in World War II, Korea and Vietnam called. And it was he and Irene who arranged memorial services and picked up the caskets when the dead boys were returned for burial.

But Leston was more than a funeral director. He was a Lawrence County councilman for twenty years, quitting after telling friends there was always a chance a man could be beaten if he stayed in office too long. He was a long-time superintendent at the Heltonville Christian Church, serving as secretary-treasurer for another twenty years.

Leston wasn't immune to criticism from time to time. No one who serves the public is. But he tried.

For more than twenty years, from the 1930s to the 1950s, each graduate of the high school received a Bible at commencement, compliments of the Jones Funeral Home. Chances are many of them hadn't opened theirs, or thought much about them, until they read or heard about Leston's death. He was eighty-four.

He had told his son Dwight and daughter-in-law Peggy he was an ordinary man who never wanted to be considered above anyone else in the community. He had asked for a funeral like anyone else would have had.

He was buried of a Sunday after an ordinary service arranged by Dwight, Peggy and his other son, Gene. It was like many of the funerals Leston had directed over the previous fifty-nine years.

He would have liked the simplicity.

Where the Customer Wasn't Always Right

Lute was a good man who was misunderstood at times by some youngsters. He appeared grouchy, especially to boys who thought life came wrapped in a smile around a package of endless merriment.

Lute owned a restaurant down by the Chicago, Milwaukee & St. Paul Railroad tracks in Heltonville. He tended to business and his wife, Emma, taught school in the late 1930s and early 1940s. It was a time when his young customers had more mischief than money, and they often hung out at Lute's place for want of something better to do. They weren't a bad lot, but they could be unruly and boisterous. Lute probably knew he needed to appear obstinate and firm, standoffish, and not eager to be their friend.

His livelihood, or at least part of it, depended on adult customers, who might not return if the youngsters became too unmanageable. Lute wasn't rude to the youngsters, but he let them know he ran the place and as far as he was concerned they were his guests.

Just because you were a customer didn't necessarily mean you were right. Lute usually had the last word. He could do that because his was the only restaurant in town.

Herbie was a high school student when he learned something about Lute's character one day in the late 1930s.

Herbie hated to part with a two-dollar bill he had, not only because it was a lot of money, but because he'd never had one before. But he wanted a soft drink, and he was out of change. He pulled a Nehi soda from the cooler and handed the bill to Lute.

Lute, who hadn't seen many two-dollar bills, either, brought back the change, ninety-five cents in coins and four one-dollar bills. Herbie looked at the change, figuring he wouldn't say anything. But his conscience got the better of him after a couple of minutes.

"Didn't you make a mistake and give me too much change?" he asked Lute.

Lute looked square at him and with eyes of ice said, "We don't make mistakes here. Whatever change I gave you was correct."

For most youngsters, that would have ended their obligation to honesty. Herbie wasn't a typical teenager, though. "You sure you gave me the right change?" he asked again.

Lute insisted he had. "Our customers may make mistakes, but we don't," he replied with finality.

Herbie took a couple of more sips of pop, waited a minute or two, then suggested that Lute look in his cash register and check the bill on top. Lute shrugged his shoulders, figuring he'd pull a five-dollar bill out and wave it at Herbie.

The color drained from his face when he saw the two-dollar bill. He looked sheepishly at Herbie, flashed a smile and said, "Sometimes we do make mistakes here."

Herbie returned three dollars, kept the $1.95 to which he was entitled and grinned from ear to ear.

The look on Lute's face was worth more than the three dollars Herbie wouldn't have enjoyed spending anyhow. And it was good to know that Lute was subject to mistakes, just like everyone else.

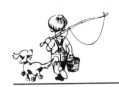

Kindred Spirits Were
in Pine Ridge, Ark.

Folks around Heltonville could relate to "Lum 'n' Abner." That's why you'd find most of them gathered around radios in living rooms at 6:30 each evening in the 1930s and '40s.

"Lum" and "Abner" were the main characters in a network radio show that took listeners on a daily fifteen-minute visit to Pine Ridge, Arkansas. It was a mythical village until Congress changed the name of an Arkansas town from Walters to Pine Ridge.

The show was comedy with realism, and the problems "Lum and Abner" encountered were like many of the tribulations the people around Heltonville faced.

Lum Edwards was played by Chester Lauch, Abner Peabody by Norris Goff. They were college graduates, but they disguised their education. They owned the Jot 'Em Down Store, the social center in Pine Ridge.

Abner liked to whine, gamble, play checkers and trade horses. Lum watched his money more closely. He was stingy and skeptical of almost any scheme Abner mentioned.

Lauch and Goff also were the radio voices of fictional Pine Ridge personalities, men similar to those who gathered at Roberts & Sons general store in Heltonville or C.E. Cummings' store in Norman. Only the names were different. There were: "Dick Huddleston," the postmaster; "Cedric Weehunt," who seldom comprehended what others were up to, and "Grandpappy Spears," who never was at a loss for words and who often beat Abner at checkers. Abner was married to "Lizbeth" and Lum was fond of "Evalena."

Lauch and Goff not only changed their voices to reflect the characters, but they wrote their own scripts and, as was obvious, they ad-libbed to make the conversation more natural. They did it so well a few people around Heltonville were convinced Cedric and Squire and Grandpappy Spears and all the others were real people.

Clem, who knew the show was believable but fictional, was a joker himself. Once when Ezra mentioned he was thinking of saving money to drive down to Pine Ridge to meet Abner and Lum, Clem said that sounded like a good idea.

Then he added, "I'm sorta partial to 'Amos 'n' Andy.' The wife and I may drive out to New York City and see them fellers." Amos and Andy were a couple of radio characters, supposedly in Harlem.

Ezra looked at Clem and replied, "I ain't got nothing in common with them. 'Lum and Abner' are just common folks like the rest of us here."

Clem never did let Ezra know he was being joshed. And Ezra never did save enough money to drive down to Pine Ridge. Clem never made it to New York City to see Amos and Andy, either.

Lovestruck Bugsy
Gets a Slicker Image

Bugsy never paid much attention to his hair or his clothes. Not until he saw Ramona for the first time one February day in the late 1930s.

Bugsy knew she had moved with her parents to a farm near Zelma and that she would be in the fifth grade, too. He watched, eager to see if she was as pretty as he had been told, as she stepped onto the bus. He was impressed. She was even prettier than he had expected her to be.

He was thankful he was wearing a cap, with ear-flaps. They helped hide his hair, hair his mother said looked like it had been combed with a garden rake. It was a mop in search of order. It had no part. What didn't plop over his eyes stood in a cowlick in front.

He looked down at his shoes and wished he had cleaned off the mud. He eased them back under the seat so they wouldn't be so noticeable.

Bugsy returned Ramona's smile, his face reddening in front of her eyes that seemed as big as saucers.

He managed to remember his name, when she told him hers. He stammered through a conversation, broken only by a couple of stops as the bus rumbled over its rural route to Heltonville.

Bugsy had mixed emotions when Ramona turned her attention from him to some others. He wanted her to continue to talk to him, but he needed time to untie his tongue and regain his composure.

It didn't help when he noticed his older sister was watching from the front of the bus. He knew she would kid him later about the attention he was paying to "that new girl."

Ramona was too busy getting acquainted that day to pay much attention to Bugsy. He did notice her looking at some of the boys who lived in town and had hair neatly combed and pressed pants instead of bib overalls.

That afternoon, Ramona smiled at Bugsy as she got off the bus. Bugsy smiled back, thinking about how he could improve his image.

He did his chores, then turned on the radio to listen to "Jack Armstrong, The All-American Boy." His sister came in, handed him a comb and said, "You should spend as much time currying your own hair as you do the horses."

She tried to part Bugsy's hair. It was like trying to divide the wheat in the

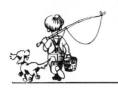

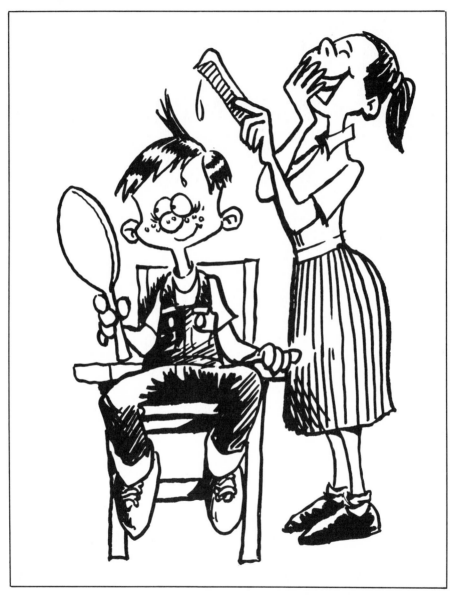

granary. She added water. That helped, but the cowlick wouldn't stay down and the hair still dropped over his forehead.

"You need some hair tonic," she said.

The next day, he ran to Roberts' general store in Heltonville and bought a bottle of hair oil for a quarter when he couldn't find Brilliantine like he had seen the barber use. He rubbed the oil into his dry scalp the next morning and slicked down his hair. His sister took one look and accused him of using a grease gun from the tool shed.

Bugsy just grinned and took another look in the mirror, admiring the straight part and the orderly look.

He used the oil for several days, then quit. His hair again was tousled and his appearance became disheveled.

Bugsy didn't answer when his mother inquired about the change in his appearance. His sister replied for him: "Ramona decided she liked an older boy in the sixth grade better than she did Bugsy."

His mother laughed. "Thank goodness. The oil from his hair was ruining my pillow cases."

She stopped laughing a few days later. Bugsy forgot about Ramona and decided he'd try to impress another girl in his class. And his greasy look returned.

Gambling on a Life
of Rewards, Doubts

Roy pulled his 1938 International truck into the gangway of the empty corn crib and stopped so the tailgate would be near one of the doors. He was delivering a load of 2-12-6 Buhner's "Happy Farmer" fertilizer from the factory at Seymour. Zeke had used the fertilizer for years and wouldn't have been satisfied with any other kind.

"You hand me the bags and I'll carry them to the crib," he told Roy.

Zeke usually took the hardest job, regardless of what was to be done. Chig had noticed that, even though he was only eight or nine at the time.

Chig propped his bike against the crib and offered to help, since his friend Tad wasn't home.

"Maybe in a year or two, my little friend," Zeke replied. "Just sit over there on the seed corn sack and watch."

It took the men the better part of an hour to unload the six tons of fertilizer.

"Pay me when you want," Roy said, calculating the bill in his head.

Zeke wrestled a worn checkbook from a pocket on the chest of his bib overalls. "I'll pay you now, providin' you don't cash the check until day after next. I gotta go into the Stone City Bank and borrow the money tomorrow."

Roy knew Zeke wouldn't have any trouble getting the money from the bank. He had a good reputation and any bank in town would loan him money, just on his word that it'd be repaid.

Roy folded the check, which Zeke had written with a stubby indelible pencil, slipped the check into his billfold and drove away.

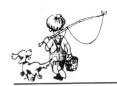

Chig looked confused at the transaction.

Zeke pulled a dusty felt hat from his head, sat down on a bag of the "bonedust," which is what he called fertilizer, and wiped away the sweat with a big blue handkerchief and said: "If you're thinking farmin' is a gamble, you're right."

Chig nodded.

Zeke said, "I ain't a big farmer, but I got a fortune in that bonedust, corn seed, soybean seed and the inoculate for it.

"Now I gotta borrow the money to pay for it. I wait until the last minute, though. Ain't no reason to pay interest any longer than I have to. The banker will wanta give me a line of credit, which would allow me to borrow anytime that I need money. But that's too temptin'. It's sorta like your dad tellin' C.E. Cummings up at Norman to give you candy whenever you go into his store."

Chig's eyes lighted up, just visualizing that possibility.

Zeke grinned. "What I'm doin' is gamblin' that the money I put into the ground will yield enough corn and beans to pay off my bills and bring me some extra cash, too."

Chig wanted to know "what happens if it doesn't?"

"Then, I'll just do my best to pay my debt and scrape by until next year and do the same thing all over again."

Chig made a mental note of what Zeke was saying.

Zeke was an optimist. "You hope you're successful more often than not and usually things turn out better rather than worse.

"And, besides, you leave this earth with what you came in with. Nothin'. The trick is to do something worthwhile when you're here."

Zeke slapped Chig lightly on the shoulders and added, "Better be getting the corn planter cleaned and greased."

Chig climbed on his bicycle and waved at Zeke.

"Maybe I'll gamble on being a farmer when I grow up," he thought to himself.

Cistern Cleaning— a Bit Demeaning!

Tyke should have suspected something when his father asked him one day at noon if he'd like to go for a dip.

"Sure would," the boy said, with mixed emotions. He was eager to have the afternoon off from chopping weeds out of the corn in the new ground, but he was worried that maybe his pa had been out in the hot June sun too long.

He needn't have been concerned about his father. It was then his dad explained where Tyke would be taking a dip—in the cistern under the screened porch of their farmhouse.

"Your mom has been complaining for days about the fact the cistern needs cleaning out. And I've noticed the water has been kind of sour when I try to shave or take a bath."

The cistern was where rainwater collected as it ran off the metal roof of the big house, into the gutter, then the downspouts. Like other farm families in the 1930s, Tyke's folks used the water for baths and to wash clothes. The drinking water came from the spring at the bottom of the hill.

As long as there were frequent rains the water stayed clear and fresh. But once the drought set in, the water began to smell differently. Three or four times a year, it needed to be cleaned, aired and freshened. That's why his dad had asked Tyke to do the chore, explaining he really needed to continue cultivating corn that afternoon.

"You can climb down into the cistern and your brother Tad can pull up with a rope what you clean out."

Tyke complained, "There may be snakes, alligators or all sorts of varmints down there. I could be eaten alive."

It didn't impress his dad, who remembered it had been just a day or two earlier when Tyke had said he wasn't afraid of anything.

After his dad returned to the field, Tyke and Tad carried in a ladder from the woodhouse and removed the heavy limestone cover from the opening over the cistern. Tyke dropped the ladder down into the dark hole, then tied a lantern onto one of the steps to provide some light.

"Here goes," he told Tad, making the last tug on a pair of hip boots. "If I'm not back in twenty minutes call the cops."

It was a line he had stolen from a Humphrey Bogart movie.

He stepped off into about three feet of water and began running a scoop shovel against the solid rock bottom of the cistern. Tad dropped down a five-gallon bucket. Tyke filled a bucket in no time, then had to wait for Tad to pull it up, run with it to the chicken lot and dump the muddy contents.

It took him maybe one and a half to two hours to finish the job. He climbed up the ladder, thinking he was through. But there was still work to do.

His mother walked out just then, reading the *Farmers Guide*. "'To clear water in a cistern, dissolve two pounds of alum in a pail of water,'" she read, then explained the water would appear muddy because Tyke had stirred it up.

She read on, "'Take a pole and stir the water in the cistern vigorously until it is in motion, then pour in the dissolved alum.

"'Take one pound of soda ash and repeat the performance. The chemicals will cause a gelatinous solution to form and settle to the bottom, carrying with it the soot and other material.'"

When she read the *Farmers Guide,* she followed the directions closely. She supervised, while Tad and Tyke carried out the work called for in those

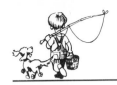

directions.

That evening Tyke's dad smiled and said, "Well, I see the alligators didn't get you, Son."

Tyke disagreed. "They must have. I feel like my bottom is draggin'."

Fake Identities Added to Dating Mischief

One year was nearing an end and some of the teenagers were in the restaurant at Heltonville wondering how to greet the next.

Tom let them talk for a while, then walked over to the table where they were sitting, placed his right foot on the chair and said: "Care to hear a personal experience that happened to me a few years ago?"

No one objected. Tom would have told the story anyhow. He was about thirty, maybe older, and he liked to talk, especially about himself. But he didn't exaggerate.

His listeners knew what he was about to tell them would be the truth.

He sloshed the contents of a Nehi soda in the bottle, watched it for a second, then took a long drink. He swallowed, savored the flavor and started talking:

"You all know Clancy, who is the same age as me. We ran around together all the time when we were teenagers."

The boys nodded. Tom went on:

"One winter we were both dating girls who lived around here. They were a couple years younger than we were and their parents didn't allow them to stay out too late, even on New Year's Eve.

"I had decided to stay home, but Clancy said we didn't have to miss out on some fun even though our girlfriends couldn't be with us. So we decided to go down to Tarry Park that night."

Tarry Park was a community off Ind. 37 between Bedford and Mitchell and was the site of one of the most popular dance halls in the area in the 1930s.

Tom took another drink, grinned at the pleasure he recalled from the past, and added:

"On the way down to Tarry Park, I suggested we not give our own names to any girls we might meet and give the pleasure of our company for the arrival of the New Year. Clancy agreed, saying that was a great idea, that it would keep our girlfriends from ever hearing about it."

Tom's listeners were becoming more curious. He paused for emphasis, then continued, "We met a couple of the cutest little fillies you ever laid your eyes on. I was preparing to introduce myself by a fictitious name when I heard the girl Clancy was with ask him who he was.

"Clancy turned red and stammered. Then you know what he did?"

His listeners shook their heads.

"He gave that girl my name. In full. That made me so mad I said I was Clancy and used his last name.

"After we took the girls home, I asked Clancy why he said he was me. He shrugged his shoulders and said, 'That was the only name I could think of at the time.'"

One of the listeners asked if the boys' girls in Heltonville ever found out about the New Year's Eve dates.

Tom said, "We never knew and we didn't care. We quit dating them and devoted our entire attention to the women we met that night."

"Were they the women you married?" someone asked.

Tom replied, "No, we married girls we met on New Year's a couple of years after that."

"No Chores, No Breakfast"

Chig awoke with a gnawing guilt. Sounds from the kitchen had caused him to sit bolt upright in bed. He had forgotten to load the kitchen stove the night before so his mom could light a fire that morning.

It wasn't a difficult chore. He had other jobs he had to do each night that were more difficult. But it was an important one if breakfast was to be on time.

Chig had learned from experience how to do the job well even though he was only eight or nine on that morning in the late 1930s. He put in newspaper first, then kindling, mostly shavings from old yellow-poplar boards. He added a few corncobs, then three or four sticks of well-seasoned wood.

His mother would awaken early, apply a match to the paper and soon have a hot fire in the stove. In a half-hour or so she would be ready to serve biscuits, gravy, sausage, oatmeal and maybe tenderloin strips if a hog had just been butchered.

Chig had asked once what would happen if he neglected to fix the fire in the range.

"Our breakfast will be late, and you won't have any at all," she replied, believably, it seemed to Chig.

He remembered that conversation as he fidgeted in bed. Breakfast was Chig's favorite meal and he couldn't imagine going to school at Heltonville

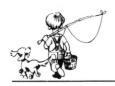

without a big breakfast.

He thought about jumping into his bib overalls and running to the kitchen to do the job belatedly. But he smelled the scent of burning wood and knew it was too late to make amends.

He dressed, tugged on his coat and did his outdoor chores, avoiding conversation with his dad or mom. Breakfast was on the table when he returned, but he didn't sit at the table. He went, instead, into the living room, picked up a school book and started to read.

His mother called from the kitchen, "Aren't you hungry, Son?"

He didn't respond. She came to the door and asked again. He looked embarrassed, but admitted he was hungry. "But you told me I wouldn't get any breakfast if I ever forgot to build the fire," he replied.

She laughed. "Everybody's entitled to be forgetful once. Let's agree that you'll go without breakfast, for sure, if it ever happens again."

Chig sat down and his mom passed the eggs, sausage, biscuits and gravy to him. He savored the breakfast, thankful he had a reprieve, that he was entitled to one mistake.

It was the best meal he ever had, he thought. He fixed the stove that night ...and every night thereafter as long as it was his task to do.

Broom Sedge Put Fire into his Step

Zeb swished a match on the seat of his overalls, watched it burst into a flame and tossed it into the broom sedge. The fire spread quickly across into the tinder-dry pasture, famished, it seemed, for something to devour.

Zeb watched the fire consume the broom sedge, an unsightly weed that was dense enough to paint the pasture in light brown. It was of no value, this broom sedge. It was a pest Zeb feared would choke out the grass which was beginning to grow green as spring approached.

The burning of the broom sedge was a spring ritual with Zeb, as it was with Ben and Clarence and other farmers who lived east of Heltonville in the late 1930s.

It wasn't unusual for the fires to run out of control, cross fence rows and leap over narrow gravel roads that snaked through the rural community.

Each spring when he mentioned he planned to burn off the pasture, Zeb's wife would remind him of the fires that had run rampant in the past. "Be careful," she admonished.

This time, he had chosen a rare March day when there seemed to be little wind. "There will be no wild fire today," he thought.

He had doused two burlap bags in the creek, just in case the fire did threaten to go beyond where he wanted it to go. He walked east, up a ridge, toward the end of the pasture a quarter-mile away, thinking he would beat the blaze.

A slight breeze skipped off his shoulders onto the nape of his weathered neck. It sent a chill down his spine, not from the cold, but from the sudden realization that even a slight wind could whip the fire into a speeding inferno.

Zeb took faster, longer steps, turning to his right to gauge the speed of the fire. It overtook him, and he noticed rabbits run ahead of it to safety.

The fire reached the end of the pasture before Zeb did. The flames lapped first at the weeds and briers at the property line, then at the rail fence.

Zeb panted, exhausted from racing the fire, and tried to smother the blaze with the burlap sacks. The fire won the first round, turning some of the old chestnut rails into ashes.

Zeb gave up battling the fire and instead removed two sections of the fence, leaving a section fifty or so yards long he saw he had no hope of saving.

The rails had been split by Zeb's ancestors, and he hated to see even a few of them burn. He watched the fire die out, then slowly headed to the house, there to confess to his wife he had again let the fire in the broom sedge outsmart him.

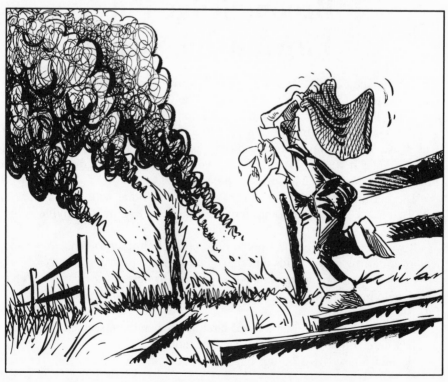

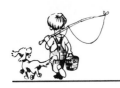

It was the last time, though. A few days later he asked the county agent how to get rid of the broom sedge. Then Zeb had lime and fertilizer spread over the pasture. The grass then grew thick, and the broom sedge never appeared again.

Tradition had given way to progress. But Zeb admitted, on rare occasions, he missed fighting the fire. But even his wife couldn't tell whether or not he was serious.

By Gum, That Log Was a Wiggler!

Lukey lived beside one of the creeks that meandered up through the hollows near Heltonville.

Some folks thought he was a ne'er-do-well, but they tended to judge a man by how hard he worked and how clean and neat he kept his property.

Lukey was content being Lukey. He didn't want to be anyone else and he never asked the world to stop so he could get on. He liked his independent isolation just fine and if he cared what others thought he never let on.

No one ever seemed to know how he made ends meet. But it was the 1930s and a lot of people had learned to stay healthy on a diet of salt pork and beans and whatever wild game they could shoot.

Lukey didn't have much: a little cabin among the trees, a crosscut saw, an ax and a minimum of ambition. He didn't use his ambition much more than he did the crosscut saw and the ax.

He split only what wood his wife would burn in the kitchen range and left the rest in big blocks he could shove through the door on the steel drum that had been converted into a heating stove.

It had been a routine Lukey had followed for years. He knew about how much wood he'd need and cut only that much.

He hadn't counted on a really bad winter, which came for a visit in December and stayed and stayed, like an unwelcome visitor who refused to leave. The temperatures were well below freezing for days, and the stove consumed chunk after chunk of wood.

Lukey took inventory of what wood was left and decided he'd ration it and, instead, carry in long pieces he hadn't gotten around to cutting. He lugged in a gum log, which would have been hard to cut anyhow, and poked one end into the stove.

The gum was eight feet long and about the size of a cross tie. Lukey would, he thought, shove the log into the stove as the end in the fire burned.

The fire had lapped at the log for maybe a half-hour when Lukey's wife, a trembling hand over her speechless mouth, pointed nervously to the log.

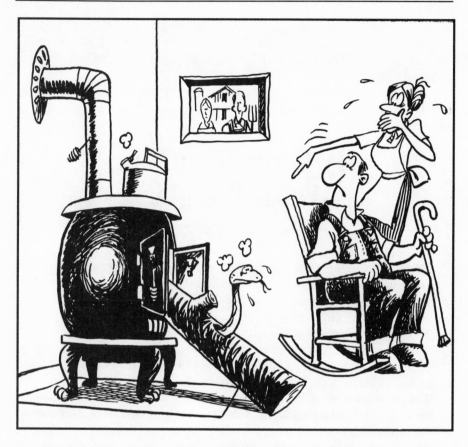

Lukey spied immediately what had frightened her. A big copperhead, thawed by the heat, was slithering from what it thought would be its winter-long bed inside the log.

Lukey trapped the snake with his cane and saw to it the copperhead didn't live to see spring or even nightfall.

A day or two later, the temperature warmed and Lukey and his wife were outside, one on each end of the crosscut saw, cutting logs into pieces of wood that would fit into the stove.

Lukey would never again leave a log sticking out the door of the stove. And he would cut enough wood to last the entire winter, no matter how cold it stayed.

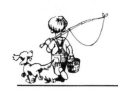

For Ben, New Deal
Was a Good Deal

Ben didn't like Franklin Roosevelt or any of his make-work projects. Ben would return home storming mad every time he traveled to Bedford on U.S. 50 from 1938 to 1940.

He'd rant and rave to his neighbor, Wes, after each visit. "Dern nincompoops," he'd bellow. "Never saw such cockamamie in my life."

Wes knew the "nincompoops" were bosses who supervised WPA workers at Otis Park at the east edge of Bedford. "Cockamamie" was what Ben thought of the ideas thought up to provide the men work during the Great Depression.

Ben would describe in detail what he had seen, then hiss, "Doubleyou ...Pea ...Aye." That meant WPA. He would then add his own definition of the acronym: "We Piddle Around."

Sometimes he'd complain about work being done on the golf course: "Just a playground for some rich folks in town."

Sometimes he'd gripe about expansion of the swimming pool: "A place for young people to walk around half-nude."

Sometimes he'd mention work on the picnic grounds: "Ain't no need to eat outdoors as long as you have a table in the kitchen."

Sometimes he raised a fuss about the two-mile stone fence being built around the park: "Don't need a fence. Ain't no livestock in the park."

But his biggest criticism came in 1939 when he learned WPA workers would build a limestone band shell in the park. "Silliest dang thing I ever heard," Ben said, pulling his felt hat from his head to let out the steam he'd built up.

"They'll have some musicians in fancy clothes play music none of us understand. Somebody should tell 'em we like music played on guitars and banjos by some boys in overalls on the back of a flatbed truck."

The band shell was dedicated that summer by Mayor Henry S. Murray, who said it would endure for at least three hundred years.

Wes teased Ben, saying, "If it lasts that long, we ought to get our money's worth."

Ben snorted, "We'll never get our money back. We pay taxes and Franklin D. Roosevelt gives the money to people to work on projects that'll never do us any good. How you figure we'll ever get $1 million worth of benefits from that?"

Wes ignored the question, knowing Ben wouldn't wait for an answer anyhow.

"I'm telling you, Wes, we been paying people to do work we don't need done," Ben continued.

Wes looked him in the eye and said, "You signed up for acreage allotments for your farm, didn't you?"

Ben nodded.

"Well, you've been getting checks for not planting corn and sowing wheat, haven't you?" Wes asked.

Ben nodded again, reluctantly this time.

Wes finished his point. "Let me put it this way. The WPA is paying men to work. You and me are getting paid not to plant crops. Which means we're getting paid not to work. Now tell me who's getting the best deal?"

Ben didn't respond, except to say he'd best be going home.

They Had a Language All Their Own

Isolated by economics and distance, some folks in sections of Southern Indiana had a language all their own in the 1930s. They had preserved the dialect of their ancestors and added colorful phrases and expressions of their own.

It was a time of the Great Depression, and many of them seldom traveled more than thirty miles from home. Except for the radio, there were few outside influences on the way they talked.

Their children learned to eliminate some of the slang in school, but respect for their elders kept them from trying to change their parents' use of words. And besides, youngsters learned quickly that the way people talked had little to do with their intelligence.

Grownups could cipher big numbers in their head, grow crops on poor land, make soap and find happiness without wealth.

It was no different around Heltonville. Barbershops, general stores, and feed mills were good places to listen to farmers talk. Uninhibited by formality, they tossed around slang as easily as they did grain in a scoop shovel. They talked mostly about men, sometimes in humor, sometimes in anger.

"He ain't worth the powder it'd take t'blow him up," one would say. Another would add, "He ain't worth the salt that goes in his bread." And someone else would call him "an ornery old coot."

A stingy fellow was "so tight he squeaks worse than a cheap pair of new shoes." They referred to a lazy farmer, who never said much or tried to fight his way out of his misery, as one who "ain't got no gumption."

There were assorted terms for the dense and slow: "He couldn't find his bottom with both hands." "His attic ain't never been finished." "He ain't got

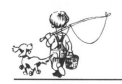
enough sense to have a fit." "The top bricks on his chimney have been damaged." Or, "He couldn't find a steeple in a cornfield."

Anyone impressed with his own importance thought "the sun rises to hear him crow." An arrogant person would "strut like a peacock" and someone would always want to "buy him for what he's worth and sell him for what he thinks he's worth."

A farmer would come in looking perplexed and explain, "I've got the jim-jams," which meant he was depressed and out of sorts. He might trip over a sack of feed and declare, "I'm as awkward today as a pregnant sow on ice." If someone suggested he sit down and take it easy, he'd reply, "I mize well," which meant he may as well.

The weather was a good topic for colorful slang. It could be "hotter than the hinges of hell," "hotter than a fox in a forest fire," or colder than various parts of a well-driller's anatomy. Clouds could mean "a real toad strangler," "a gullywasher" or a "goose drownder" was on the way.

Anything or any person that was a pest, a big bother or irritating was called a "joner." Frustrating problems or chores could be "joners," too. "Joner" may have been shortened from "Jonaher," but nobody seemed to know for sure.

Anyone who disagreed with a comment might be told, "If you don't like it, lump it." A youngster who spoke up with an opinion that didn't set well with the older men was sometimes told, "You're born, but you ain't dead yet." That meant he still had a lot to learn.

The men would leave one at a time, telling the others, "be seein' you'ns." The others would reply, "Not if we see you'ns first."

* * *

Postscript: Television and transportation have diminished the size of America and now rural and urban folks use the same language. And the color has gone from most conversations.

Back Creek Men Taught Life Lessons

It wasn't much of a road, less than four miles long, a link between Ind. 58 and U.S. 50. Most folks called it Back Creek Road. A few referred to it as Possum Hollow Road.

It has a number now, which isn't nearly as descriptive. And it has been blacktopped and widened, a concession to motorists.

In the 1930s and '40s the road was a mixture of creek gravel and crushed stone that pinged the undersides of cars in a clanging melody.

The road was straight and smooth for about a mile south of Ind. 58. Then it went down into a narrow valley and back up another 45-degree grade before following a cut into the hills and dropping back into Back Creek bottom.

The ten men who lived on Back Creek Road were as rugged as it was. They were as different in character as the terrain the road covered.

Boys who grew up among those men learned from each of them, gaining wisdom they could use in whatever highways they chose to travel after leaving Back Creek Road.

They learned from Roy, a trucker and farmer, a man who made frequent trips to the stockyards in Indianapolis. Roy knew a lot about life outside Heltonville and Norman, and shared what he knew with anyone who cared to listen.

Roy knew the value of fun and laughter.

Wes, who lived down the road, knew the importance of hard work and the pursuit of excellence in whatever he tried to do. He worked at the stone mill from 4:00 p.m. to midnight but was always the first farmer out in the field the next morning.

He taught the boys the work ethic, honesty and integrity.

Thornt lived on a little plot of ground, raising a big family by working in town or wherever he could find a job.

He showed the boys there was more to life than a big house and a fine car. He taught them they could have self-respect regardless of how poor they might be.

Clyde lived a quarter-mile south of Thornt. Most of the time he had a steady job in town. When he wasn't working there, he helped on the farms as a hired hand.

He was outspoken. He taught the boys to have an opinion and to express it.

Oval lived across the road on a place he farmed when he wasn't working in town. Oval didn't seem to let many things bother him, knowing what didn't get done one day would still be there to do the next. He'd just as soon stop and talk as he would to go on working.

The boys learned patience from him.

Saul, who was Clyde's father, lived in a little house down in the valley. He shared the wisdom of his age with the boys. The peace he had found within himself was evident to them.

Willie, his other son, lived just down the road. Willie was the boss of a crew of timbercutters. Willie worked hard, played hard and, occasionally, it was said, got the two mixed up.

But Willie taught the boys that life was to live ...within certain guidelines.

The Wrays lived back off the road in the fertile bottoms. There were Wes, the father, and Smith and Harry, his sons. They lived quiet lives as shepherds of stock and stewards of the soil, and anyone was a better person for having known them.

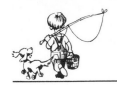

There were other men down the road the boys didn't know as well, but each added to a storehouse of wisdom that would last a lifetime.

The men are all gone from the road now. Each year, the leaves on the trees along Back Creek Road take on their fall brilliance. But the characters who once lived there were more colorful.

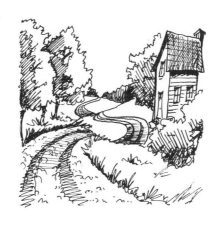

GROWING UP

Winter Is "Recess" for Young and Old

Ben was a man at peace with his environment. He had learned, over seventy-plus years, that life was a series of peaks and valleys. Good, he knew, usually followed bad.

Ben had spent his adult life on a little farm east of Heltonville, working with a team of horses after most of his neighbors had bought powerful Farmall, John Deere, and Allis-Chalmers tractors.

There was no point, he reasoned, to adapt to the new. The shadows were lengthening on his life and his days were too short to spend them learning new ways. He kept busy, though, working and thinking, often doing both at the same time.

One of those times came on a mid-winter Saturday about 1940 when the temperature was in the single digits. He had hitched his horses to a sled and used it to bring two shocks of fodder from the snow-covered cornfield to the barn.

He tugged the shocks into the gangway, unhitched and unharnessed the team. It didn't bother him when Tad walked up while he was talking to the horses. Horses, he often said, understood him better than most people.

Ear-flaps dangled from Ben's cap. He wore a denim jacket over overalls and a flannel shirt. His yellow and gray gloves had double thumbs so they could be worn on either hand. A buckle was missing from each of his high-top overshoes.

Ben nodded, friendly-like, when he turned and saw Tad. "Fixin' to shuck the corn," he said, nodding to the stalks in the barn. "You might just as well sit and gab with me while I work." Tad was a neighbor. He was just eleven years old, but Ben made him feel like an adult.

Ben fitted a shucking hook over the glove on his right hand, stooped down on his knees, and started husking the ears from the stalks. He flipped each ear toward a feed bin, seldom making an errant toss. He stopped once, holding a big ear in one hand, a nubbin in the other.

"These two ears are like life," he said. "Some things turn out well, others not so good."

One of the horses snorted, emitting a cloud of steam. A cow bellowed softly.

Tad eyed the two ears and nodded to acknowledge he understood. He hunkered down into his jacket against the cold and said, "Seems like a long time until spring."

Ben looked up, stopped for a moment, and said, "Don't rush through life, son. Enjoy each minute you can. Winter ain't all that bad. It's a time to rest up

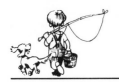

from the year that's done past and get ready for the year that's a-comin'.' "

Tad didn't respond. Ben went on. "Just think of it as a half-time of a basketball game. It's a time to stop and take a look at where you've been and where you're headed."

Tad said, "Sort of like a recess at school, huh?"

Ben nodded and continued to separate the corn from the stalks. When he finished, he carried some of the fodder to the mangers in the barn. The animals wasted no time sampling it.

Tad tugged the collar of his coat around his neck and pulled the sock cap over his ears.

"Guess I'd better be headin' home," he said.

He walked to the big doors at the end of the barn, then walked back to where Ben was. "Reckon the cold winter weather will make us enjoy spring more," he said.

Ben nodded. A grin crept across his wrinkled face. It had been a morning well spent. He could have done the work anytime. An opportunity to share his knowledge with a youngster was rare.

Grandma's Maple Candy Was Sugar-lickin' Good

The good times came for Mrs. J. after the work was done at the sugar house. The sap had been boiled into syrup and poured into pails. Most of it would be sold to customers from town, who would soon come, each to buy a gallon, maybe more.

The rest wasn't for sale. Not at any price. It was Mrs. J.'s personal stock, and it would be used to bring smiles to her grandchildren, who came each weekend to find treats no general store carried.

Mrs. J. was stooped at the shoulders and her silver hair was pulled back into a bun. She looked older than she was. Years of hard work on the farm near Heltonville had done that to her.

Her hands shook, letting the teacup chatter against the saucer when she carried her coffee to the table to sit for brief spells on busy mornings. An apron covered the print dresses she wore, giving her a place to rub the palms of her hands as she worked in the kitchen. A big smile covered her face, hiding six decades of hardship.

Her grandchildren hadn't yet been told about her being widowed young and raising her children, these youngsters' parents, alone. All the youngsters knew was the happiness she gave them, especially each March in the 1930s.

She would wait until they showed up on Saturday morning to pry the lid off a pail, pour some of the syrup in a pan, and heat it over the wood stove. She then beat the warm syrup and poured it into a muffin tin.

The grandkids watched as she placed the filled muffin tin outdoors to cool. It would take some time for the syrup to harden, but the wait would be worth it. There were magazines like *Collier's, Saturday Evening Post, Country Gentleman,* and *Farm Journal* to read while they waited.

Their eyes glanced up from their reading frequently until she brought in the first pan, turned it upside-down, and banged it against the table top. The sugar cakes fell out, round and unbroken. Mrs. J. handed one to each of the youngsters.

They ate slowly, savoring each nibble, extending the preciousness of the moment. Mrs. J. handed each of her visitors two more cakes as they left.

Tad, who was six, maybe seven, would take one of his to school in his lunchbox the next Monday. He would make sure some of his pals saw it. They had turned down his efforts in the past when he tried to trade a fresh tenderloin sandwich for a Milky Way, Tootsie Roll, or Mr. Goodbar they brought with their peanut butter and jelly sandwiches.

This time things would be different. He slowly removed the sugar cake from the wax paper, making sure the others watched.

"Grandma made it," he said, holding it up between his thumb and index finger.

Someone said, "Trade you these caramels for it."

Tad shook his head.

Don offered a Three Musketeers bar.

Tad turned that down.

Tad licked the top, then the bottom just to show the sugar cake wasn't for sale. Then he broke it in two. He could taunt them again the next day with the other half.

They had the last laugh, though. Mrs. J. made another batch when Tad mentioned the following Saturday what he had done. She broke the cakes into quarters, wrapped them up, and handed them to Tad.

"Take these to school Monday. And learn to share with others what joy you get in life," she said gently.

A Windy Kid on a Windy Day

Gordy carried a knife in one overall pocket, a string in the other, a smile on his face, and endless imagination in his head.

He was never at a loss for words. The knife let him win games of mum-

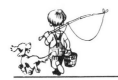

bletypeg and carve an assortment of items he used to amuse himself despite the isolation of his farm home.

He seldom came to school at Heltonville on Monday mornings without stories about what he'd done over the weekend. One Monday, he'd made a bean flipper. The next week he'd tell about making a bow from a hickory sapling and arrows from sassafras shoots.

He seemed even more excited than usual one Monday after a windy March weekend. He couldn't wait for William Wright to dismiss the fourth-grade class for morning recess so he could tell all his buddies.

"Made me a kite Saturday," he told Cecil and Tad.

They waited, knowing he'd continue his monologue without being asked. "Cut two sticks about this round," he said, holding up the little finger on his right hand.

"Peeled off the bark and measured the sticks so one would be just a mite longer than the other. Then I notched each where they crossed, the longer one up, the shorter one across," he said, not hesitating between words.

Cecil and Tad tried to visualize what he was describing.

"Then I tied some heavy string from one corner to the other, sorta forming one triangle at the top and one at the bottom. Once that was done, I found me a big piece of brown paper that had been wrapped around some bologna Dad brought home from the general store," he added.

Cecil and Tad were anxious to toss a softball around, but Gordy kept talking.

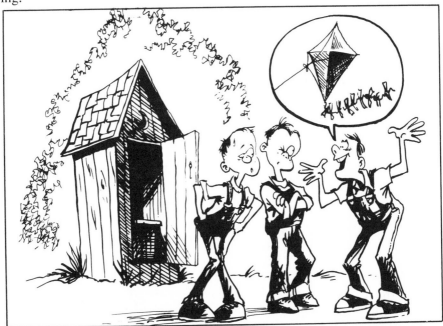

"Folded the paper over the string and pasted it down."

Cecil wanted to know what he'd used for paste.

"Made it from flour and water," Gordy answered.

Cecil and Tad had made flour paste before. They knew it would hold the creased, brown paper snugly.

Gordy caught his breath and continued, "Once the paste dried, I took some crayons and decorated the paper. Even signed my name like an artist would down at the bottom."

Tad asked if he added a tail to the kite.

"Yep," Gordy said. "Took a bunch of rags Mom was saving to make a quilt. Tied 'em together for about six feet, then added a pair of socks at the end."

Tad and Cecil fidgeted from one foot to the other, knowing recess would end before they had a chance to go to the outdoor toilet if Gordy didn't finish his story soon.

"Then I tied on the string and lifted the kite up into the wind," Gordy said proudly. "It was the best homemade kite I ever saw."

Cecil said, "Well, how did it fly?"

The excitement faded from Gordy's face. "I don't know," he replied. "I never did get it off the ground. Musta been too windy. It just kept flopping in the wind, then nose-diving into the ground. It did that until I got tired of running and quit trying."

His friends laughed. Gordy was unperturbed. "The fun was in making it," he yelled, following them to the outhouse.

Farm Life Was Like Fun in the Park

Bunky had looked forward to late April when he'd be free for the summer. He had been in school for eight months, and he was weary of the daily regimentation.

Like most eight-year-old boys in the late 1930s, he was as restless as a gnat. He lived in Heltonville and had explored the hills and hollows in town until there was little new for him to discover.

After a few days, conversations at the barber shop seemed the same. The excitement of watching the freight trains pass through waned. Games of tag and andy-over became routine.

Bunky jumped at the chance when Tad suggested he spend a day on Tad's family's farm east of town.

"Go ahead," his mom said. "It'll be a new experience."

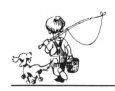

Even she would have been surprised at the experiences that awaited Bunky. Bunky had just arrived at the farm and propped his Western Flyer bike on the kickstand when Tad yelled, "Come on. We're going to ring some pigs."

Bunky watched over the woven-wire fence, his fingers stuck in his ears, as Tad's father put the rings in the noses of the squealing pigs. The rings, which actually were wire triangles, would keep the pigs from rooting the ground in the hog lot, Tad explained.

Once that job was done, Tad's father hooked the disc to the tractor and · asked the boys if they'd like to ride on the draw-bar as he worked the soil.

The dust covered Bunky's clean clothes, but he didn't seem to mind. He looked at home on the tractor.

They rode for a while before Tad mentioned some wild strawberries might be ripe in the woods next to the field. They found the patch, but no ripe berries.

"Betcha we can find some mushrooms, though," Tad said. Then he walked to a poplar tree and spotted some big, yellow morels.

"Eat these raw?" Bunky asked.

Tad laughed, then told him he'd have to wait until they were fried by his mom.

They walked back toward the house, a dozen big mushrooms in Tad's striped railroader's cap. The boys paused on the hillside to watch a colt romp awkwardly after its mother.

Bunky almost ate his weight at dinner, savoring his share of the mushrooms. It was his first farmer's meal. There would be more in the summer ahead.

He spent the afternoon on the farm. He and Tad curried the horses, drank warm milk from the cream separator, and slopped the pigs, which already had grown used to the rings in their noses.

Bunky looked tired, but still excited, as he rode off on his bicycle.

"Come back anytime," Tad's mother told him.

It was an invitation Bunky had hoped for. He returned often. He watched as the horses' hooves sank into the finely worked soil as they pulled the corn planter.

He helped put up hay, harvest wheat, mow fence rows, hoe in the garden and build fence. He learned to milk cows. And in the afternoons, he splashed in a pocket of water that formed a swimming hole in the creek.

He saw the corn grow from seed to stalks and watched the ears form. He noticed how quickly the pigs grew and observed how the once-ungainly colt had become graceful.

All that was new to Bunky, but not to Tad, who mentioned one day he wished he lived near a park in town close to a playground.

Bunky grinned. "This entire farm is a playground. Ain't nothing like this in any park I've ever seen."

Tad knew he was right. The farm was his personal park. It just took his young friend from town to let him know how fortunate he was.

He'd Been Born but He Wasn't Dead Yet

Chig was at that age when he thought he had learned about all there was to know. It was a stage most ten-year-olds go through.

He listened impatiently when his dad tried to tell him something. When Chig seemed disinterested, his dad would utter a mild profanity and declare, "Son, you're born but you ain't dead yet."

Which meant there were still a lot of things the boy had to learn about life.

Chig nodded, knowingly and smugly, when his dad tried to tell him how to dismount from a moving vehicle. A farm boy needed to know how to jump off a hay wagon or a farm truck picking up tomato hampers.

"Ain't nothing to it," Chig replied.

His dad knew Chig would have to find out for himself, perhaps painfully.

Part of that pain was obvious one April afternoon in 1939 when Chig walked down the county road from Ind. 58 east of Heltonville. He was bloodied and battered. The patches on the knees of his overalls were torn and gravel dust covered most of his body.

"Looks like you been chewed up by a rock crusher," his dad said. The tears welled up in the corners of Chig's eyes, but he didn't cry. His dad suggested he sit down and tell him what happened.

Chig began slowly. "Well, I was walkin' up 58 from Billy's house when Andy stopped and said, 'Jump on the runnin' board and I'll take you up to the corner.'"

Andy lived in Norman and drove a 1935 Ford.

Chig went on, "Well, I hopped on and gripped the inside of the door. I thought Andy would stop and let me off. Instead, he says, 'I'll slow down to about five miles an hour and you can jump off. That way I won't have to stop completely.'"

His dad bit his right index finger. He wanted to laugh and feel compassion at the same time. "Go on," he said.

Chig tried to brush the dirt from his overalls, but the cuts on his hands were too painful. "Well, he slowed down and I jumped off at a right angle. I felt like I was on a Ferris wheel and merry-go-round at the same time. Seemed like I was running sideways and forward all at once.

"Before I knew it, I was nose-down in the gravel. If Andy saw what hap-

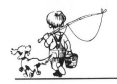

pened, he didn't bother to back up and see if I was OK."

His mom came out and used a wash cloth to clean Chig's wounds and coat them with iodine and Mercurochrome.

A few days later, his dad taught Chig how to jump off a moving wagon. "Always jump forward and hit the ground running in the same direction as the wagon. Otherwise, you'll fall for sure. The faster the car or wagon you're on is moving the faster you'll need to run."

Chig learned quickly. Or so it seemed.

A few weeks later, he walked down the road, holding his left arm like it was in pain. He started talking before his dad could ask what had happened.

"Tried to hop the train outta Heltonville. I just stuck out my right arm and grabbed on to one of those iron bars at the back of a boxcar."

"Darn near jerked my arm off. I held on, though, and made a perfect exit by running forward into the grass up by Zelma."

His dad said, "Tomorrow I'll start teaching you how to board a moving vehicle."

Chig dropped his arm and started laughing. "I just made that up. I didn't try to hop a freight car. But if I did, I'd know you had to run along beside it before you tried to jump on."

His dad grinned and patted Chig on the back. "Good thinkin', Son. Just don't tell your ma you fibbed to me."

Chig looked down at the scars on the palm of his hand that remained from his bout with the gravel when he'd leaped from Andy's car.

There were other things he would learn for himself later. But he thought at the time he would listen to his dad in the future.

He did for a couple of weeks. But he didn't pay any attention to how his dad told him to load a hay wagon. He lost half the bales before he reached the barn.

His dad started to bellow, but he laughed instead when Chig looked up from reloading the hay and said: "Like you said, Pa, I've been born, but I ain't dead yet."

Lads Flipped Over Homemade Weapons

A bean flipper stuck in a hip pocket gave a boy a sense of importance. No youngster in the late 1930s would have been without one when winter surrendered to spring and the outdoors offered adventure limited only by a lack of imagination.

Some people called them slingshots, but to boys around Heltonville they

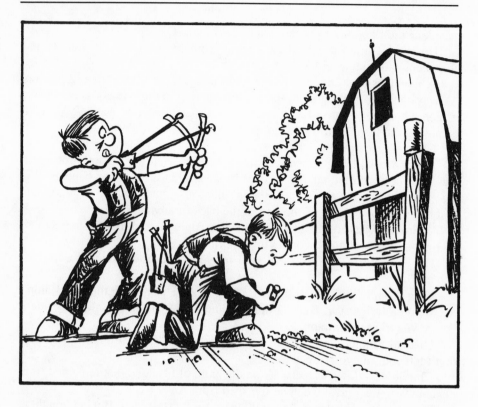

were bean flippers, weapons to be used to propel beans, pebbles and other missiles. The flippers could be bought at the store, but the manufactured ones weren't as good as those fashioned by the boys themselves.

An eight-year-old with a knife and any skill at all could make one. At least Chig and his friends had no trouble making them.

The first thing they looked for was a stock shaped like a Y, which could be found on almost any hickory sapling. An ideal stock had a base about three-quarters of an inch in diameter with the yoke shaped evenly. Once the stock was found, the bark was removed and rings cut around the two prongs an inch down from the top.

Then from an old inner tube the boys cut strips five-eighths of an inch wide and about twenty-four inches long. The boys then needed pieces of leather which would form the seat for the missile. Chig found the tongue of a shoe to be the best possible kind of leather. It was soft and pliable and easily cut to a two-by-three-inch rectangle.

A slit was cut into each end of the leather and the rubber strips inserted about an inch, and tied securely. The other ends were then placed in the cuts made in the prongs of the fork and anchored with the string.

Once the flippers were made, they were tested immediately. Chig liked to

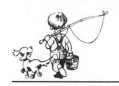

shoot rocks against the metal roof on the barn and listen for the echoes to carom off the hills in the distance. The pigeons scattered, scared by the noise.

Tad aimed at a Velvet tobacco can on a fence post. He missed.

The boys were testing their flippers when Chunky rode up on his bicycle. He had a big grin on his face as he pulled a slingshot from his pocket. "See this?" he asked.

It was a question that needed no answer.

"Came from a store in Bedford," Chunky said proudly.

Tad and Chig weren't impressed. "Doesn't look very strong," Chig said.

The fork was shaped from three strands of heavy wire coiled around each other. The flipper wasn't anything like the ones Tad and Chig had made.

"Try it out," Tad said.

"Done so already," Chunky replied. He fired a shot against the barn. The rock he used plunked off the side, almost lazily.

"That ain't nothing. Pull it back as far as it'll go and let loose," Chig said.

Chunky picked up a piece of gravel and pulled the rubber pieces as far back as he could. One piece of the rubber flipped loose from a prong, leaving Chunky with the fork in one hand and the rest of the flipper in the other.

He looked kind of embarrassed, wrapped the rubber around the fork, shoved it in his pocket and said: "Didn't like the dang thing, anyhow."

Chig and Tad wasted no time helping him make one as sturdy as theirs.

Every Sunday Was Grandma J.'s Day

If Grandma J. knew it was Mother's Day, she never let on. She was too busy at her home farm near Heltonville.

It was just another Sunday to her. There were chores to be done. . . cows to be milked, cream to be separated, livestock to be fed. And cakes, pies and cookies to be made.

Her son and three daughters, and their big families, would be there later. She would be disappointed if they didn't show up for dinner, even though it meant hours of preparation on her part. She expected them all to visit after church at least one Sunday each month in the late 1930s.

Mrs. J. didn't go to church very often. It wasn't that she wasn't religious. Church just didn't fit into her routine. And she didn't care for formalities. Sometimes her daughters would urge her to attend services with them, but she always had an excuse.

She got her religious inspiration by reading some of the Scriptures each evening by lamplight. It gave her something to think about before she dropped off to sleep.

By the time her "brood" arrived on Mother's Day Sunday, she had two tables set, one for the grownups, one for the kids.

Years of hard work had stooped her shoulders and slowed her step. She resented any implication she couldn't take care of herself, or her guests, just because she was old. Her daughters knew better than to bring dishes for dinner. She would have been offended.

When one of the daughters offered the bouquet she received at church for having the most children present, Mrs. J. said, "I have all the flowers I need. You just take that home and enjoy it."

She insisted all her guests be seated and eat, bringing out dish after dish for them to pass around. She didn't sit down until she made sure all the food had been served.

Later, she declined when her daughters insisted she relax and let them wash the dishes. Enjoying the conversation, she dried dishes while they washed.

It wasn't until all the work was done that she sat down in her easy chair in the big living room. The youngsters were outside, the girls sunning in the yard, the boys playing hide and seek in the big barn. It was a special moment, a time to enjoy. No words were needed to accent the joy of togetherness.

She nodded off from time to time, but her guests didn't mind. She deserved a few moments of rest. And it meant they, too, could doze off briefly.

The stillness didn't last long. The youngsters came bounding into the house and Mrs. J. rubbed her eyes and headed back to the kitchen. She knew they were ready for more of her chocolate cake.

Afterward, the men agreed it was time to leave for home. "The cows will be waiting to be milked," one of them said.

Mrs. J. insisted she share the leftovers with each of them. Each daughter thanked her with a big hug. It was not until then that they wished her a happy Mother's Day.

She looked both embarrassed and pleased as they departed. After all, she reasoned, every Sunday is Mother's Day when your son and daughters and grandchildren make you feel important . . . needed, even if you were old and bent with age.

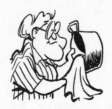

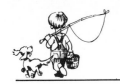
Graves Awaken Boys' Dreams of the Frontier

In an earlier time, May 30 would have been Decoration Day. Later, it would have been Memorial Day. But times change, Congressmen seek longer and longer weekends, and traditional holidays are moved to Mondays.

It was May 30 in the late 1930s when Dale and Tad explored the grave sites in what had once been a family plot. There were four, maybe five tombstones in the tiny abandoned cemetery, not more than a hundred yards or so from Dale's house.

Some people said it was the Frank Hunter family graveyard. Others called it the Fullen Cemetery, probably because it was near where the old one-room Fullen school had stood.

Whatever its name, few people came to remember the dead, or for any other reason. Time had darkened the limestone monuments to dark gray, but the two boys could still read the faded dates and letters. For them, the graveyard was a history book. The tombstones were the page markers.

There was the grave of Francis Hunter: "Born April 16, 1801. Died Jan. 23, 1885."

Dale and Tad imagined what it had been like almost 140 years earlier when Francis Hunter was born and what he had done as a boy their age. They visualized the white man meeting the Indians, settling on the land and clearing the giant poplars, changing woods into fields.

They would learn later their imaginations were short of reality. Francis Hunter, who was called Frank, had married Jane Harper, the daughter of Jennie Roundtree, a Cherokee Indian princess.

Frank and Jane had met when an Indian tribe camped by the falls in a creek that cut through the farm where Frank grew up. And they had lived in a log cabin on the site where Dale's grandparents lived. Jane was buried in the cemetery, too.

William F. Hunter had served in the Civil War with Company A of the 97th Indiana Infantry Regiment. A small American flag was on his grave, and on the spot where Madison Clampitt, another war veteran, was buried.

Clampitt had married Minerva Hunter and served in the Army when the United States waged war with Mexico in the late 1840s. The boys assumed Minerva and William were brother and sister and that Frank and Jane were their parents.

Dale and Tad knew little about history, but that didn't stop them from recreating battles in their minds, and images of Clampitt coming home to Minerva to resume life in the wilderness. They could imagine giant trees on the hills being felled and logs being shaped into new timbers for a home, corn being planted in fields newly cleared by oxen, water being carried from a nearby spring and the face of a wilderness being slowly hewed into what would be called civilization.

Now forgotten were the efforts of those who had given new shape to the small world Dale and Tad knew. Only the monuments stood as reminders of who these pioneers were and when they lived.

Neither boy said much as they stood lost in time. Their solitude was broken by a voice from the back door of Dale's house.

"Dinner time," his mom yelled.

The boys' thoughts returned to the present. But those thoughts would return, especially on Decoration Days to come, to the little cemetery. And Dale and Tad would return, too, from time to time, each for his own private memorial.

No One Could Match Indy's "Wild Bill"

Tad was never quite sure why he chose "Wild Bill" Cummings as a hero. Maybe it was because his mother's maiden name was Cummings. Maybe it was because his older brothers idolized the race driver. Maybe it was because "Wild Bill" was a Hoosier.

Whatever the reason, Tad was no older than five or six when he picked Cummings as his favorite driver. Tad acted out the part of the driver himself, sitting behind the steering wheel of a 1929 Overland, moving his lips in an attempt to create the sound of a race car he had never heard.

"Wild Bill" had won the Indianapolis 500-Mile Race in 1934, and no one had been happier than Tad's father and older brothers. They often talked about Cummings, especially each May before Decoration Day.

They'd never been to a race. The Great Depression kept them from saving enough money to buy tickets. But it didn't keep them from reading about the races or about the men who drove in them.

They shared stories about the drivers with the men who gathered at the general stores, blacksmith shops and feed stores in Heltonville and Norman. By 1936, Tad was seven, old enough to try to absorb all of what was said about "Wild Bill."

He heard the stories about how Cummings had become interested in speed when he rode a motorcycle on his first job as a grocery delivery boy in Indianapolis. And how Cummings became one of the best drivers around the dirt tracks of America.

When Tad asked how Cummings got the nickname "Wild Bill," he was told a lot of different stories. Some men said it came from the way Cummings

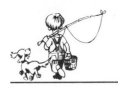

rode his motorcycle, some said it was the fearless way he drove.

But no one knew for sure. And "Wild Bill" never explained the origin, Tad's brothers said. At least not in any interviews they had read.

Cummings had followed up his 1934 victory with a third-place finish in 1935, but his fortunes turned sour in 1936. He didn't complete a lap and was the first driver out of the race.

"Clutch problem," one of Tad's brothers explained.

That didn't change how Tad felt about "Wild Bill." Tad was old enough to read the sports page of the *Bedford Daily Mail* a year later. He scanned the brief items from the Indianapolis Motor Speedway under an Indianapolis dateline each day, looking for any tidbit about "Wild Bill."

His brothers told him "Wild Bill's" luck was sure to change for the 1937 race. "It has to after last year," one of them said.

They were right. "Wild Bill" qualified at 123.343 MPH to start the '37 race from the pole position in the Boyle Products Special.

The dry cell battery on the family radio was too weak for Tad to listen to the race. It wasn't until that night he heard Cummings had finished sixth, despite completing the entire 200 laps.

"There's always next year," one of Tad's brothers said.

Cummings started from the sixteenth position in 1938 and went out of the race with radiator trouble on the seventy-second lap.

Tad thought to himself, "Next year, maybe."

But there would be no next year. "Wild Bill" Cummings died the following February after his passenger car crashed through a guardrail not far from his home southeast of Indianapolis.

There would be other drivers and other 500-Mile Races. But there would never be another "Wild Bill" Cummings. At least as far as Tad was concerned.

Farm Fathers Needed No Annual "To-do"

They had names like Jake, Wes, Ben, Homer, Roy, Clyde, Clarence, Joe, Oval and George. They were farmers and husbands.

And fathers, too. Fathers who were embarrassed when their daughters made a big to-do over them on the third Sunday in June.

Their sons were too much like their dads to be sentimental on Father's Day.

The men appeared tough and hard. Their skin had been bronzed by the sun of summer, weathered by the raw winds of winter, but their looks were deceiving. Inside, they were putty that could be molded to accede to any justifiable request.

On most Father's Days, the men would hem and haw after opening their gifts. They'd say their wives and daughters should have spent the money for something for themselves.

The men cared about their wives and daughters, but it was their sons they taught the lessons of life and with whom they shared wisdom gained in the tormented decades of World War I, the turbulent 1920s and the depressing 1930s. Most of the men had never been farther from Heltonville than Iowa to the west or Ohio to the east, but their knowledge seemed boundless to their sons.

On weekdays, the men wore faded felt hats and overalls that allowed them to run their thumbs up and down the inside of the bibs as they talked. They sometimes swore and used barnyard language around each other, but never around women or children.

In mixed company, they took on an aura of gentility that masked their masculinity. On Sundays they wore brown pants and blue denim shirts. They sat together in the back rows at church, harnessed uncomfortably in ties their wives insisted they wear.

They coughed nervously when the preacher talked hellfire and damnation, unconscious confessions to transgressions perceived as sin. In truth, the men were as God-fearing as the pastor.

They were good men, who dug graves at the cemetery for the dead, shared their tools, swapped help without worrying about who was spending more time helping whom, and put their families' welfare above their own.

They could turn casual encounters into lasting friendships. No one in their midst remained a stranger long.

The men had seen things when they were still new. Things like the automobile, farm tractors, combines, electricity and talking-picture shows.

It likely was for that reason they spent more time teaching their sons lessons of the mind than of appearance. They taught their sons to be careful with their money, to borrow only when necessary and to repay their debts as soon as possible. The Great Depression had made them more aware of the virtue of frugality.

They were not teachers or child psychologists, and they were unaware of the education they were passing on to a new generation. Most of what the sons learned was from observation, watching fences being built, corn shucked, wheat threshed, livestock tended and crops cultivated.

Some of the knowledge came from what their fathers said, axioms like, "If it's worth doing, it's worth doing well" and "If you work for someone, give him a good day's work regardless of what you're paid."

And they sometimes learned philosophy: "Yesterday is a setting sun. Tomorrow is a sunrise. Today is a time to work and live, to make tomorrow better than yesterday, to sow the seeds for a harvest later."

Chances are, their sons never considered Father's Day special. But their fathers were.

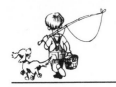

Special Comforts
of a Picture Show

A boy could learn a lot listening to a conversation between Zeb and Clem. Eavesdropping was a form of education for Chig when he was ten. That's why he sidled up close to the two men one Sunday morning in the summer of 1939 so he could hear what they were saying.

The exchange took place outside the rural church they attended near Heltonville. The location prevented the two men from using most of the descriptive phrases they sometimes worked into their salty dialogues. That didn't keep Zeb from being animated, though. Some folks said he wouldn't be able to talk if his hands were tied.

The topic was the weather. It had been hot, as summers in Southern Indiana always are. The temperature had been in the low 90s, and electricity hadn't yet reached farm homes.

Zeb was saying, "The wife saw the story in the *Bedford Daily Mail* about the Von Ritz and Indiana theaters in Bedford getting their new air-conditioning systems. The things cost $10,000 each and are supposed to have the effect of fifty tons of ice melting daily."

Zeb went on, "We were trying to get some sleep the other night upstairs, where there is no ceiling or insulation under the roof. The sun had baked the bedroom all day, and it was like an oven.

"It was so hot we tossed and turned and turned and tossed half the night before falling asleep.

"The next night at supper, the old lady suggests we go to Bedford and see a show. 'It'll give us a chance to relax in air-conditioned comfort,' she says."

Clem, who knew "the old lady" was Zeb's wife, asked what Zeb's response had been.

"I told her," Zeb explained, "that I'd lived through the summer of '36 when it was a lot hotter than it is now. That's when we had ten straight days above 100 degrees and three straight days above 110."

Clem said he remembered. "I used to go back into the caves south of Heltonville to cool off," he said.

Zeb laughed. "I mentioned that to my wife, but she said she'd advanced past the cave-woman stage."

He said he also had suggested that they just drive to Norman, where C.E. Cummings showed free movies outside his general store on Saturday nights.

"She didn't like that idea, either," Zeb said. "She thinks those movies are old ones. She said she preferred to watch more sophisticated shows," he added.

Clem shuffled from one foot to the other. "So what finally happened?" he asked.

Zeb looked exasperated. "Oh, she won, as usual. We drove into Bedford Friday night and went to the show at the Von Ritz."

Clem asked, "What did you see? That movie with Tyrone Power and Jean Arthur?"

Zeb looked embarrassed, which was unusual for him. "I don't know," he said. "The place was so comfortable I went to sleep before the movie started.

"Best two hours of sleep I've had in a month."

The church bell rang about that time. Clem and Zeb walked up the steps. Chig followed slowly. There was no air-conditioning inside.

Baseball Scores Were for the Newspapers

It looked, at first glance, like the usual crowd had gathered for the Sunday afternoon baseball game on the diamond at Homer Duncan's farm. Most of their friends already were there when Tad and Tyke rode up on their bikes. So was the usual group of men, too old to play, too young not to watch the others.

A stranger was to make the afternoon different from other Sundays in the summer of 1939.

The diamond, scalped, dusty and shadeless, was on Ind. 58, midway between Heltonville and Norman. The Heltonville Merchants were to face a team from Jackson County that afternoon.

It soon was obvious that the stranger was backing the visitors. He wore a denim shirt, long sleeves rolled up on his skinny bronzed arms. He removed his brimmed hat from time to time to fan himself. He appeared to be sixty, maybe older.

He yelled continuous encouragement for the Jackson County team, but he clapped when Ed Cain, Bish Wagoner or one of the other Merchants made a good play in the field.

It was between innings when he bought an RC Cola from the ice tub, flipped a nickel to the vendor and started a conversation with Tad, Tyke and the other nine- to eleven-year-old boys.

They were surprised at his knowledge of baseball. He talked about run-and-hit, hit-and-run, bunt situations, curve balls, fast balls, pivots on double plays, hitting the cut-off man, base-stealing and fielding techniques.

He did so while sipping his soda and watching every pitch. He was still talking when the manager of the Merchants passed a can through the crowd. The boys dropped in a nickel each. The stranger pulled a wilted one-dollar bill

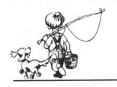

from a worn pocketbook and let it float into the can without comment.

"Visitors don't usually chip in," Tyke observed.

The man replied, "If you're going to watch, you oughta pay. Doesn't make any difference where you are."

Heltonville led by a run going into the top of the ninth inning. The visitors had runners on first and third with two outs when the batter lofted a fly ball. Dale Harrell moved back from his second-base position to make the catch, then lost the ball in the sun. The ball hit the palm of his glove and bounced about ten feet in the air. Earl Lantz, or maybe it was his brother Raymond, coming in from the outfield, caught the ball on the carom.

The game belonged to the Merchants.

Tad thought the stranger would be upset about his team's loss. He wasn't. He clapped his wrinkled hands and said, "Good backup. Smart playing."

He read the surprised look on Tad's face, knowing it called for an explanation.

"The game was meant to be fun. There are no losers when you play as hard as you can," he said. He thought for a minute, then added: "The only reason they keep score is for the newspapers."

The boys never learned the stranger's name, but they never forgot what he had to say that humid afternoon.

They Who Bake
Also Serve

None of the women seated in the pews up near the pulpit seemed able to keep her mind on the morning sermon. Mettie couldn't. Neither could Float, nor Nellie, nor Grace. Adie couldn't. Nor Edith, Onie, Doris, Pearl nor Mabel. Nor Ellie nor Laura.

They weren't hungry, but they were looking forward to the noon meal. It was the second Sunday in July, the day of the annual basket dinner, a day-long homecoming for anyone ever associated with Mundell Christian Church, a rural congregation southeast of Heltonville.

Deacons and elders, who made most of the decisions for the congregation, were all men. And so were the preachers who came and went in the 1930s and '40s.

But it was the farm women, quietly and with an air of gentility, who kept the men in line. The women were content, most of the time, to stay in the background, teaching Sunday school classes and preparing the sacraments each Sunday . . . and the basket dinner once a year.

Once the last amen of the morning had been said, the women marched each Sunday . . . and the basket dinner once a year.

Once the last amen of the morning had been said, the women marched hurriedly, in single file, from the sanctuary down two short flights of steps to the church basement.

There, they tied on aprons, some with fancy stitching, sewn especially for the day. They opened the wicker baskets in which they'd brought their covered dishes and they wasted no time removing the contents.

Within minutes, two thirty-foot tables were covered with an assortment of food no restaurant could duplicate. The women handed plates and silverware to their husbands and youngsters. They would wait until others had gone around the tables before filling their own plates.

Boys ten and eleven, with big appetites, eyed the delicacies and fidgeted through a visiting preacher's lengthy message that seemed even longer to them.

As soon as the prayer ended, the feast began. It was a smorgasbord of plenty, homemade or home-baked, except for a few loaves of bread. There was an assortment of meat—beef, ham, pork, chicken—prepared in a dozen different ways. Chicken dumplings. Meat loaf.

There were sliced tomatoes, green beans and peas fresh from gardens, roasting ears from fields, slaw, mashed potatoes, baked beans, Navy beans, pinto beans.

And there was dessert. Chocolate, white, lemon, angel food and devil's food cakes. The minister bypassed the devil's food cake and took a piece of angel food cake instead.

And there were pies. Apple, strawberry, peach, rhubarb, raspberry, blackberry, lemon, gooseberry, mince and other kinds, too.

The bigger the helping a diner took, the bigger the smile on the face of the woman who fixed it. The less food left, the better. An empty dish, pie pan or cake tin, was a badge of approval.

Only a few men bothered to learn who had fixed what, but that didn't bother the women. Their reward came in pleasing others. The women praised each other after the men had traipsed outside to relax under the shade trees, traded recipes and helped each other find the dishes they had brought.

Sometimes the preacher would return to the basement for a sip of tea before the afternoon services. He'd mention, "Well, you won't have to fix this much food for another year."

And someone would always remind him, "You forget the threshing crew will be around in a few weeks." It wasn't a complaint. It was a promise of another bountiful meal. And sometimes the preacher would show up to say grace . . . and to eat with the crew.

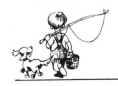

Geography Opened Up a Big World Outside

A late-summer ritual had been completed. Tad and his brother had returned with their parents from the annual back-to-school trip to Bedford. They had bought all the books they needed and all the new clothes their parents could afford.

The new clothes looked uncomfortable, especially the shoes, after a bareback, barefoot summer. The new overalls would remain stiff, the legs swishy, until a couple of boilings in the wash kettle. The collars on the denim shirts were rigid and scratchy.

Tad gave the clothes scant attention, placing them on top of a dresser in the upstairs of the big farmhouse. He romped downstairs and went quickly through his third-grade textbooks. They looked interesting, but his time with them would come later when Miss Hunter assigned homework.

He placed his books in a neat stack, noted their fresh smell and opened the sack that belonged to his brother, who would be in E.O. Winklepleck's fifth-grade class. Tad leafed through the arithmetic book, then opened a U.S. geography book. The pages clung together, reluctant to surrender the knowledge they contained.

Tad peeled open each page, his curiosity growing. Each chapter took him to a new part of the United States. He moved across the face of the nation, from New England, down the Atlantic Coast states, to the South, into the Midwest, across the Great Plains, down to the vast Southwest and up the Pacific shore.

He saw names he couldn't pronounce, places like Montpelier, Savannah, Schenectady, Tuscaloosa, Cheyenne, Wichita and Sacramento. He tried to record the maps to memory, to imprint the locations of Chicago, Philadelphia, Washington, Kansas City and St. Louis. They were places he might see sometime. Cities like Seattle, San Francisco or Los Angeles seemed too far away for him ever to visit, even in his imagination.

He read about the mountains and the rivers, the Corn Belt and the Cotton Belt, and saw pictures of unfenced wheat fields in Kansas and open ranges in Wyoming. They were different places than the small fenced fields and barnlots of the Southern Indiana he knew.

He looked at the irregular boundaries of each of the forty-eight states and wondered how they came to be.

He sat glued, his travels limitless. He journeyed far from the limited world he knew, a world that reached to Bedford on the west and Seymour on the east, Bloomington on the north and Mitchell on the south.

He remained on his journey across the nation until his brother called out,

"Hey, want to ride to Norman and get an ice cream cone?"

Norman was three or four miles away. It had seemed like a long bicycle ride until that afternoon. Now it was just a short distance. After all, Tad had just seen the entire country narrowed to eight-by-eleven-inch pages.

First Day Back Was a Jarring Experience

It was a weekend of mixed emotions. Excitement and anticipation were tempered with apprehension and melancholy.

It was always that way on the first weekend in September in the 1930s and '40s when youngsters prepared to return to school at Heltonville after Labor Day.

It was a time of transition, a time to cast off the freedom of summer and accept the restraints of autumn. It had been a good respite, that summer of 1939, but another school year offered a new beginning amid a commotion of change.

Tad, Pokey and Bill looked renewed, tanned and refreshed by a summer of work and play. They were eager to meet their new teacher in the fifth-grade classroom on the third floor at the school, but they were reluctant to part with the carefree days they had grown to enjoy.

They had been to school the previous Friday to enroll and to pick up their book lists.

The school bus they rode was new, the yellow made brighter by the sun. The black "Pleasant Run Township" sign was not yet coated with the red dust of the gravel roads. The seats were hard, uncupped, the leather fresh and firm. No initials had yet been written on the backs of the seats. No dirt, debris or note paper littered the floor.

Each of the boys had gone to Bedford on Saturday with their parents to buy new books and new clothes. The stores were crowded, as they were each year on that day, with parents and youngsters all spending money they'd scrimped to save since school ended in the spring.

Books were bought first. Boys could make do with old clothes, but books were vital. What money was left over went for overalls, denim shirts and shoes for Tad and Tyke and for an assortment of clothes for their sisters.

The girls were more fortunate. Their mothers made many of their clothes with craftsmanlike care on the treadle sewing machines at home.

Once the shopping was done, it was time for Tad to stop at Marley's barber shop. The barber tugged a comb through the twisted mop of hair, then trimmed it closely above the ears. The newly revealed pale neck accentuated the tan on Tad's face.

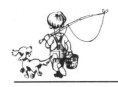

On the way home that afternoon, he opened his new books, the aromatic pages clinging to one another, seemingly hesitant to free even a hint of the education to come. The books were clean, the pages free from scribbling, the covers waiting to absorb fingerprints.

Tad thought about school most of the weekend, but waited until Tuesday morning to tug on his new Big Mac overalls and cram his feet into his new shoes. The shoes creaked, pinching his toes. The legs of the overalls swished with each step he took.

He managed a part in his hair, with an assist of Vitalis, picked up his lunch pail, its paint unchipped and its sides free of dents, and headed out to the road to await the bus.

He boarded the bus and bade goodbye to a summer he would relive now only in memory.

Savoring Pleasures of Autumn's Passing

Ben was in the autumn of his life, Tad in the springtime of his. That may have been why Ben, the man, chose a late September day about 1940 to talk to Tad, the boy, about the seasons and their relationship to life.

It was a warm, sunny afternoon when Ben waved to Tad as he got off the bus after a day at school in Heltonville. Tad walked to the field where Ben was cutting and shocking corn.

The green was fading from the grass in the pastures, the sumac was turning red and the leaves were yellow and red on the hardwood trees in the distance. Walnuts that had fallen onto the gravel road had been hulled by passing cars.

Fall was in the air.

Ben asked Tad, who was in the fifth grade, about his day at school. The boy replied that he would have preferred to spend the time outdoors, knowing winter would come all too quickly.

"It's too bad fall couldn't last all year," Tad said.

Ben shook his head. "We really wouldn't want that. The seasons are a lot like our lives. They each represent stages through which we all must pass. We can no more change those phases of our lives than we can the seasons. And I'm not sure we'd want to if we could."

Tad looked puzzled and asked Ben what he meant. Ben pulled the felt hat from his head, used it to flick away a bee, then explained, "Spring is a time of innocence, a time when life is green and fresh and vulnerable. It's a time of simplicity and hope and expectation, a time to grow, a time to look ahead."

He paused, looked at Tad and said, "Enjoy your springtime, Son."

Ben went on, "Summer is a time in life when you lose your youth and become a man. It's a time of maturity, a time to store the fruit of your labor for the fall and winter ahead."

Tad wanted to know if Ben was in the summer of his life.

"Afraid I've passed that stage," Ben said. "I'm into autumn. It's almost time for me to enjoy the golden years, to relax and enjoy the fruits of my seventy years, to let the wrinkles line my face and work just enough to keep my elbows and knees from getting rigid."

Tad doubted Ben would stop working, even in the winter of his life. The boy hesitated, reluctant to ask about winter, knowing the answer.

Ben volunteered: "Winter is when the cycle is completed. The years go on, but our lives are complete."

Tad stared at him with awe and admiration.

Ben smiled and said, "Think of life as this stalk of corn. It started out as a seed, grew and branched out. The tassels formed and pollinated the silk, an ear grew and the stalk matured and died. But it left an ear of corn, enough grains to start life anew next spring.

"That," he said, "is what life is all about."

Tad nodded as if he understood.

Ben looked contented, like a man who had almost fulfilled his mission in life and was satisfied with his accomplishments. He put his hat back on and walked slowly east toward his home, the sun setting behind him. And Tad bounded up the hill toward home.

A Civil War Fought by the Red and Gray

Chances are there were some things Bob and Marshall liked better than squirrel hunting, but they didn't talk about those things in public. Instead, they talked about squirrel hunting to anyone who would listen.

Bob was a son in the Ray Roberts & Sons general store in Heltonville in the 1930s and 1940s. Marshall was a young teacher at the school up the hill from the store.

They hunted together almost daily each year after the season opened August 15, traipsing the wooded hills to find the heaviest squirrel population. Sometimes they got the legal limit of five squirrels each. Sometimes they returned home with none.

But it was the hunt, the enjoyment of being in the wide-open spaces, that they liked.

It was common knowledge Bob had a bag of unlimited excuses he used to beg off from work at the store. He spent the excuses one at a time as the sea-

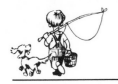

son passed, inventing a new one now and then.

Being a teacher, Marshall didn't have to be excused from work early in the season. He could hunt each day. But after school started, he could hunt only on Saturdays. After school started, Bob hunted alone . . . and he never forgot to remind Marshall when the hunting went well.

No one knew for sure, but they figured Marshall must have doubted one of Bob's stories, which instigated an incident early one September. It had been an ideal morning to hunt. A rain had fallen, making it possible for Bob to walk into the woods quietly. He managed to bag two squirrels, one red, one gray.

He drove to the school and parked on Ind. 58, almost beneath Marshall's sixth-grade class on the second floor. Bob knew it wouldn't be long until Marshall would walk to the window and look out across Fred Dulin's house to

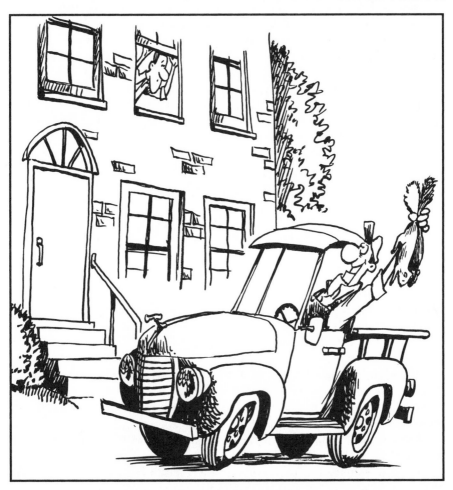

the wooded hills beyond and wish he were hunting.

Bob knew Marshall's habits well. When Marshall came to the window, Bob tooted the horn on his truck, saw Marshall look down and pulled the gray squirrel from the truck and held it up. Then he held up the red squirrel, then the gray again, then the red, and the gray again. Marshall figured that meant Bob had the limit for the day.

Bob waved at Marshall and drove down to the store, probably laughing on the way. He wasted no time telling about what he had done. What effort Marshall had made to concentrate on his teaching duties was lost, at least for a couple of hours.

He didn't find out he had been duped until some time later. By then some of his students had heard about what had happened, and one of them, Jack, liked to take a grain of truth and turn it into a bushel of fun.

He said, "We'd been talking about the Civil War when Mr. Axsom walked to the window and we heard the horn blow."

Axsom was Marshall's last name.

"Mr. Axsom seemed to lose his train of thought. He got so excited seeing those two squirrels he mentioned their colors. Half of us in class will grow up thinking the Civil War was fought by the red and the gray instead of the blue and the gray."

Everybody knew Jack was making the story up, but they laughed anyhow. So did Marshall when he heard it.

Autumn Was a Time for Reflection

Autumn, it seemed, was a season of joy for farm wives around Heltonville. They still awakened before dawn and worked past dusk, but now and then, in this intermission between summer and winter, they took time to relish a life that sometimes was more difficult than joyful.

There was still work to do on those October days in the late 1930s. Overalls, heavy with dust, had to be soaked in hot kettle-water and agitated in a gasoline-powered washer. Clothes needed to be mended and ironed, chickens tended, milk separated, meals cooked, pies baked, school lunches fixed and children steered in the right direction.

But it was a time, too, to appraise the life they had made for themselves and their families. They seldom were disappointed.

Their husbands looked at the hay mows and corncribs, counted the livestock and checked the cost-income ledgers to label a year bad or good.

The women gauged a year's success by other things. Material things, like

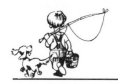

the supply of canned goods in the cellar, potatoes in the bin, chickens in the hen house and the amount of butter, egg and cream money hidden in a pitcher in the corner cupboard.

But success was also gauged by things not material, things like the health of children and husbands and the women's own spiritual well-being.

On their way home from school on Bus 7, Tad and Tyke and the other youngsters noticed the women on warm days. Some still worked in gardens that had surrendered to grass. They gathered the last of the tomatoes, saving

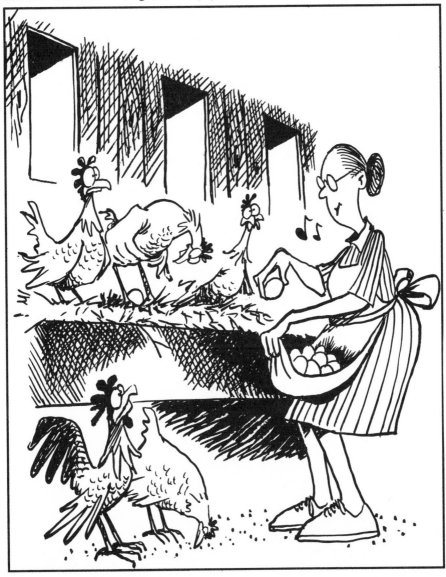

even the green ones from the first freeze, and pulled a few turnips, just ripening.

They needed no bucket, no basket. They shaped big pockets in their aprons, holding out the front as they walked toward their houses.

Other wives cut the last of the flowers, then cleaned out the beds, spreading grass clippings to cover the soil for a winter's rest.

Some women gathered walnuts that had fallen on the gravel roads or on the dry pastures. Still others sat on their front-porch swings, needlework in their lap, stopping often to gaze across the hills at the reds and yellows in the trees.

Tad stepped off the bus on one of those fall days, did a 360-degree inventory of nature's fall landscape and ran toward the house where his mother was seated on the porch step.

She was singing, "God will take care of you," and she seemed to believe each word.

Snowy days and freezing temperatures and hardships borne on the winds of winter lay ahead. So did wash days in freezing temperatures and chores through drifts of snow.

But so did warm evenings around the stove, club meetings and quilting bees. And church each Sunday morning and evening.

Tad's mother seemed happy and content. Tad didn't interrupt. He waited until she quit singing before telling her about his day at school.

Delicious Apple Was His Just Dessert

Pokey was hungry, and the apples were the biggest, reddest and shiniest he'd ever seen. They were in a bushel basket at the entrance to a little grocery store on the east side of the courthouse square in Bedford.

It was late afternoon on an autumn Saturday in 1939. Pokey had eaten a bag of popcorn and a Tootsie Roll while watching the double feature at the Lawrence Theater, but he was still hungry. Like most growing ten-year-olds, he seldom had a shortage of appetite.

Pokey shuffled from one foot to the other, waiting for his dad to end his conversation with another man at the edge of the sidewalk. Pokey eyed the apples. He could imagine the crisp, sharp sound of the first bite and the sweetness of the taste.

He looked away, scanning the courthouse across the street, trying to forget the apples. But the basket was like a magnet, drawing his eyes back.

Pokey's rigid willpower began to soften. He looked at the store, at his dad, up and down the sidewalk and into the store. No one, he thought, was

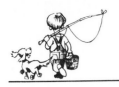

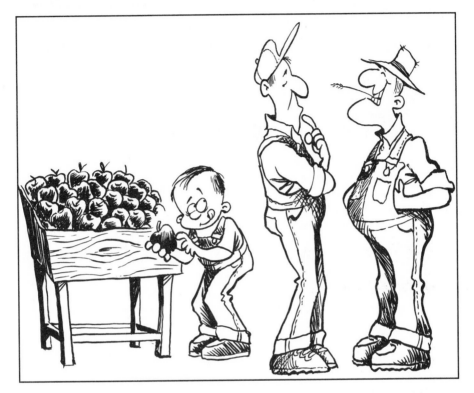

watching. He picked up the apple and rolled it around in his hand.

He wanted to bite into it, but his hand wouldn't react to his hunger. He replaced the apple in the exact spot from where he took it. Conscience had defeated desire.

He sheepishly kept his head down and walked to the car, afraid someone had seen him beat temptation. His dad finished his conversation and followed him.

The sun was dropping behind the courthouse, and it was time to head home to do the chores, but his dad drove west instead of east toward Heltonville. They were out of town before his dad spoke.

"I saw you almost take that apple," he said. "If it looked that good to you, we'll just drive out to Applacres and buy a bushel."

Applacres was on Ind. 37 toward Mitchell. There were enough apples there, Pokey thought, for every boy in America to have one. There were bushels on bushels of Red Delicious, Grimes Golden, Cortland and other varieties.

"Show me the best bushel you have left," Pokey's father said. "My boy here just did something to make me proud."

The clerk recommended the Red Delicious. Pokey lugged the basket of apples to the car. His dad paid the clerk and tossed an apple at Pokey.

It was even redder and bigger than the one in the basket at the store.

Pokey bit into the apple as they drove out Ind. 58. It exceeded his anticipation.

His dad watched him out of the corner of his eye. "Chances are, that apple tastes better than the one you picked up in town. And it won't awaken your conscience and gnaw at your insides," he said.

He was right on both counts, Pokey decided, chewing each bite to prolong the flavor.

Getting Educated Outside School

Gordy had trouble keeping his shoelaces tied and his hair combed. And he wasn't the best student in William Wright's fourth-grade class at Heltonville.

But he seemed to know a little bit about a lot of things, and he didn't hesitate to let others know how smart he was. He gave the impression that the sun rose each day to hear him crow.

Gordy was likable, despite his impetuousness, which is why Tad invited him to his home one night a few weeks after school started. Tad figured he could withstand Gordy's verbal volleys for a few hours.

The school bus had just pulled away from the school when Gordy started identifying the turning leaves.

"Sumac," he yelled, pointing to the red hues in bushes along Groundhog Road. "Gum," he cried out, spying blushing red leaves off in a wood.

He spied an assortment of colors—crimson, ruby, sienna, scarlet, vermilion—and matched the tinges and tints with the trees. It was obvious he had paid more attention to what his dad had told him about the outdoors than he had to what Mr. Wright had tried to teach him about arithmetic and social studies.

It wasn't until the bus pulled up the lane where Jake Cummings lived that Gordy stopped talking.

"What's that?" he asked, looking out on a field that looked like a fence-row-to-fence-row carpet of white. The flowers hid the ground and shielded the green plants from which they grew.

Gordy's friends smirked. It was one of the few times Gordy admitted to them there was something he didn't know.

"Write down the date," one of them said. "This might never happen again."

Tad and the others took turns telling Gordy about the field that looked as soft and serene as a puffy cloud on a still day.

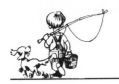

"It's a field of buckwheat," Tad said.

Gordy admitted he'd never heard of buckwheat.

Tad explained, "It can be seeded after wheat is harvested, so farmers can get two crops in one year if they want. It blooms in September and can be harvested later, just like wheat."

The others told Gordy that the seeds were triangular, "like beech nuts," that buckwheat could be ground into flour or turned into feed for livestock.

Tad added, "It makes a good bee pasture, too."

"Whatcha mean by that?" Gordy asked.

Dale answered, "My grandpa says the heavy blooms, or flowers, whatever you want to call 'em, last for a month and provide more nectar for honey bees than any other crop."

The conversation about buckwheat was still going on when Tad and Gordy got off the bus. Tad and Gordy mentioned the blooms to Tad's father later that afternoon.

Gordy gushed, "Buckwheat is planted after the wheat harvest and can be used for flour or livestock feed and makes a good place for bees to gather nectar."

Tad let his eyes roll up into his forehead to signal his dad he was in for a verbal marathon on the virtues of buckwheat. His father cleared his throat and said, "I don't have time to listen right now. Gotta finish the chores."

The next day Gordy gave the other boys in class a dissertation on the value of buckwheat as a field crop.

Mother Nature Offered Between-meal Snacks

A farm boy around Heltonville had no trouble finding a snack between meals in September, and he didn't need to ask his mom to fix it.

Mother Nature saw to that in the late 1930s and 1940s. She provided pawpaws, persimmons, butternuts, hickory nuts, walnuts and hazelnuts. And apples and pears that grew unattended on trees in abandoned orchards.

Almost any boy liked apples and most of the nuts that could be found on farms and in woods. Pears weren't as good as apples, but they were tolerable. Pawpaws and persimmons required special attention to be savored. Premature taste tests could sour a boy on both for a year, maybe a lifetime.

Persimmons could be found in a few yards, but the best ones seemed to be around places where houses once stood before their occupants surrendered to the Great Depression and moved on in search of prosperity elsewhere.

Tad swore off persimmons after biting into one that hadn't fully ripened. His mouth had puckered with bitterness and he spat instead of swallowing.

"Worst damn thing I ever tasted," he said, knowing he could use mildly profane language with his dad.

His dad laughed. He taught Tad how to tell when persimmons were ripe, and how to scatter straw under trees to keep the persimmons from bruising as they fell.

Persimmons were for the entire family. Tad picked up gallons each fall for his mother to squish through a colander and make puddings from an assortment of recipes.

The pawpaws were only for Tad, his brother and his father.

Years of walking the hills and hollows had provided Tad's father with a mental map of the best spots to find pawpaws, firm and full.

"Indiana bananas," he called them. "Like bananas," he told his son, "they need to ripen in the shade. The trick is to pick 'em while they're green, spread them out in the grass, and let them ripen under the fall sun."

He checked the pawpaws each day or two until they were ripe, then spread them out on a table in the smoke house. He'd pull open one end and ooze the pawpaw, which almost turned to mush, into his mouth, spewing out the seeds. He limited himself to a couple of pawpaws a day to prolong the joy of their taste.

The bitey taste wasn't as palatable to Tad, but he learned to like pawpaws, especially after his dad told him a dozen or so times:

"You'll never go hungry, Son, no matter how poor you are, if you learn to appreciate the things God provides free."

Rooster Rustlers Got Egg on Their Faces

He who cackles over a roasted rooster doesn't cackle long. Lute saw to that after an incident one autumn evening in the late 1930s.

Herbie had just left the high school gym at Heltonville after basketball practice. He hadn't yet urged his tired body to start the three-mile trot to his home on Henderson Creek when some friends stopped him at the bottom of the hill near the railroad tracks.

They wanted to know if he'd like to join them in a chicken roast. Herbie accepted the invitation, thinking the food might give him enough energy to sprint home.

"Who has the chicken?" he asked.

His friends said they hadn't caught one yet. They were listing the homes in town where chickens were kept, when someone looked across the street into the restaurant Lute ran.

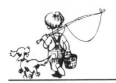

"I got it," the youth said. "Let's snitch Lute's pet rooster."

The vote was unanimous.

The rooster was more than a pet to Lute. It was almost like a friend. Lute sometimes held it on his lap and stroked the feathers until they were sleek and shiny.

It was a fondness the perpetrators forgot in the meanness of the moment. One of them kept an eye on the restaurant, making sure Lute was at work, while the others caught the rooster.

They plucked the feathers as best they could, then roasted the rooster over an open fire. Lute locked the front door of the restaurant about the time they started to dine. He sauntered over to the fire.

"What you boys doing?" he asked. It was a question that needed no answer. "It's been years since I had chicken cooked over an open fire," he added, enjoying a mental image from the past.

One of the youths asked him if he'd like some chicken. He took a piece, chewed on it for a while, then asked, casually: "Where did you boys get the chicken?"

One of them replied, "We'd rather not say. Someone might ask you if you knew who stole their chicken and you would have to lie. It's best you don't know."

Lute accepted the explanation, tossed the remains of his piece into the fire and said, "That was the worst chicken I've ever tasted."

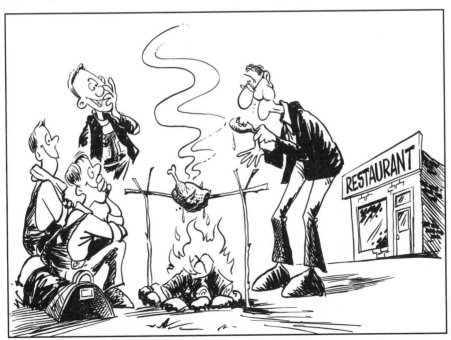

Herbie and the others bit their lips. They kept from laughing until Lute went into his house after telling them how much better roasted chicken was when he was a boy.

It was just as well. Lute didn't think it was a laughing matter the next day when he found his pet rooster was gone. He added two and two and came up with four.

His temper didn't ebb for days. His memory of the pet rooster died even more slowly. He banned Herbie and the others from his restaurant for the next six months and then begrudgingly allowed them to re-enter.

What's an Election Between Friends?

Maybe it was because:
• People had more faith in their fellow man.
• Candidates were closer to the voters.
• Folks weren't as critical as they are today.
• The tempo was slower and elections weren't as ho-hum.
• There was a lack of phonyism and cronyism.

Or maybe the passage of time has dulled the memories, and things were no different then than they are today.

Whatever the reason, there seemed to be a touch of excitement when township trustees were to be elected in Lawrence County in the 1930s and '40s. The races almost always were contests between friends, not between Democrats and Republicans.

The candidates seldom threw mud and almost never talked about their opponents, partly because they never could figure out who was related to whom and couldn't take any chances on offending possible allies.

At least that's the way it was in Pleasant Run Township, the area at the northeast corner of Lawrence County.

Township trustees had a lot more to do then than now. They were the major-domos over the school system, administered what little poor relief there was, saw that some cemeteries were kept clean, collected dog taxes, wrote checks to farmers whose animals were destroyed by dogs, assessed property and let people cry on their shoulders.

Dr. Jasper Cain did all those things. So did the trustees who followed, men named Ed Stipp, Jack Clark, Thornt Clampitt and "Doc" Bartlett.

The only time you knew they were Republican or Democrat was at election time. Politics never played much of a part in their decisions, or if it did not many folks knew about it.

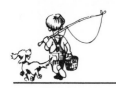

The trustees all had a kind of respect not associated today with what would be called "minor" offices. When a farmer mentioned he was going to drive out to Hunter's Creek to see Jack Clark, young people envisioned it somewhat as they would a visit to see the Pope today.

The trustees reigned supreme on the first and fifteenth of every month during the school year. Those were the days they'd drive to Heltonville to pay the teachers.

The teachers would warn their students to be on good behavior, and no one made a sound when the trustee walked into the classroom, sorted through twelve to fifteen checks, placed one on the teacher's desk and smiled. The teacher would smile back, not to make brownie points, but as a matter of gratitude because jobs in classrooms were hard to find.

Nobody ever got rich being township trustee back in those days. The job paid six hundred dollars a year with a little extra on the side for rental of office space, which more than likely was a desk off in the corner of the kitchen of a farmhouse.

A youngster who asked a trustee once why he ran for the job was told: "Somebody has to do it, and, besides, I like the prestige."

Then the trustee winked and laughed, to make sure the lad wouldn't think he was taking himself seriously.

Maybe because the trustees didn't take themselves seriously was why the voters did. It wasn't unusual for seventy to eighty percent of the eligible voters to show up at the Pleasant Run East and Pleasant Run West precincts to vote. It was a kind of tribute to the quality of men who sought offices.

Farm Wives Forced Sweeping Changes

Some of Jeb's neighbors laughed when they saw the patch of broomcorn he'd planted on his farm near Heltonville.

"Just what we need. A broom farmer in the community," Clem roared.

Jeb didn't let a little ribbing bother him. "When my wife, Maudie, tells me to raise cane I raise cane. If she tells me to raise broomcorn, I raise broomcorn," he replied, only partly in jest.

Clem said, "I don't pay much heed to my old lady," winking at Jeb to indicate he might not be telling the truth.

Jeb grinned and said, "Broomcorn doesn't take much work and it does save us a few pennies."

It was the late 1930s and a few pennies meant a lot to farmers who had managed to survive the long years of the Great Depression.

The broomcorn flourished. It looked a lot like sorghum, except for the panicles at the top. They were large and loose, dozens of long straight branches arising from a short main axis.

When the broomcorn matured, Jeb cut off the heads from the stalks. The stalks were then fed to the livestock, who savored the sweetness.

The tops were left to dry. They had been stored for a few days when Jeb showed them to Clem.

"If you'd left the stalks on, you could have used them as the handles and you'd have a broom. All you have now are little whisks and no handles," Clem said.

Jeb explained he planned to take the tops to Jackson County to a broom maker. "Won't cost me a cent to have the brooms made. I'll trade him some of the tops for his labor."

Clem snorted. "What you can't beg or borrow, you barter."

Jeb knew he was being taunted. He ignored Clem.

The brooms were finished a month later. Clem and his wife spotted them in a corner of Jeb's porch one Sunday when they were visiting.

"Sure wish I could buy brooms like that," Clem's wife, Millie, said. "The ones I buy at the J.C. Store in Bedford aren't nearly as good and they don't last more than a month."

Jeb handed her one. "I had this one made just for you," he said, making sure the gesture wasn't lost on Clem.

Millie thanked him, then looked at Clem and announced, "Next year, we'll raise our own broomcorn."

Clem turned red in the face, cleared his throat, looked at Jeb and said, "When your wife tells you to raise broomcorn you raise broomcorn. Think you could loan me the seed?"

"Sure," Jeb replied.

He waited until he and Clem were alone to have the last laugh.

"Bah, Humbug" to Holiday Switch

Jed wadded up the *Bedford Daily Mail,* flung it on the worn carpet and called out to his wife.

"Maudie, he's done it again."

Maude was out in the kitchen doing the dishes. She yelled back, "Who's he and what's he done again?"

Jed didn't try to hide his rancor. "He is Roosevelt. As in Franklin Delano Roosevelt." He let the words roll off his tongue in an attempt at imitating the

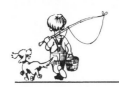
President's cultured accent. "And he's decided to change the date we observe Thanksgiving."

Maude wiped her hands on her apron as she came into the living room. "Not even FDR and his highfalutin friends would do that," she said.

"Well, he has," Jed said, picking up the paper and jabbing his finger at the story. "It says here Roosevelt has moved up Thanksgiving a week to the third Thursday in November."

Maudie wanted to know why. Jed read some more, then said, "He says it'll help business by giving Americans a week longer to shop before Christmas."

It was 1939, and times were still hard, even though the nation was gradually climbing out of the pits of the Great Depression. Jed and Maude lived on a farm outside Heltonville. They had managed to survive and raise a family without taking part in any of FDR's relief programs. And they had grown tired of all his social engineering schemes.

"Damnedest thing I ever heard of," Jed kept saying. "Now he knows more than the Pilgrims."

Maude went into the kitchen and returned with a big glass of milk for Jed, thinking that might keep his ulcer from acting up. He drank the milk, then said, "Folks barely have enough money to buy more than one or two gifts for their kids. And old Delano is waving his fancy cigarette holder like a magic wand, giving them an extra week to do it."

Maudie patted him on the shoulder. "If folks don't have any money to buy anything, why do they need an extra week not to do it?" she asked.

Jed didn't answer. He flipped on the radio. "Lum 'n' Abner" made him forget about FDR for a while.

The next day he announced his family would observe Thanksgiving on the fourth Thursday, "FDR be damned."

The rest of the nation, except a few other traditionalists, had its big feast on the third Thursday.

The Saturday morning after that, Maude said, over breakfast, "Reckon we'll be going into town today to start our Christmas shopping. Can't disappoint the President."

Jed stammered and stuttered and acted like he was going into town to ask attorney Bob Mellen to start divorce proceedings.

Maude finally laughed and said, "Well, I suppose we can wait another week."

"Darned right we can," Jed said. "Wouldn't give FDR the satisfaction of starting today."

* * *

Postscript: President Roosevelt's decision to move Thanksgiving up a week never won wide approval. Congress later made Thanksgiving a nation-

al holiday and decreed that starting in 1942 the day would be observed on the fourth Thursday in November. Nobody was happier about that than Jed and Maude.

Breaking Even
Was Good News

Zeke was too busy making a living for himself and his family to worry much about a profit and loss statement. That's why he waited until the weekend before Thanksgiving each year to find the bottom line for his farm operation.

It was a time to figure his outgo and his income, a time to appraise what he had accomplished, a time to determine what he had done right and wrong. And a time to determine whether his own Great Depression was nearing an end.

He had been too busy during the growing and harvesting seasons to keep daily records. It would have been easier had he done so, but he farmed days and worked nights at the stone mill near Heltonville.

Instead, he stashed receipts and records of what he had been paid into a shoe box tied with a rawhide string and kept atop the corner cupboard in the kitchen. The contents were his alone. Neither he nor his youngsters dared look inside.

The stubs in his checkbook told him what he had spent when receipts were lost.

Zeke did his figuring on Saturday if the weather was too nasty to be outdoors. If the weather was good he did chores on the farm and delayed his bookkeeping until Sunday afternoon.

He worked alone in the sitting room, the door closed, coming out from time to time for a fresh cup of coffee. No one interrupted him, not for a phone call, not for a visit by the pastor, not for any emergency less than death.

In case anyone asked, his wife, Millie, said he was engaged in a study of his assets and liabilities. "He's trying to figure out what we have to be grateful for before Thanksgiving," she would add.

Sometimes it appeared there would be little reason to be thankful.

Like one year around 1940, when Zeke came out of his isolation, holding a lined sheet of paper in one hand, the shoe box in the other.

Millie asked for a report.

"It appears we about broke even," Zeke added.

Millie frowned:

Zeke smiled. "But we had a good time doing it," he said.

Millie wondered how he could have had a good time working ten hours a

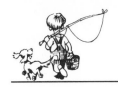

day on the farm and eight hours a night at the stone mill.

Zeke ignored her remarks and added: "Our bank balance doesn't show it, but we have something to be thankful for next Thursday."

Millie wanted to know what he meant if the bank balance didn't show any profit.

Zeke grinned again. "Well, it doesn't show the job I've got at the mill that pays me $26.27 a week, the hogs we're fattening for slaughter, a barn full of hay, three cribs full of corn, a laying house full of chickens, a cellar full of canned goods, five milk cows, two good teams of horses, a new Farmall H. . . ."

Millie interrupted him. "And a houseful of happiness," she added, with emphasis.

Neither had to tell the youngsters that was worth more than money in the bank.

Best Defense Against the Winter Blues

Zeke knew winter soon would come, blustering relentlessly from the north. His big house, perched unprotected atop a hill, offered little defense against the fingers of frigid air that wriggled into each crack and crevice.

But Winter 1938 didn't send cold shivers down his spine, even though the house had no central heating or insulation from the cold. This time he was prepared for whatever ill wind that bounded across his farm east of Heltonville.

He had built a new fifteen-by-thirty-foot building, setting aside part of it for a washroom for his wife and a playhouse in the loft for his youngsters. He divided the open space that was left into two sections. One part was filled with dried wood, split into small pieces for the kitchen range. The other part was stacked nearly to the rafters with ash, white and red oak, beech and hickory for the big stove the family huddled around on cold winter nights.

Zeke called the woodhouse his security blanket.

"Let winter come," he told his son, Tad. "We have enough wood to last until May. And it'll stay dry, under cover from the rain, snow and sleet."

Tad remembered the perspiration that dripped from his brow on the hot days when they had cut and stored the wood. "That'll be two heatings we'll get from each stick of wood," he said.

Zeke grinned, then said, "And when Ma tells you to bring in wood for the range, you won't have to pick up ice-coated sticks and try to split them as they slip through your fingers. That's already been done. All you'll have to do is fill the woodbox."

Tad replied, "Just so she doesn't ask me to do it while I'm listenin' to Jack Armstrong, the all-American boy, on the radio."

Clem, a neighbor, walked up about that time. Zeke showed him the wood-house, opening a door to expose the wood, then took him through the wash-room and up the steps to the play loft.

"Too bad you don't have a stove out here," Clem said. "That way you could exile the youngsters to the loft when they get obstreperous."

Zeke stuck his hands in his denim jacket, laughed and said, "Might do that, 'cept this place would be more comfortable than the house if it had heat in it."

Clem eyed the woodhouse in detail, then said, "You may be right. Looks to me like you built a mansion to keep your wood dry. You spent a lot of money just to make things easier for your wife and kids."

Zeke reminded him that winters could be long when you're cooped up with an unhappy woman and a houseful of kids arguing over who's going out to get the next load of wood.

Clem still wasn't convinced Zeke's money for the woodhouse had been well spent—until his wife found out about it. The next year Clem had a new woodhouse, almost as nice as Zeke's.

Loyal Supporter in a Lost Cause

It had been a week when reverie turned to reality, a week when emotion and euphoria peaked slowly, then waned suddenly.

It was always that way during the week of the high school basketball sectionals.

Teams from small schools went to the big-city gym in pursuit of a miracle. Some managed an upset or two, few lived out a dream of a championship.

Nora's parents were familiar with the scenario. They had witnessed it all before. Now they had observed it as the parents of a cheerleader.

Nora had led yells for the Heltonville team that 1938-1939 season. She was eighteen, a senior. She should have known the season would end, that there would be no trip to the regional.

But she refused to think about an eventual loss, even if the Blue Jackets had to face Bedford in the first round. The fact Bedford had been in the state finals the year before didn't dampen her enthusiasm.

Instead, she smoothed out her blue and white corduroy outfit, ironed the blouse and polished, then repolished, her white boots before relacing their white strings. She reshaped her cap, a crown formed from a piece of card-

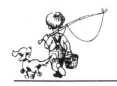

board and covered with corduroy.

Her uniform and those of the other two cheerleaders, Cora and Mabel, were made by their mothers, their handcraft necessitated by economics.

Nora had spent the week rocking the big farm house as she practiced yells—yells like:

Razzle zazzle, zizzle zip
Come on, team, let'er rip
And:
Bottle of pop
And a big banana
We're from
Heltonville, Indiana.
And:
We are the blue,
We are the white.
Come on, team
Fight! fight! fight!
And:
When you're up, you're up
When you're down, you're down
When you're up against Heltonville
You're upside down.

Plus others that went "zickety boom rah, rah" and "rammy dammy, zickety zammy."

When Friday arrived, Nora was as well prepared as coach Marshall George's basketball team.

The cheerleaders led the yells as the team went through its warm-up routine. The noise they generated from two hundred or so fans was just a murmur compared to the reverberations created by the Bedford cheer block.

As expected, Bedford took an early lead. Within minutes the outcome was no longer in doubt. Only the margin of Heltonville's loss was unknown.

The cheerleaders kept yelling, but their cause was lost. Bedford went on to win, 43-14.

Nora's mother could read the loss in her daughter's eyes when she returned from the game that night. Nora yanked off her boots, tossed her pillbox hat onto a chair and told her parents the sad story of the game.

She grumbled a few non-profane epithets against Bedford as she slumped into a chair, appearing as if her life as she had known it had ended.

Her mother need not have been concerned about Nora's depression. Her thoughts of the defeat disappeared the next morning when a boy called for a date. Nora spent as much time primping for him as she had spent primping for the ball game the previous day.

And Bedford, despite its rout of Heltonville the night before, seemed like a good place to go on a date.

THE GOOD YEARS

A New Car Was
Hope and a Risk

Optimism, tempered with restraint, was replacing pessimism. It was the summer of 1940 and the economy was creeping up from the bottom of the Great Depression. The wheat harvest had been good and the prospects for a good corn crop looked even better.

Zeke didn't make snap decisions or spend money on whims. But his mental calculations indicated the year's profit from his farm near Heltonville would allow him to buy a better used car than the rattletrap he'd been driving.

He'd been burned in the past, it seemed, each time he'd traded cars. He wasn't about to let that happen again.

He picked a Saturday morning to drive his 1935 Chevrolet to Bedford. His first stop was at a service station where he had a thick film of red clay dust washed from the car. He wanted to make it presentable in case he decided to trade.

He then drove to a used-car lot on U.S. 50 and told a salesman he wanted to look around, "alone. Don't need any help to tell whether or not I like a car," he asserted.

The salesman didn't mind. Zeke was wearing a dusty pair of bib overalls and a sun-faded felt hat and didn't appear to be a likely prospect to buy a car.

Zeke hadn't walked past more than three cars when he spotted a gray 1937 Buick. It was love at first sight. He had to look up the salesman, who reluctantly let him take the car for a drive out U.S. 50 East.

When he returned, Zeke asked, "How much?"

The salesman said, "That's a pretty expensive car. We're asking $375," he said.

Zeke pointed to his old Chevy and asked, "How much to boot?"

The salesman said $325. Zeke said $275. They settled for $300.

Zeke said he'd have to go to the bank to get the money. The salesman looked skeptical. Zeke didn't look to him like he could talk the bank out of a loan.

Zeke returned in about ten minutes and counted out fifteen twenty-dollar bills. "Took this out of my checking account," he said, just to prove to the snooty salesman he had liquid assets.

Once the paperwork was completed, Zeke switched license plates and started to leave.

"That's a mighty nice car to drive around gravel roads out in the country," the city-slicker salesman said. "It ought to be driven on long trips over good roads."

He didn't know Zeke planned to take his family to Washington to see the

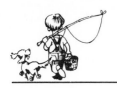

nation's capital in a couple of weeks. And Zeke didn't tell him. If the sales-man thought he was a clod, it didn't bother Zeke.

After all, he had the Buick and the salesman was left with the old car Zeke no longer wanted.

* * *

Postscript: America was at war eighteen months later and cars became scarce. Zeke was happy he had the Buick. He kept it until World War II ended.

Happiness and Tractor Both Began with "H"

Zeke had owned a farm tractor for five years, but he was as excited as an eight-year-old with a store-bought kite that April morning in 1940.

His new Farmall H had arrived at his farm near Heltonville. He watched the truck driver back up to a creek bank, unchain the tractor and drive it onto the bluegrass pasture. It ran as smoothly as the Singer sewing machine Zeke's wife used.

Zeke looked over the "H" while the trucker drove the old F-20 tractor onto the truck. Zeke had traded it in, reluctantly. It had served him well, even though it had a crank instead of a starter and wheels with lugs instead of rub-ber tires. And it had no lights, power lift, power takeoff, or other extras like the new tractor did.

It had been ideal for a field of new ground, where sapling stubs could have punctured a balloon tire. But it couldn't be driven out on Ind. 58 where signs every mile cautioned, "Tractors with lugs prohibited."

The truck was barely through the gate before Zeke was aboard the "H." He stepped on the starter and the tractor sang out, each cylinder in tune. It was music to Zeke's ears. He drove the tractor to the tool shed, backed up and hitched the plow to the drawbar, tying a trip rope to the seat.

A grin spread from ear to ear across his weather-wrinkled face as he drove to a field. One of his sons hurried ahead to open the gate.

Zeke steered the "H" through the gate and drove fifty yards or so across the end of the field, turned to the right and pulled the trip, letting the plow slice into the clover sod. He shifted gears easily. The tractor hummed, despite the weight of the two twelve-inch plows as the points ripped off the loam, rolling it over the moldboard, exposing the cold underside to the warm sun.

Zeke set his eyes on a fence post at the opposite end of the field so the fur-row would be straight. He gripped the wheel, occasionally turning back to make sure the plows were going six to seven inches deep into the earth.

The upturned soil looked dark and rich and smelled as fresh as the April air. Zeke's big collie followed in the furrow, curious about what was happening. Red worms wriggled from the ground to warm in the sun. For some, the heat was a death sentence. They vanished quickly into the beaks of birds that swooped down for a fresh meal.

Zeke yanked the rope when he reached the end of the field and the plow raised slowly from the earth. Zeke locked the wheel and turned sharply before tripping the plow. Again it dug into the ground.

He pulled his dusty felt hat over his forehead, shielding his eyes from the sun that bounced off the bright red paint on the tractor's gas tank. Zeke stayed aboard the tractor the rest of the afternoon, reluctant to stop even at 6:00 to do the milking.

He ate supper quickly, found a big piece of cloth in the garage and walked back to the tool shed. He used the cloth to wipe the dirt off the tractor, trying to maintain the newness as long as possible.

His wife joined him after doing the dishes. She walked beside him to the field where he had plowed. "Best job of breaking ground I've ever done," he told her.

They walked hand-in-hand back to the house, but not before taking one last look at the new "H." It was spring, a time for renewal, a time for happiness. And nothing could make a farmer happier than a new Farmall H.

Nature Answered Great Questions

Rural youngsters were taught at school. They were educated on the farm.

Their educators were their fathers, men wizened by their experience and willing to share their intelligence with others. Theirs was a wisdom chiseled from the land, whetted by nature and honed by a belief in something bigger than themselves.

To most youngsters, their fathers were their idols, their role models, their confidantes, allies in good times and bad.

But sooner or later, the boy would reach out for independence in search of answers to questions he thought were beyond his father's knowledge. It was a time all youngsters experienced, a belief they had grown wiser than their fathers.

For Tyke that time came when he was ten or eleven. It came gradually, it seemed, as he listened to older youths and sat in on conversations at general stores and restaurants where he had biked for a Royal Crown Cola or an Eskimo pie.

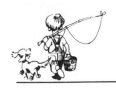

He was at an impressionable age, free of skepticism and doubt. The spoken words he heard from others, he accepted as fact.

He relayed some of the things he had heard to his dad one day, then questioned the value of church and the things that were taught there. His dad looked hurt, but he didn't make a big speech or quote Scripture or repeat any of the sermons the preacher delivered.

He just said quietly, "Let's go for a walk, Son."

They walked together, climbed over a slat gate into the corn field where the corn was ankle-high. It had been a good spring and the wind whipped the leaves on the small stalks into a sea of dark green.

Tyke's dad said, "Take a long look at this field and tell me this is all the work of me and you alone. Or the accumulation of all the help others have given us."

He looked skyward, then said: "We don't make the rain or the sun or perform the magic that can turn one grain of corn into a stalk that produces one or two ears, each with 400-500 grains."

They crossed another fence into a field of red clover, lush and awaiting the mower. A bag of seeds, none bigger than a speck, would yield a hundred bales or more of hay.

They walked to the orchard where the earliest apples were taking shape. Tyke's father talked about the seasons, how each spring brought new life that yielded its produce in the summer, relaxed in the fall, went dormant in winter and was reborn once again in a never-ending cycle.

They watched a young mother bird brings worms to her nest of young, a newborn calf find sustenance, instinctively, from its mother.

Tyke's father talked about the land and the things on it. Tyke seldom interrupted to ask questions. He was learning, too, just listening.

As they returned to the house, his dad said, "Well, you still doubt there is Someone greater than me, or you, or any other human being we'll ever encounter?"

Tyke said, "I don't now."

His dad figured that was about the best present he could have ever asked for on Father's Day, which was just a couple of days away.

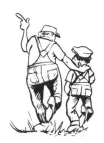

Plowing the Way to Better Things

Chig was twelve when he learned that some of life's more enjoyable experiences often come at unexpected times. He wasn't much bigger than a home-made bar of lye soap, but like most farm boys his age he thought he could handle a big Farmall tractor.

His dad wasn't as sure. Chig persisted in his pleas to drive the tractor until his dad suggested a compromise.

"If you can show me you're a man, I'll let you drive the tractor when we work the ground before planting corn," he said.

Chig wanted to know how he could prove he was a man.

"Know that two-acre offset over on the west field?" his dad asked, not waiting for an answer. "If you can take the team and plow that with a walking plow, it'll prove to me you're tough enough to operate the tractor."

His dad expected Chig to decide to wait another year to drive the tractor rather than plow with horses. He was wrong.

The next morning, Chig harnessed Dolly and Bird, the sorrel horses his dad treasured, and fastened the traces to the doubletree on the plow. He flipped the plow on its side, flicked the reins and drove the horses to the field.

His dad followed, feeling a bit guilty. He took the lines and drove the horses to open the first furrow. He showed Chig how to loop the reins around his neck and hold the plow.

"Be careful," he said. "This job is as tricky as licking honey off a thorn."

He walked off, then yelled, "And be sure to let the horses rest now and then."

Chig was alone in an unfamiliar world with only the horses to talk to. He grasped the handles of the plow and lifted them slightly so the point would dig into the sod. He felt a sense of authority when the team responded to his command to "giddup."

The plow point ripped a twelve-inch strip loose from the earth, eased it up onto the moldboard which rolled it over, covering what was left of a clover crop from the summer past. Chig made a couple of trips through the field before checking the depth of the furrow. His dad would be pleased to know it was seven inches, like he had wanted.

The work went well. Chig stopped to rest every half-hour or so, needing a breather more than the horses. The smell of the mellow overturned earth gave a freshness to the April air, a fitting welcome for a new growing season. Birds glided down on the freshly plowed ground, plucking worms that had squiggled through the dirt in search of a warm place in the sun.

Chig's arms grew tired as the morning wore on, but he didn't quit. Nor did

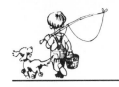

he linger long at lunch, when his parents expected him to surrender, admitting the plow had beaten him.

He declined a suggestion that he wait until the next morning to return to the field. Instead, he trudged on that afternoon and again the next day, until the plot had been plowed.

His dad pointed out how the dead furrow could have been filled back in a little better, but added, "otherwise, I couldn't have done a better job myself."

Chig couldn't remember when he'd ever been happier with himself. His dad told him to forget the chores that evening and "go visit your friends."

Chig's arms sagged from his shoulders. "The only friend I have right now is the bed," he said.

He forgot the soreness in his arms and legs the next morning when his dad told him to disc one of the fields. With the tractor.

All Occupations
Had Their Rewards

Conversation seldom paused to catch its breath at the barber shop in Heltonville. If there was a lull, someone always brought up a topic to stimulate debate.

No subject generated bigger arguments than money. Big money. Like the amount made by movie stars and big-league baseball players.

The men who visited a barber shop about 1940 eked a living off their farms, earned twenty-five to thirty dollars a week at the stone mill, survived on the two dollars a day they earned from the WPA or managed to feed a family with the earnings from hewing crossties or cutting timber.

Five hundred dollars was a fortune to them. A thousand dollars was something only a few rich folks had.

To Tad and other ten-year-olds, a dime was big money, and a quarter seemed like a lot to spend for a haircut.

Tad was waiting for his turn in the barber chair one Saturday morning in January when Jim looked at him and said, at a brief respite from the chitchat: "Son, you ought to think right now about being a baseball player or a movie actor."

Tad smiled, not knowing what direction the man was steering the conversation.

The man went on, "Yep! You could make yourself a mint. Just read in the paper about how much the New York Yankees will pay Joe DiMaggio this year. Nobody seems to know for certain, but the paper said he might make upwards of $80,000."

Tad didn't have to reply. The men who filled the bench along the side of the shop did that for him.

Sid was the most vocal. "I don't care how good DiMag is. Ain't nobody worth that kinda money," he said. "Besides, that's more than the president makes."

Clem cleared his throat in protest. "DiMaggio hits for a better average than Franklin Roosevelt. And he makes fewer errors."

By then the debate was raging.

Frosty said, "A man's worth ought to be based on his value to his employer. If DiMaggio can bring a hundred thousand fans to the ball park, he ought to be paid for it."

Jiggs disagreed: "I read the other day where Gene Autry was making a hundred thousand dollars or so. That's too much money for ridin' a horse, pluckin' a guitar and singin' Western songs."

The barber stopped to whet his razor on the strop and said, "Part of that's for having to kiss his horse Champion instead of his girlfriends in the pictures."

Jiggs, who was in the barber's chair by that time, laughed with the others. "And Gene Autry doesn't make as much as Clark Gable, who kisses women instead of horses," he argued. "Like I said, no one is worth $100,000 or more just for playing a game or appearing in front of a movie camera."

Most of the men nodded in agreement. Frosty wasn't one of them. "If you could fill the Von Ritz or Indiana theater in Bedford, you'd be worth a bunch of money, too."

The barber stopped work, cleared his voice, looked at Tad and said, "Son, I suggest you become a barber instead of a baseball player or a movie actor."

His customers looked bewildered until he added: "I fill this place every Saturday morning, so I should be making more money. Startin' right now, the price of a haircut is going up from twenty-five cents to thirty-five cents."

He looked like he meant it.

Until a grin spread across his face and unmasked his pretense.

Jiggs and the others decided it was time to change the subject.

That's the Way the Ball Bounces

Maebeth had spent at least ninety minutes preparing for her Saturday night date with Bernie. She had marcelled her hair with curling irons, applied rouge and lipstick and pulled on the homemade dress she had entered in 4-H competition the previous summer.

She was anxious for Bernie to arrive. He had promised to take her to Bedford for a movie and a sandwich and Coke later.

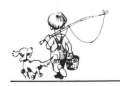

She had returned to her room for some last-second primping when Bernie arrived. Maebeth's brother, Chig, ushered Bernie into the living room of the farmhouse near Heltonville.

"Did you hear Mitchell won this afternoon?" Bernie asked. It was March 30, the day of the 1940 Indiana high school basketball finals.

Chig, who was eleven, said he'd heard the score on the radio. Mitchell had beaten the favorite, Fort Wayne South, 23-20, that afternoon and would meet Hammond Tech for the championship that night.

Bernie said the game would be like David against Goliath. Hammond was a big city compared to Mitchell, a town of three thousand or so eight miles down Ind. 37 from Bedford.

Chig listened as Bernie talked about seeing the Bluejackets in the sectional and about players like Roy Ramey and Duane Conkey. It was obvious Bernie was more interested in basketball that night than he was in a movie.

That's why he sat back down after Maebeth entered the room. She suggested a couple of times that they'd best be on their way. Bernie kept talking about basketball.

"Time to turn on the game," he told Chig about 8:00. The static on the battery-powered radio was clearer than the voice of the announcer once the game started. Mitchell stayed close early in the game, trailing 8-7 at the end of the first quarter.

Bernie and Chig yelled and clapped each time Mitchell scored. Maebeth frowned and glowered at them.

"Still time to make the second show," she said.

Bernie didn't answer. He jumped up and pumped his right fist when Marvin York scored a basket to put the Bluejackets up 9-8.

It would be Mitchell's last lead of the game. Hammond Tech led at the half 15-9.

"Goodbye, Mitchell! Game's over," Maebeth said. "We might just as well go."

Bernie said there was still time for Mitchell to come back and win. Maebeth stomped off into another room where her parents were reading, her dad the *Farmers Journal*, her mom the Bible lesson for her Sunday School class.

Mitchell managed but one basket in the third quarter and Hammond Tech widened the difference to 22-11.

Maebeth came back in, banged down a pan of warm popcorn and suggested coolly that maybe they should just wait for the midnight show.

Bernie still didn't surrender. He said a ten-point lead didn't mean the game was out of reach. It was, though, for Mitchell. The game ended. Hammond had won, 33-21.

"Finally," Maebeth said. "Now can we go?"

Bernie said, "Let's wait and see who wins the Gimbel Award. Maybe someone from Mitchell will get it."

He was right. The award went to "Red" Conkey.

Maebeth waited. Bernie waited, too . . . for the scoring summary. He didn't pay much attention to Maebeth until the announcers finally signed off from Butler Fieldhouse.

"Ready to go?" he asked.

She looked him in the eye. Her voice didn't quiver, despite its chill. "I'm going up to my room. And I'd suggest you go on home."

She didn't speak to Bernie again for a week. And she only agreed to go out with him the next Saturday night when she was sure there were no basketball games to be heard on the radio.

Making the Best
of a Bad Situation

Tad roamed the farm free and happy once school was out, unrestrained by the need to dress well. He wore no shirt or shoes. The bib and galluses on his overalls outlined his tan.

Tad's apparel changed only on Sundays when he wore a pair of dress pants and an open-neck sports shirt to church. He had one suit, which he wore only when his mother ordered. Knowing his dislike for formality, she did that on rare occasions.

One of those times came one June about 1940 when a relative died. "You'll have to wear your suit to the funeral," Tad's mother told him.

Tad's face turned a blustering red. "That suit is wool. I'd rather wrap myself in barbed wire and go as a mummy," he said. "Wouldn't be any more scratchy than wool on a hot day."

His mother overlooked his complaint. "You don't hear your brother Tyke complaining, do you? Besides, it may cool off for the funeral," she said.

Tad waited as long as he could before the funeral to knot his tie and pull on his suit. The skies turned gray just before he entered the church. Tad thought the clouds might cool the air.

He chose a seat next to the window, thinking any breeze would ease his discomfort.

A downpour started about the time the minister gave a eulogy to the deceased. The temperature dropped, but the humidity rose. Tad squirmed in his seat, too embarrassed to scratch. He ran his right index finger inside his starched shirt collar to ease the snugness. He used his left hand to dab his handkerchief, soaking up perspiration on his forehead.

The prayers, songs and sermon seemed endless to Tad. He spotted a fan and used it, reading the advertising about the Day, Carter & Roach Funeral

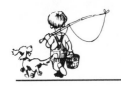

Home at Bedford, hoping to take his mind off the wool that gouged at his legs.

Once the services ended, Tad hurried outside, expecting the air to have cooled. It hadn't. The sun came out and turned the rain to steam.

Tad wanted to run to the car and shed his pants, but his mother grabbed his hand to prevent his escape. He stood by the grave until the casket was lowered and he shuffled his feet while his parents waited for flowers to be laid in place.

Once in the car, Tad voiced his misery. Tyke, who was two years older, laughed at him, saying, "I have wool pants on, too, but it didn't bother me. Wanna know why?"

Tad did.

Tyke pulled up his pants. Long underwear, damp from the heat, covered his legs. "That kept the wool from scratching," he said.

Tad wanted to know why Tyke hadn't told him to wear long johns.

"Better if you learn from experience," Tyke said.

Learning the Price of Independence

Tad couldn't have been happier. He was eleven and it was July 4, 1940. He had some new clothes, enough coins to clink in his pocket and a ride to Freetown.

Freetown was a town about eighteen miles on Ind. 58 from Heltonville. "Freetown. A free town," Tad thought to himself. He hadn't yet read much about the Declaration of Independence, but he knew it marked the beginning of freedom for Americans.

As Tad waited for Bogey and his parents to pick him up, he counted the coins in his left front pocket. They came to $1.30. Tad pulled a wadded and wilted dollar bill from the thin wallet in his back pocket and looked at it.

He knew $2.30 was a lot of money. But he had earned it punching wires on a hay baler for his uncle at $1.50 a day. His parents had convinced him he should put most of what he made in an account in Stone City National Bank at Bedford.

"Save it," they told him, "and you'll have money to spend when school starts."

It was wise advice, he would learn that day.

At Freetown, Bogey and Tad jumped out of the car and headed for the carnival area. They each paid ten cents for three chances to knock over milk bottles from a milk stool. They were unsuccessful. They tried again, then again without toppling a single bottle. They would learn later the bottles were weighted with lead.

Tad had spent thirty cents of his money.

The boys stopped at a scale where the attendant promised a prize if he couldn't guess Tad's weight and age within close parameters. Tad forked over a dime. The man hit his age on the mark and was off only a pound on his weight.

Forty cents of Tad's money was gone.

Tad stopped at a basketball shoot. He paid a dime for three shots, made one and received no prize. He tried again, watching all three shots carom off the rim. He tried again, making one shot.

He had spend seventy cents in about twenty minutes.

He and Bogey moved on to test their strength. Bogey tugged another dime from his pocket and traded it for a rubber sledge, pushed his shirt sleeves up under his arm pits, flexed what muscles he had and brought the hammer down, expecting it to smash a piece of metal high up to a bell.

He was disappointed when it didn't get halfway to its mark. He was more disappointed when he turned around and heard some girls his age giggling over his lack of strength.

Now Tad was down eighty cents. He drifted over to a man using what appeared to be halves of three English walnut shells and one marble.

"Guess which one I put the marble under and win thirty cents for a dime," the carnie said.

Tad lost twelve straight times, accepting a challenge to double, then triple the amount he'd win. He didn't know money could go so quickly.

He had now lost two dollars. He was both angry and hungry.

He spent his last thirty cents on a couple of sandwiches and a soda.

And it was only noon.

Bogey's parents loaned Tad fifty cents and suggested the boys spend the afternoon on the rides instead of games of chance. They did.

Tad told his parents what had happened when he returned home. His mom scolded him for being so foolish. His dad said, "Now, Mom! It's July 4 and a boy has a right to learn that independence doesn't come cheap."

Tad nodded, then added, "Guess you're right. But I didn't expect to have to pay $2.80 for it."

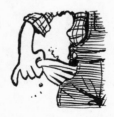

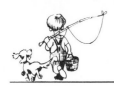

Church Meetings Were Food for the Soul

Rural churches were more than places to worship. They were social centers, places to meet old friends and make new ones, places to be married, places to celebrate the birth of infants and to eulogize the dead.

They provided playgrounds for new generations, graveyards for generations past. They were sanctuaries for those needing aid and comfort and for those in search of a meaning to life and death.

The busiest day of the year came in mid-summer. Some churches called day-long observances "homecomings." Others referred to them as "reunions" or "basket dinners."

At Mundell, southeast of Heltonville, the second Sunday in July was an "all-day meeting." It was a day Dale, Tad, Tyke, Billy, Ray and the other youngsters eagerly awaited in 1940, not because of the morning and afternoon services, but because of the basket dinner at noon.

The boys fidgeted through the opening of services, waiting for superintendent Nolan Bowman to announce they could go to their Sunday School classes. They behaved themselves in Miss Cummings' class, knowing she might tell their mothers if they acted badly.

That, however, was all the regimentation they could take. They didn't return to the sanctuary for the sermon when Sunday School classes ended, fleeing instead to the outdoors to romp under the shade trees. They kept their voices low, lest an adult leave the church to muffle their shouts.

An hour later, the men came from the church, leaving their wives inside to set the tables in the basement.

No one had to be called twice when the food was ready. Dale, Tad and their pals shuffled their feet during what seemed like a lengthy prayer, knowing young people would be allowed to go through the line first.

They didn't keep the people behind them waiting long. They piled their plates with fried chicken, ham, beef, corn-on-the-cob, apple butter, homemade biscuits and everything else except vegetables.

They used their free hands to hold tall glasses of lemonade, then stepped outside to find a cool place to eat. They always went back for seconds. The third time was for desserts—a big slice of apple pie, a scoop or two of banana pudding, a piece of chocolate cake.

"They're like threshing machines," an adult laughed. "There is no end to how much you can feed them."

That wasn't quite true. The boys eventually surrendered, reluctantly, knowing there was more food than they could devour.

They dozed for a time, rousing themselves when songs filtered through the walls of the church. They moseyed through the cemetery before crossing the rail fence to explore Charley Mark's poplar grove.

When the congregation left the church, the boys climbed into the back seats of their parents' cars, knowing chores were ahead. Tad looked through the basket his mother had brought, knowing the women would have shared any leftovers. There were pieces of pie, cake and a big cup of banana pudding.

Tad was delighted when his mother told him, "You can have some of that for supper."

Tad was even happier when his mom reminded him the ice cream social at the church would be that Wednesday night.

He was in heaven. And he hadn't heard a word of either sermon that day.

Willkie Was Also a Barefoot Boy

Had Wendell Willkie not been a Hoosier, Tyke would have noted the nomination of the Republican presidential candidate and thought little more about it. But Tyke was twelve years old that summer of 1940, a boy in search of an idol.

He had a few heroes to whom he could relate. Baseball players like pitcher Bob Feller, a farm boy like Tyke, and infielder Billy Herman, who had grown up at New Albany. And Ken Maynard, a cowboy star who had lived in Columbus before heading for Hollywood.

But Tyke was beginning to realize there was more to life than baseball games and westerns. He came to that realization after reading newspaper reports and listening to radio accounts of the Republican nomination for president.

Few people around Heltonville mentioned Willkie's name before the Republican convention in Philadelphia. Those who did, spoke only with skepticism. Willkie had no chance of winning, they said. He would be done in by better-known candidates like Thomas Dewey, the crime-busting district attorney from New York, Sen. Robert A. Taft or Sen. Arthur Vandenberg, whose names were household words.

Tyke hoped they were wrong. He wanted Willkie to win the same way he wanted Indiana University to beat Iowa in football and Illinois in basketball.

His innocence gave him a loyalty to his state and the people it produced, a loyalty without doubt or demand. It didn't bother him when Willkie was referred to as "the barefoot boy from Wall Street." Tyke went barefoot that summer himself. And as far as he knew, Wall Street was no different than 16th Street in Bedford.

And the pictures he had seen of Willkie made him look like he had slept in

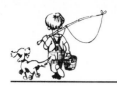

his suit while waiting for his hogs to be sold in the stockyards up at Indianapolis.

But Tyke figured there was nothing wrong with a rumpled look. It made Willkie appear more like a man of the people than Tom Dewey, who always had a tailored air.

And Tyke's fondness for Willkie grew even stronger when he learned Willkie had grown up in Elwood, which wasn't as big as Bedford, and owned farms in Rush County.

The convention voting started on Thursday, June 27, and Tyke would have stayed up all night if his parents had let him. He missed the "We Want Willkie" chants in the convention as the Willkie bandwagon rolled over Dewey, Taft and Vandenberg.

It wasn't until the next day he learned Willkie had upset the old-line Republican alliances, winning the GOP nomination for president on the sixth ballot. Suddenly Tyke's hero belonged to the nation, or at least that part of the nation that was Republican.

The skeptics around Heltonville and Norman said they had thought all the time Willkie would win. Even Tyke's father, who cared little for Franklin Roosevelt's social engineering or his desire for an unprecedented third term, was happy. "Maybe the Republicans have finally got someone who can throw the 'Great White Father' out of the White House," he said.

He found Tyke a Willkie-McNary button to wear and the boy seldom went anywhere without it that summer. He followed the campaign closely, figuring there was no way Willkie could lose the election.

But he did in November.

Tyke's father comforted him, saying, "It's not the end of the world. We can survive four more years of FDR . . .maybe."

But it was three or four months before Tyke told the barber to quit cutting his hair like Wendell Willkie's.

A Sweet Reward
for Hard Work

Hired hands didn't slack off in the hot August afternoon sun when they worked for Wes. It wasn't because Wes was a slavedriver. He expected them to earn their money, but he knew each man's limitations. And it wasn't because he paid them a few cents more than the going rate for farm labor around Heltonville in 1940.

The men worked hard, whether it was putting up hay, filling the silo or hulling clover seed. They knew their rewards would come at the end of the day.

Wes never let them leave for home without inviting them to sit a spell outside his spring house. The men sipped some of the cold water, then doused themselves with a dipper. They walked to a nearby creek, squatted and washed the dirt and dust from their arms, before plopping down in the shade of the beech trees that ringed the spring house.

Once they were comfortable, Wes carried out a big watermelon that had chilled in the basin of the spring. It was a ritual the men had come to expect.

He took his big pocket knife with the long blade, cleaned it with a leaf of grass, and thrust it into the melon that he'd bought in the White River bottoms near Medora. The melon split with a cracking invitation.

Wes played no favorite. He carved out the heart of the melon and divvied it up so each of the men could share in the moist sweetness.

The men let the melon dissolve slowly, savoring it, knowing it was a luxury in taste that came all too rarely. They knew there would still be a couple more slices of the melon for each of them. But those pieces wouldn't be as tasty as the heart.

Once the last piece of the melon had been finished, the men tossed the rinds into a bucket for Wes to feed to the hogs.

Wes had returned from the spring house, his arms loaded with roasting ears stacked like sticks of wood. He made another trip inside and came back with a bucket of tomatoes.

As the hands gathered their corn and tomatoes, Wes pulled his wrinkled checkbook from the bib of his overalls. He searched his pockets for a stubby, indelible pencil, then wrote each of them a check for their day's work.

The men folded the checks twice, slipped them into their worn wallets and thanked him.

"Not at all," he replied. "Can I count on you fellers to help me again sometime?"

They nodded. Then one of them would always add, "providin' you got some melons in the spring house."

Wes appreciated the humor. He knew they'd be back if they hadn't found steady work.

The men got in their rattletrap cars and drove off, stirring brown clouds of dust to drift behind them.

Wes watched them go. Their day's work was finished, but he still had to do the milking and feed the livestock.

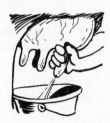

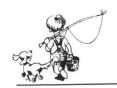

No Use Barking About Dog Days

Any hint of a breeze had died, its obituary written by stagnant air that rested lazily over the farm, days on end.

The sun baked relentlessly. Scum formed on farm ponds, causing the cattle to turn up their noses and look for fresh water downstream from the spring. The pastures had turned brown and the dairy cows gnawed on ragweed, which ruined their milk. Hogs sought shade, their wallowing holes long dried to dust.

Grass cooked by the heat crackled beneath the bare feet of youngsters as they walked to the creek to seek relief in what water was left in their swimming holes. Only weeds and crabgrass thrived.

Farm wives stopped working from sunup to sundown and took refuge on the porch swing, fanning themselves with *Country Gentleman* magazines.

These were the dog days of August 1940, maybe 1941. No matter! Most Augusts were the same.

The only thing that made this one different was Jim. Jim was a carpenter Tad's father hired to build a corn crib.

As with most men of character, Jim was quiet. He let his intelligence ease out, rather than try to influence his listener with what he knew.

His wisdom seemed limitless to a boy of twelve. Tad was helping him mix mortar for the crib's concrete-block foundation, the heat dripping from his sun-browned brow.

"Dog days are for dogs that don't have to work," Tad said.

Jim said, "Dog days have nothing to do with lazy dogs, which is what most people think. They're called dog days because this is the time when the Dog Star rises and sets with the sun."

He explained this star was the brightest in the Canis Major constellation and told Tad where to look for it. Jim wiped the perspiration from the sweat band on his felt hat and said, "That ain't real important. What is important is how you view dog days."

Tad wanted to know what he meant.

"Think of it as nature's vacation season. Only the sun is working. But that's 'cause it gets some time off during the winter.

"It's like life. When you get to middle age, like me, you sometimes get burned out. So you take it easy, relax a bit, back off and take a look at where you've been and where you're headin'. You can go on when you get your second wind," he added.

Tad pulled the hoe through the mortar mix and wondered how that related to the seasons of the year. Jim explained that, too: "The year was born in the newness of spring, like a lamb in still cold weather. But it made it. The lamb grew and the grass greened; the flowers bloomed, and the crops did well.

"By July the year was in its maturity. In another month or two, fall'll be here, the autumn of life, and by winter, the corn and beans and gardens will be buried in snow.

"Seasons are like life," Jim said, knocking the mortar off his trowel against a concrete block.

He took a drink from the water keg and said, "It's best we quit talking and get back to work."

That night Tad's sisters complained about the heat.

"Enjoy it," Tad said. "It's just a phase of life."

Boy and Ice Cream Won't Be Separated

You could take a boy out of the country, but you couldn't get him past a store that sold ice cream—at least if that boy was Chig, or one of his friends who grew up around Heltonville around 1940.

They lived in an area not yet reached by electricity. And without electricity, there was no refrigeration...and no ice cream stored in the freezer. That made trips to C.E. Cummings' general store in Norman and Roberts' store in Heltonville a special treat on summer evenings.

Chig usually went for a double cone, a ten-cent bargain with chocolate on one side, vanilla on the other and a strawberry dip mounted in the center.

He perfected the art of eating a cone, twisting it slowly, savoring each turn, letting not a drop melt, run down the side and drop to the ground. He straddled his bicycle outside the store as the cone slowly disappeared.

His buddies, Tad and Tyke, used their dimes for nickel cones, which they would enjoy before buying five-cent ice cream sandwiches that melted almost as soon as the boys walked from the store out into the heat.

The trips were enjoyable and Chig was looking forward to another bike ride to town one August evening when his dad said he had to go to Norman on business.

"Want me to bring you back some ice cream?" he asked.

Chig said, "You bet. A quart of vanilla."

His dad laughed, figuring Chig intended to share it with his buddies a quarter-mile down the road. He was surprised when Chig, who was no more than ten at the time, was still alone when he returned.

He pulled from a sack the quart of vanilla, made by the Johnson Creamery at Bloomington, and said, "You'll never be able to eat all of this, but it's yours to try."

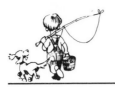

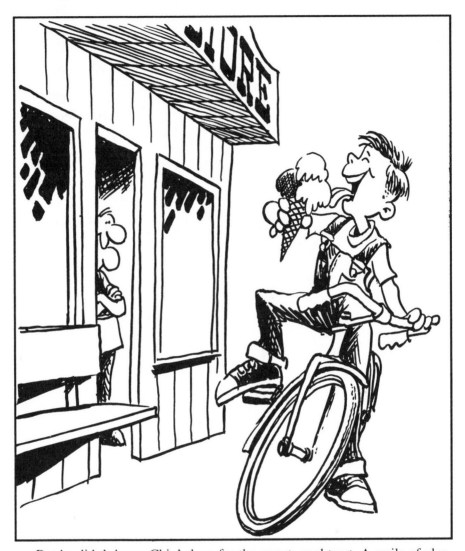

But he didn't know Chig's love for the sweet, cool treat. A smile of pleasure followed each spoonful until Chig was scraping the sides of the cardboard carton. When he was finished, he held a corner of the container to his mouth and sipped the cream that remained from the melt-down.

His dad, who had seen the coming of the automobile, the farm tractor and the airplane, was seldom surprised by anything, but he shook his head in disbelief at his son's appetite for ice cream.

"Never saw anything like it," he said.

He would have been surprised a year or two later when Chig was old enough to earn some money working for neighboring farmers. Chig stuck a few coins in his pocket and rode his bike to the restaurant in Heltonville.

"Gimme a giant chocolate malt and a strawberry sundae with an extra dip of ice cream," he said.

Lute, who ran the place, looked at him and asked, "You expecting someone else to help you?"

Chig shook his head. "Nope. Gimme the sundae first, then the malt."

He ate the sundae, then sipped the malt while a couple of customers looked to see if the bib of his overalls would split from the galluses and the buttons explode from the sides.

Chig had the double treat a couple of more times before summer ended. He then cut back on ice cream to half a pint a day, which he ordered each noon when he went to the restaurant from school.

"Gotta get in shape for the basketball season," he told Tad, who bought the other half of the pint Lute had divided.

True Veteran Stayed Behind the Scenes

He was quiet and reserved. He never talked much about himself, except for bragging sometimes about his kids.

He kept out of the limelight even though he dabbled in township politics. He had two or three different nicknames and even some of his friends didn't realize what his real name was until he ran for trustee.

He gave no clues that he was a veteran of World War I who had seen action in the trenches of France and had been at the front when the Germans used poison gas against Allied troops.

He farmed north of Heltonville in the 1940s so Tad and other youngsters who lived on farms east of town didn't know him too well. Tad probably would never have known about the man's war record if he hadn't been with his dad one Saturday morning in Heltonville.

Tad's dad called the man "Doc." Tad listened to the men talk about corn yields, President Franklin Roosevelt and other topics before one of them mentioned Armistice Day.

"Going to the parade in Bedford?" asked Tad's pa, who had been too old for World War I.

"Doc" said he didn't know. "Can't decide whether to bring myself to go or not."

Later, after the conversation was over and Doc had left, Tad asked his father, "What'd he mean 'bout bringin' himself to watchin' the parade?"

It was then his dad revealed what he knew about "Doc's" service in "the war to end all wars," about the mustard-gas attacks, about shrapnel, about

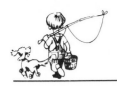

shell shock, about Flanders' Field, about the armistice of November 11, 1918, and about the observances held each year to remember the Americans who had fought.

"We're going to the parade, aren't we?" Tad asked his dad.

School would be out that day and his dad kidded him, "Figured we'd shuck corn if the weather is nice. I can use your help."

Armistice Day turned out brisk and bright and his dad postponed the corn harvest and said, "Let's drive to town and watch the parade."

Tad hadn't understood the solemnity of Armistice Days until then. He watched men and women stand at attention for the American flag. His eyes scanned the crowd for "Doc."

Tad didn't spot him, but he saw men like "Doc," tall and bowed at the shoulders and rugged of features with faces of creases. He watched them wipe tears from their eyes as veterans' units passed.

"Doc" wouldn't have cried in public. Maybe that's why he didn't show up, or why, if he did, he chose to view the ceremony from a place where he wouldn't be seen.

Tad told his dad on the way home, "If I was a veteran I'd want people to know about it."

His dad said, "Maybe you would, maybe you wouldn't. Real men don't always boast about what they've done."

Tad concluded "Doc" was a real man.

* * *

Note: Armistice Day was changed to Veterans Day in 1954.

Learning About
the Good Things

If Tad's mom had told him once, she'd told him a hundred times: "Be thankful for what you have." But like most nine- or ten-year-old boys, he thought other families had more of the good things in life than did his.

He didn't know what wealth was, but he knew some folks seemed to have more riches than others. His comparisons were based on what he'd seen when he visited homes in Heltonville.

It was a few days before Thanksgiving around 1940 when his mom suggested he think of the things for which he could be thankful. He promised he would, but then asked, "What are you thankful for, Mom?"

Before she could answer, he said, "You don't have an electric washing machine like the women in town."

She smiled and said, "No. But we do have a Maytag with a gasoline engine which gets clothes just as clean."

Tad said, "You don't have a 'frigerator or even an ice box."

She replied, "No. But we have a good springhouse, where we can keep milk and butter cool."

He said, "We don't even have electricity."

She answered him, still unperturbed, "No. But we have an Aladdin lamp and four or five coal-oil lamps."

Tad kept talking. "We don't have a coal furnace."

His mom responded, "No. But we have a good heating stove, a wood-house full of oak and beech, and besides wood is cleaner than coal."

His dad walked in about that time, but didn't interrupt.

Tad said, "We don't have any indoor plumbing."

His dad was perceptive enough to catch the drift of the conversation. He answered that time.

"Yes," he said. "But we do have an outhouse without any cracks and a wood-plank path to it."

Tad turned to his dad and said, "You don't have a cornpicker, like some farmers."

His dad replied, "No. But I got two good hands and can shuck a load of corn faster than anyone else around."

Tad was like an overheated gasoline engine. He didn't stop easily. "Well, we don't have as much money as some people do."

His dad said, "No. But we have other things. Milk cows. Some beef cattle. Cribs full of corn. A barn full of hay. Some good land."

"And we all have good health. We go to church on Sundays and we don't owe anybody anything we can't pay back."

Tad didn't respond, so his dad added, "And I'm thankful I got two boys who get up early enough to help me do the chores before they go to school."

Tad smiled at the praise, grabbed a milk bucket and headed for the barn. He thought about what his parents had said. He sometimes wished he could afford to do some things other kids his age did, but his mom never had to tell him again to be thankful for what he had.

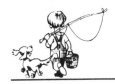

Wish Books Didn't Have Everything

The Thanksgiving leftovers were gone and it was time to look ahead to Christmas. That, for most farm families in 1940, meant looking through the big catalogs. Wish books, some folks called them.

Spiegel's, Sears Roebuck & Co. and Montgomery Ward & Co. catalogs could be found in almost every home around Heltonville and each offered hundreds of pages of items at reasonable prices.

The catalogs provided an alternative to shopping in town for Zeke and Millie. Zeke wasn't comfortable in crowds, especially those who packed the stores in Bedford on the Saturdays before Christmas. He farmed and worked at the stone mill, too, and couldn't shop any other day.

The less time he spent buying Christmas presents, the better, or so he said. He was pleased when he saw Millie looking through the big Sears catalog, making notations on a piece of lined Golden Rod notepaper as she searched for bargains.

She went through the book by sections, looking in women's wear and jewelry for presents for their daughters, men's wear and sporting goods for their sons. She skipped the home furnishings, kitchen and laundry and home-modernization sections. There would be no money for any of those things until next year.

She tore from the back of the book an order form that promised "We guarantee to please you."

The order blank had places for the catalog number of the article wanted, the quantity, the name, color, size, price and shipping weight.

She waited until Zeke left the room to fill out the line for a pair of "Hercules sanforized bib overalls made from the finest blue blood denim." She filled out another line for a denim jacket, made of the same material. The price for each item was $1.29.

For her sons, she ordered sanforized heavy chambray shirts at forty-eight cents each. She mentally calculated the total after each item, then figured she could afford to buy each of the boys hightop "Indian Pac" shoes, with nine pairs of hooks. The price was $1.98 each. She didn't know it, but the boys would have picked the same shoes if they'd had a choice.

She debated between ordering them Red Ryder carbine air rifles for $2.98 each or Buck Jones Daisy BB guns for $3.25, Bob Feller model baseball gloves for $2.98 or an official basketball, with laces, for $3.98.

She chose the gloves and basketballs, figuring they were safer.

Millie ordered some items for the girls, making sure each of the youngsters would receive items of equal value.

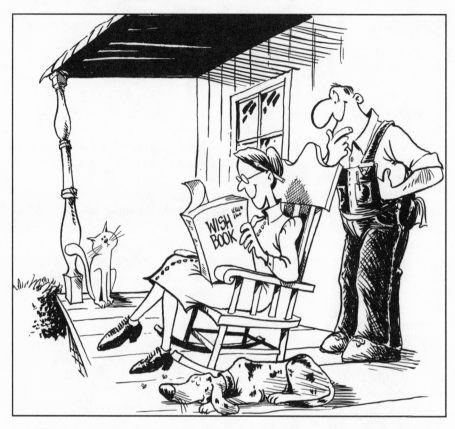

The items took about two-thirds of the order form and Millie reluctantly added up the total, knowing Zeke wouldn't be too happy if it was too much.

"Comes to $35.70," she said, handing Zeke cash from her butter and egg money to pay for the things she had ordered for him.

He grumbled before pulling a stubby indelible pencil from the bib of his overalls and wrote out a check. "Seems like a lot, but at least I won't have to take you to town to shop."

It took courage, but Millie replied, "Afraid you're wrong about that. I still have some items I need to buy in town."

Zeke stammered a few words he didn't learn from the preacher, but it was an act. He didn't want Millie to know he had to go to town, anyhow, to buy her Christmas present.

Some things were just too important to leave to a clerk in a big mail-order house in Chicago, even if he did have to fight the crowds in town.

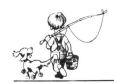

The Major Leagues of Mushroom Hunting

If mushroom hunting had been an organized sport, Pat would have played in the major leagues. At the time Ted Williams of the Boston Red Sox was making hitting a science, Pat was proving that mushroom hunting is an art.

He could find mushrooms when and where no one else could. He brought in sackfuls in a few hours in 1941 when others returned empty-handed from a day-long search around Heltonville.

Some people would have spied on Pat, hoping to see where he found the big yellow morels, but they knew he would be able to elude them in the Henderson Creek hills.

Pat would only smile noncommittally when the envious used devious means and trick questions in an attempt to find his secret. It was only to Tyke that he offered any explanation at all for his success.

Pat stopped at Tyke's house one afternoon, carrying a brown bag full of mushrooms.

"Where've you been?" Tyke asked, knowing better than to expect a direct answer.

Pat ignored the question, but he did pull out a three-by-five-inch Spiral notebook from the right hip pocket of his overalls. He handled it with care, like it was an ancient manuscript of undetermined value.

Pat was about nineteen, several years older than Tyke. He appeared like a teacher, ready to impart vital information to a student.

"This little book holds the mystery of the mushroom. I have to be careful none of the pages come out," he explained.

He leafed through the book quickly, then returned to the front.

"What this is," he said, waving the book in the air, "is all the information I've recorded about mushrooms."

Tyke looked impressed. "What kind of information?" he asked.

Pat said, "Lots of information. I have written down the dates, times, places and number of mushrooms found each year.

"And what's more, I have recorded the temperature and the humidity, the soil conditions and the number of days since the last rain. If I ever find a soil thermometer, I'll list the soil temperature, too.

"I'd die before I'd give up this book," he added.

Tyke laughed. "You may, if anyone else finds out about it. But do you really think all that information helps?"

Put pulled a big sponge from the bag, patted the sack and said, "What do you think?"

Tyke smiled. The answer was obvious. "You've told me everything I need to know about mushrooms but where to find them. Gonna tell me that?"

Pat grinned, and answered, "Like Confucius, or somebody, said, the best route through life is the one you find yourself."

Tyke looked puzzled. Pat added, "Same goes for mushroom hunting. You'll remember the ones you find yourself a lot longer than the ones some-one shows you."

Pat turned to walk back to the road.

"You forgot your mushrooms!" Tyke yelled.

"Didn't forget 'em. They're yours. You'll have to find the next mess your-self."

Horses of a Different Color

Tad didn't know the man who was dominating the conversation that Saturday morning at Jerry Jones' feed mill in Heltonville. He was a stranger talking a language alien to Tad.

It was the first Saturday in May 1941, and the men had discussed the war in Europe, corn planting and grain prices until the talk turned to the Kentucky Derby that afternoon.

"Yep! I bet a wad of dough on Whirlaway in the Kentucky Derby today. Them 8-1 odds look awful good to me," the man said.

Thoroughbred racing was foreign to Tad. His was a world of draft horses, mules, jacks and jennies and nags retired to pasture. The only thoroughbreds he knew were hounds farmers around town used to chase foxes and tree rac-coons.

Tad knew even less about parimutuel betting or odds. Tad, who was eleven, had never been to Louisville, which was just seventy miles away, let alone visit Churchill Downs, the race track the stranger mentioned from time to time.

He wasn't alone in his lack of knowledge. Few of the farmers paid much attention to horse racing. "That's a sport for rich folks," his dad had told him once.

One of the men asked, "How you gonna bet if you're not at the race?"

The stranger said he had sent his money down with a friend. "Told him to put it all on Whirlaway."

Someone wondered, "What'll you get back if the horse wins?"

The stranger did some mental calculations, then replied, "At eight-to-one odds I stand to get back eighty dollars for every ten dollars I bet. If I bet a hundred dollars, and I ain't saying I did, I'd get back eight hundred dollars. But the odds could drop if a lot of bettors put their money on Whirlaway

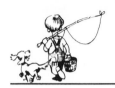
before the race starts."

Some of the men whistled their amazement. Tad's father shook his head. "I don't believe in gamblin'," he said. Some of the others agreed with him.

The stranger scanned the circle of men with his eyes, put his hands in his back pockets and said, "You're all farmers. And you're gonna be puttin' in your crops in a week or so. And plant a few acres of tomatoes to sell to Morgan Packing Co.

"What you're doing is bettin' it'll rain, your crops will flourish and you'll get back two dollars, maybe three dollars, for every dollar you spend to put the crops in the ground. Right?"

The men looked at each other like maybe the stranger had a point. Tad's dad said, "You're right as far as you go. But I got more faith in my land and in the Lord providin' rain and good weather than I got in some horse I've never seen and in some rider who ain't no bigger than a sack of Jerry's flour."

"Amen," said one of the men who went to the same church.

The stranger brushed the dust from the feed grinder off his pants and smiled.

"A difference of opinion is what makes a horse race. See you fellers in a week or two."

The men watched him leave, then resumed talking about farming. They didn't mention the Kentucky Derby again.

* * *

P.S. Both Tad's father and the stranger were winners that year. Whirlaway won the Derby, returning $7.80 for each $2.00 bet. He went on to win the Preakness and Belmont Stakes with jockey Eddie Arcaro. It was a good year for farmers, too. The crops returned Tad's father's investment . . . and a good profit to boot.

Telling Time Without a Watch

Years in the sun had bronzed Clem's face and lined it with streams for the sweat to flow. He was about sixty-five, that summer of 1941, when Chig, who was twelve, learned to know him.

They were two generations apart, a man who knew the answers to many of life's lessons, a boy who was eager to learn them. Wisdom and curiosity blended the old and the young into a solid friendship.

They were brought together by necessity: Clem needed someone to help him on his farm near Heltonville; Chig needed spending money.

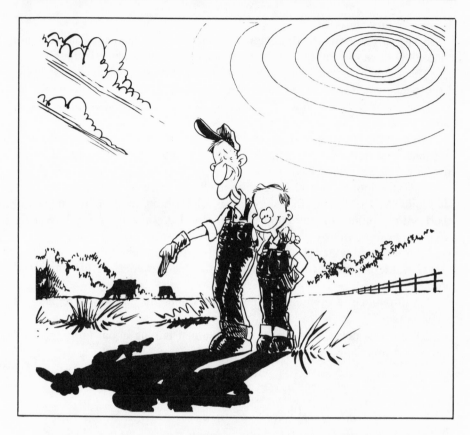

"He can help you anytime I don't need him," Chig's dad had told Clem.

The first occasion came one June day when Clem sought help in shocking bundles the binder had dropped as it cut swaths through a golden field of wheat. Chig had shocked grain before, but Clem showed him how to do the work more easily. They worked for what seemed hours, Chig wondering when they would quit for lunch. He hesitated at first, then gathered enough courage to ask, "When do we stop for lunch?"

Clem said, "At noon." He stood upright. "It's only 10:30 now."

Chig was amazed Clem could tell time without a watch.

Clem smiled. "Don't need a watch. I have a clock right here," he said, pressing his right index finger to the side of his forehead.

He told Chig to face north. "Think of the spot right in front of you as twelve on a clock. Consider nine o'clock where your left arm extends. Three o'clock where your right arm reaches. Drop your arms and see where your shadow falls."

Chig did as he was told. His shadow fell midway between nine and twelve.

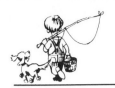

"What happens if I don't know which way is north?" the boy asked.

Clem smiled. "Just remember to get up early enough to see where the sun comes up. That'll be east."

As an afterthought, he said, "In case you're out at night, better take a watch."

He took a drink from the wooden water keg, handed it to Chig and said, "We best be gettin' on with what we're doing."

They worked for a time before Clem asked, "What time do you think it is now?"

Chig turned to the north, looked at his short shadow and said, "My stomach says two o'clock, but the sun shows it's a few minutes 'til twelve."

Clem grinned, "We'll take the sun's word for it."

They walked a quarter-mile to Clem's house. His wife had dinner on the table. The clock said 11:58.

Chig was happy he had correctly read his shadow. He was happier to see the food.

It was the first of many things Chig was to learn from Clem that summer. He forgot some of those things, but not how to read the sun's clock.

* * *

P.S. Chig had to readjust his mental clock when the nation went on Daylight Savings Time during World War II. He quit for lunch at·11:00 a.m. by the sun, noon by the kitchen clock.

"Twins" Shared Their Differences

Folks around the Mundell community southeast of Heltonville called them the twins.

They were born on the same July day in 1929, but they weren't brothers. Kin was an only child. Tad had two brothers, four sisters.

Kin wore new clothes. Tad wore clothes handed down from his older brothers.

On the surface, they appeared to have little in common, except their birth date. Maybe it was those contrasts that tightened the bond between them as they grew up a couple of miles apart.

Kin lived with his mom and dad in a house on his grandfather's farm. His dad, who worked in Bedford, was an hourly employee, bringing home a fixed amount of money each Friday. That meant the family had money for a movie on weekends and an occasional dinner at a restaurant.

The house Kin lived in was small, neat, always painted and in good repair. It had electricity provided by a Delco generating system.

Tad lived with his parents in a big, rambling two-story house on a farm where his dad wrestled drought, erosion, wind and hail in a continual fight to reap a profit from each crop.

Tad didn't know what an allowance was. His parents gave him spending money only on special occasions. He earned any other change he had doing whatever a boy could when he was seven, eight, nine and ten.

About the only time they dined out was at church dinners.

The farm house had no electricity, but it was always well maintained, even if it wasn't as new as Kin's home.

Kin and Tad rode the same bus to school in Heltonville, had the same teacher, attended the same Sunday School class, visited each other almost every Sunday and stayed overnight as often as their parents permitted.

That gave Kin a chance to be a tumultuous part of a big family, Tad an opportunity to observe the relative calm of a small one.

They argued, as all boys do at times, but they never fought. They tried to outdo each other in school and in other competition. As friends, never as antagonists.

In time, they assumed their association would last a lifetime. But that was before they realized the universe extended beyond the ten-mile radius that was their world.

That time came one warm summer day in 1941 when Kin plopped his bicycle into the ditch in a hay field where Tad and his dad were working. It was one of the few times Tad had seen him look downcast.

Kin explained why.

"We're moving," he said, shuffling his feet into the clover stubble. "Dad's got a job at the ammunition plant at Charlestown. We'll be moving there before school starts."

Tad took on the same sad look.

They spent a few more weeks together, admitting their envy of each other's home life. They promised to write each other about school and to exchange visits the next summer. It was a promise neither kept. They saw each other a few times in the next few years, but they gradually grew apart.

Each found new friends and new interests. But chances are they still remember each other on the July day they add another year to their lives and think back to those summers a half-century ago.

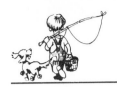

His Tomatoes Were Money in the Bank

The big boys laughed when Bugsy showed up one August morning to pick tomatoes for Clarence.

Their jokes about his size echoed off the tin roofs on the barns in the distance. Bugsy didn't mind. He had been called "Runt" so long he thought that was his name. And he knew if the boys didn't like him they would ignore instead of rib him.

He was eleven, but he looked no older than eight. He didn't weigh much more than a bar of homemade lye soap and he was as frail as a weed in a windstorm. His railroad engineer's cap rested loosely on his ears and his overalls had been rolled up to keep from dragging the ground.

He wore a pair of shoes with loose soles that flapped as he walked. His appearance belied his courage. He wasn't afraid of the bigger boys or of hard work. Bugsy lived on a nearby farm and Clarence knew Bugsy had true grit when he was given a job to do.

When the laughter died down, Clarence looked at each of the boys who had come to work and said, "OK, you all know I pay by the crate. The more crates you fill, the more you'll make."

Bugsy nodded, plopped his five-gallon pail between two rows and started to pick. He kept his head down, looking up only when he stood to empty the bucket. The other boys talked. He didn't join in. He didn't even pay attention. He just concentrated on filling bucket after bucket.

He stopped at the end of the row for a drink of water. A couple of the other boys had finished a row first but that didn't bother him. He resumed picking while they tarried.

He worked throughout the morning, stopping only long enough at noon to eat the lunch his mom had fixed.

He was halfway down another row before the others finished playing pitch-and-catch with green tomatoes. He slowed his pace when the sweat in his shirt steamed from the mid-afternoon sun. But he didn't stop.

The boys finished the field about 5:00 p.m. and Clarence paid each one as

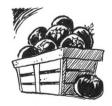

they finished their last crates. None left until all had been paid. They were curious to see who made the most money.

They didn't laugh when Clarence announced, "Today's big money-maker is Bugsy." To make his point, Clarence stretched out the name like an announcer at a prize fight.

Bugsy slipped the money into a front pocket, trying to keep a smile from splitting his face.

His tormentors applauded. He appreciated that almost as much as he did the money.

For Moms, Smoking Wasn't Stylish

It was a man's prerogative if he wished to smoke back in the early 1940s. It was a woman's flirtation with scorn.

A mother could tolerate, with reluctance, a son who sneaked a smoke of long green behind the barn or rolled his own cigarette from a bag of Bull Durham or from a can of Prince Albert.

If she happened to find a pack of Marvels in his shirt pocket, she'd be disappointed. But she could understand that.

What she couldn't understand was young girls who smoked, or even hinted they'd like to. Good girls, farm wives around Heltonville said, wouldn't be seen with a cigarette in their hands.

One of the wives, or so it was told, once walked up to a young woman in Bedford and asserted, "Young lady, I'd rather commit adultery than smoke."

The young woman replied, supposedly, "So would I, but I only have thirty minutes for lunch."

That not only perturbed the mother, the story goes, but it made her even more committed than ever to do anything in her power to keep her daughters from ever smoking what some folks called white cylinders of sin.

It wasn't easy. Especially in 1941. Glamorous movie actresses smoked on the silver screens, their cigarettes lighted by their suitors.

Tobacco companies went all-out to lure women smokers. And they did it with slick, colorful ads in the wide selection of general-interest magazines that found their way into homes.

The advertisements often showed attractive singers, actresses and other celebrities extolling the virtue of a particular brand.

There were Chesterfield ads in *Collier's* and other places of:

• Marion Hutton with sequins on her red dress, cigarette in hand, and type that read "Marion Hutton in Glenn Miller's 'Moonlight Serenade' broadcasts today's most popular numbers.

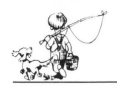

"There is a greater demand than ever for Chesterfields. Smokers who have tried them are asking for them again and again, and for the best of reasons. Chesterfields are cooler, better-tasting and definitely milder . . . So tune in now for your 1941 smoking pleasure. They satisfy!"

• And of Marjorie Woodworth, "Chesterfield's girl of the month in the Hal Roach hit, 'All American Coed.' A United Artists release."

• And of a beautiful model with a sales pitch that read: "Double and redouble your pleasure with the smoker's cigarette, Liggett & Myers Tobacco Co. Right combination. World's best tobacco."

• Lucky Strike used models, too, along with slogans like "LS/MFT, Lucky Strike means fine tobacco. In a cigarette, it's the tobacco that counts."

• And there were ads for Old Golds promising that "Apple Honey" would help guard Old Golds from cigarette dryness.

• And for the impressionable youth, there was a young-looking Johnny, with a promotion that pleaded, "Call for Philip Morris, America's finest cigarette. You can't avoid some inhaling, but you can avoid worry about throat irritation even when you do inhale."

Pokey's sister tore out some of the advertisements and kept them in her room, thinking maybe she'd try to convince her mother that smoking for women was in style.

But she never did. She could confide a lot of things to her mom, but never her desire to try cigarettes.

He Drove Model T
Straight to H

Ben didn't cotton to new-fangled contraptions. The simpler things were, the better, he reasoned.

He was still driving a Model-T Ford in the 1940s. And he never did get around to buying a farm tractor. What field work he did in his twilight years was behind a team of horses.

Ben was a kindly sort—friendly most of the time . . . except when he was cantankerous. Most neighbors knew better than to whet his temper when he already was in a bad mood.

His fuse was as short as a bobtailed dynamite stick.

Ben lived with his wife, Ellie, on a small farm south of Ind. 58 and east of Heltonville. They were nearly self-sufficient. About the only time they drove the ten miles to Bedford was to buy a few things they couldn't grow or make at home.

They did attend church, but they missed Sunday services often enough to cause the minister to worry about their salvation. But, then, he fretted a lot,

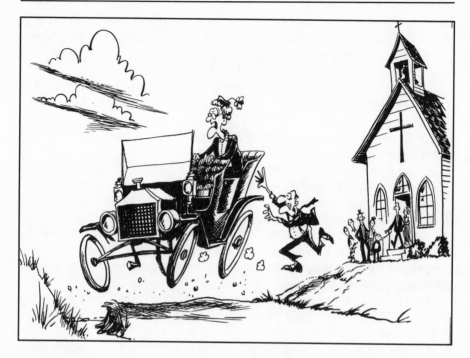

anyhow, over the final destination for members of the congregation.

The last time Ben and Ellie went to Mundell, a rural church nearby, was in 1940, give or take a year or two.

Ben parked the Model-T in the church lot, backing it into a spot to make sure he had room to crank it to a start later. Ellie walked up the steps and joined the women inside. Ben waited outside for the bell to ring, talking with other farmers about crops and the weather.

After the services, Ellie remained inside to talk. Ben visited with the men a few minutes and then began to shuffle from one foot to the other. His neighbors knew he was getting perturbed when he pulled out each suspender and let it pop back against his perspiration-darkened shirt.

It was obvious he was ready to head home and that Ellie's dallying was to blame for his impatience. His face had turned red by the time Ellie walked down the steps. He followed her to the car, then set the spark and the gas levers and fidgeted with some other instruments as she eased into the back seat where she always sat.

Ben walked to the front of the car, grabbed the crank, and gave it a twist. Then another. The car lurched forward. Ben jumped to the side to avoid being hit. The car went across Powerline Road, which ran beside the church, banged against the clay bank and stopped, still chugging as only a Model-T could.

Ellie looked scared.

Ben ran as fast as his aging legs would take him to the car, jumped in and

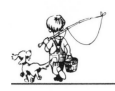

shifted into reverse. He backed out quickly and headed for home, his bronze face by now even darker red.

But he didn't get away fast enough for the congregation to keep from hearing Ellie give him a piece of her mind. Ben didn't look at her. He just stared straight ahead, letting Ellie vent her embarrassment.

Neither Ben nor Ellie ever came back to church, at least not for Sunday services. And the minister never had the nerve to call on Ben or Ellie to ask them to return.

A Lesson Learned from a Fallen Hero

Chig had looked forward to the 1941-42 basketball season, counting the days as he practiced his shots in the barn. He had just turned twelve and his parents had told him he could attend all of Heltonville's at-home high school games that season.

He, Billy, Ray and other youngsters who lived east of town had seen a few games the previous year, walking the five miles home when they couldn't find a ride.

They chose their heroes on the team and tried to emulate their shots and mannerisms in their barnloft games. Chig tried to pattern his play after "Boob" Henderson, a guard who could shoot well from out on the floor and handled the ball like a magician.

Only teachers and sports writers referred to Boob as Loren. Chig never knew how Boob got his nickname, but he knew it was used more with affection than with humor. Boob was a friendly teenager who could turn a casual encounter into a lifelong friendship.

Adults told Chig the team should be even better than the year before, even though Pat Bailey, the leading scorer, had graduated. Boob, they said, could offset the loss with help from Lester Neff, Herman Chambers, Dale Norman, Gerald Denniston, Bob Hillenburg and the other players.

Some fans counted on Boob scoring fifteen to twenty points a game, and leading the team to victory after victory. Their hopes, and Chig's high expectations, ended almost before the season started. Chig heard the news one Saturday morning before a game that night. Boob, hunting the previous afternoon, had injured his hip as he tried to climb over a fence.

The injury didn't appear too serious at first. But Boob would not play that night. The news grew worse the next week. Boob's playing days appeared to be over.

And then the analysis was final. The injury was permanent and Boob would always walk with a limp.

Chig's enthusiasm for basketball waned. He went to the games, watching the team play Shawswick, Tunnelton, Needmore, Williams, Fayetteville, winning some, losing some.

His disappointment continued until he was in a group one night at a game when Boob started to talk. Chig mentioned he missed watching Boob play.

"Life doesn't always turn out the way you want it to. You can't build tomorrow on yesterday. And remember things could always be worse," Boob said, showing wisdom beyond his years.

It was like Chig's dad had said, "What's done sometimes can't be undone." Chig figured he could make it through the season if Boob could.

Chig chose another hero, but things weren't quite the same. And, as Boob had said, things could be worse. The U.S. entered World War II that December, the gym burned the following April and the school had no basketball team in 1942-43.

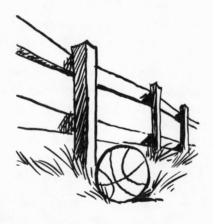

HOMEFRONT

The War
Next Door

It is December 5, 1941, and Herbert Dale Harrell is on the destroyer Flusser in the Pacific.

Fate has distanced him, temporarily, from Pearl Harbor. A few days earlier, the Flusser had been at Pearl Harbor and Seaman First Class Harrell was pulling duty on a captain's boat, a little gig with a crew of three that escorted officers from ship to shore or from shore to ship.

The previous Saturday night, the captain's boat had plied the harbor, taking officers and their ladies to dances aboard a battleship. Harrell watched the officers and the women board the ship. He viewed the dancing across the water from the deck of the Flusser and listened to the music of the dance band.

In the parlance of Southern Indiana, the couples were, he thought, "putting on the dog." Chances are he let his mind think of guitar and banjo music he was more accustomed to hearing back in Heltonville, Indiana, where he had grown up and graduated from high school.

Any threat of war seemed as remote as it had a year earlier when "Herbie" Harrell enlisted in the Navy in search of his future. He had seen envoys from Japan receive a royal welcome at Pearl Harbor on a stop from Tokyo to Washington. Any hint of animosity was lost in the pomp and ceremony.

A day or two after the dance, the Flusser left port as a screen for carriers sent on maneuvers around the Midway Islands.

Looking back, Dale would think that "somebody from higher up must have told someone to order the carriers out to sea."

It would prove to be a wise move.

Once the carriers are at sea near Midway, the Flusser is ordered to return to Pearl Harbor for patrol duty. In two more days, the Flusser will be within radio range of Honolulu. The men will be looking forward to a few hours of shore leave.

But the serenity of the sea will end. And there will be no time for enjoyment on shore. The men on the destroyer will learn on December 7, via the ship radio, that Pearl Harbor is under attack from Japanese planes.

Harrell will remember in the years to come the constant reminder via radio, "This is not a test. The Japanese are attacking Pearl Harbor . . . This is not a test. The Japanese are attacking Pearl Harbor."

The Flusser is ordered to join up with other ships in the Pacific. It will be a few more days, about December 11, before the Flusser returns to Pearl Harbor to refuel.

The men will see the havoc of the December 7 bombing. And the scene will be recorded in Harrell's mind, never to be erased. There won't be a dry eye on the ship. Seamen with tattered tattoos and tales from a hundred ports will weep.

It will be years before there again are dances aboard U.S. Navy ships on Saturday nights.

There will be no more duty for Seaman Harrell on a captain's boat. The war has seen to that.

* * *

Postscript: Dale Harrell has retired as a rural mail carrier and now lives on a small farm near Heltonville where, among other things, he experiments with new colorations of Indian corn.

World Outside Hits Heltonville

Don paid more attention to what was going on in the world than most seventh graders did. It was obvious before December 8, but it became even more so after that.

Principal Loren Raines had solemnly called the upper six grades at Heltonville into the assembly that morning. He wanted them to listen over the radio as President Roosevelt addressed the nation.

The Japanese had savaged Pearl Harbor in a sneak attack the previous day. Roosevelt called December 7 "a day that will live in infamy" and asked Congress to declare war against Japan. Congress agreed.

The country had no alternative. But the attack on Pearl Harbor and the decision to go to war left a lot of unanswered questions in the minds of the seventh graders.

They mentioned those questions at lunch. Tad asked, breaking the string on his lunch which was wrapped in a newspaper, "Wonder if anyone from around here was at Pearl Harbor yesterday?"

Don said, "Herbie Harrell has been on a destroyer. He could have been."

Cecil, eating a peanut butter sandwich, wondered about how well-prepared the United States was to wage war.

Don said the country had been building up its army since the Germans invaded Poland in September 1939. "Draft started in October last year, but a lot of guys enlisted before that. Read someplace that Lawrence County had an enlistment rate of one man a day last year."

Bob wanted to know what had happened to William Howard Thompson, a

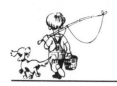

son of the restaurant owner who had graduated from Indiana University.

"He's in the Army Air Corps," Don said. "He has been an instructor pilot and now he's an assistant flight commander at a flying school in California," Don added.

Leonard asked, "Wonder where th Coach is?" Everybody knew he meant Cladie Bailey, another IU grad who grew up near Heltonville and coached basketball before being called to active duty as an ROTC officer.

Don said, "If he's an Army officer he may be in the Pacific soon."

The boys talked about the work at Burns City and Charlestown and mentioned men who had taken jobs at the two facilities. Burns City was a powder storage base in Martin County, west of Bedford. Work had started there in October 1941. Charlestown, about sixty miles southeast, was the site of a new smokeless powder plant. It was started before that.

Tad mentioned that Lawrence County had been on daylight saving time since the previous May and asked Don if he thought that would help in the war effort.

Don said, "From all I've read, wars are fought night and day, so I guess an hour's daylight won't make any difference."

The others laughed for one of the few times that day.

They would continue their discussions of the war for four years. And, as usual, Don could answer more questions than anyone else in the class.

* * *

Postscript: Heltonville's William Howard Thompson served throughout the war and now resides at Bakersfield, California. Lt. Col. Cladie Bailey was killed in 1944 in the Philippines; he was the highest-ranking officer from Lawrence County to die in the war.

War's Realities
Come Home to Chig

Christmas and New Year's had been a time of mixed emotions and now they were gone. It was now 1942 and the country was at war.

Chig had received Christmas presents as usual, but even a twelve-year-old boy sensed there had been less merriment than normal in what usually was a season of joy.

There had been no signs of Christmas at all in parts of the world. And the new year looked bleak for Americans.

The Japanese had attacked Pearl Harbor three weeks earlier and threatened to expand its hold over more of the Pacific. A half-world away, Adolph Hitler and his Axis associate, Benito Mussolini, ruled most of Europe and parts of Africa and continued to spread terror and their misguided belief in a superior race.

Chig read news stories of the fighting and tried to visualize what war was like. Real comprehension was beyond his limited knowledge and experience.

His folks told him there would be time later for him to fret about war and destruction, that it was time for him to think about returning to school, to get on with the business of life.

"Don't rob yourself of your boyhood," his mom told him.

It was good advice, but the signs of war were ever-present and Chig couldn't ignore them, even if he wanted to. The year passed slowly, agonizingly so.

In mid-January, the Japanese launched a massive attack against American and Philippine forces on the Bataan Peninsula. The valiant Bataan resistance ended in April, but Gen. Douglas MacArthur promised once again from his headquarters in Australia that he would return and avenge the loss. It was the kind of pledge a staggered America needed to restore its confidence.

That same month, the hardships of war came home to Chig in terms he could understand. The school and gym at Heltonville burned on graduation night when the thirteen seniors were to receive their diplomas.

The nation had mobilized for war by then and a new school would have to wait until peace came. Chig and other eighth graders spent the rest of the school year in classrooms in church basements and lodge halls. The school would have no basketball team that season and would play all games on the road for years after that.

Rationing came and Chig no longer could sprinkle his toast with sweetness or coat his oatmeal with sugar.

Chig's parents kept telling him darkness was always the blackest before dawn, that things would get better.

They were right. Allied forces began to pursue the Nazi forces across North Africa later that year and the U.S. scored some victories against the Japanese.

But the war was far from won. Men, Chig knew, would die in battle. Others would be wounded, others taken prisoner.

That would make inconveniences like shoe rationing, which would come later, seem insignificant.

Chig knew he was at least secure in his isolated world. He had started the year as a twelve-year-old boy. He would feel sixteen, maybe older, before it ended.

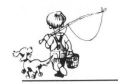

A Boy Grows into a Man

Biceps had begun to form in Chig's arms, making him think he was more man than boy. He was twelve or thirteen, young enough to think he was beyond pain or harm, old enough to know no fear.

It was a phase most boys around Heltonville went through. It was to his parents' credit that they humored his brashness, rather than ridiculed it.

They reasoned he would outgrow that phase in life when he wore his cockiness like a decal.

That's why his dad didn't protest when Chig announced one morning he'd fill up the new 1941 Farmall H and grind feed for the livestock by himself. His dad was apprehensive, but reluctant to inhibit Chig's desire to work.

His dad just stayed close enough to help if Chig got into trouble.

Chig mounted the tractor after breakfast and drove to the 500-gallon gravity-flow gasoline tank mounted about eight feet off the ground. He reached for the nozzle to insert it into the gasoline tank.

The handle slipped from his grasp and crashed across his forehead, whacking his nose. Chig felt the pain but made sure the nozzle was clean and began to fill the tank.

The pain continued. Chig rubbed the back of his right hand across his forehead and noticed the blood. It didn't appear, he diagnosed, anything a man like himself should be concerned about.

He thought no more about the wound, driving the tractor up to the hammermill in the granary. He noticed the pain again as he squinted shut his left eye to align the pulley on the Farmall with the one on the mill.

He could endure pain, Chig assured himself once more.

He shoveled corn, wheat and oats into the mill and it responded by beginning to crush, spewing clouds of dust to settle over Chig and the clothes he wore.

He finished the chore before lunch. His dad walked to the granary as soon as he heard the tractor stop. He complimented Chig on a good morning's work.

Then he noticed the wound projecting through the dust coating on Chig's forehead.

"What did you do to yourself?" he asked.

Chig said it was nothing, "just a little accident with the nozzle on the gas tank. Takes more than something like that to stop us men, doesn't it?"

His dad nodded, but said, "You'd better go wash up and find out how bad you're hurt."

Chig cupped his hands in the pan on the washstand outside the house, bent over and doused himself. He raised up, looked into the mirror tacked onto the outer porch wall and saw the ravine the sweat had cut into the caked blood as it ran from his forehead. He looked a disaster after the fact.

No one knew if he also saw the big gouge on his nose before he fainted. His parents revived him quickly, happy his wounds were more superficial than significant.

Chig rested the remainder of the day and showed no after-effects the next morning. The cuts on his forehead and nose healed, but the scars remained.

His folks thought the scars gave Chig the looks of the man he thought he was.

Twisted Cedar Helps Courage Take Root

It stood there alone, twenty-five years later, a memorial to the 1917 tornadic winds that ripped through the area.

It was just a cedar tree, old, gnarled and void of beauty, worthless except maybe for fence posts.

But it seemed to have a personality, one it revealed only to those who paid it close attention. Boys, who grew as the tree did, considered it a friend, not out of pity because of its handicap but because of its rugged endurance.

The cedar leaned at a seventy to seventy-five-degree angle, slanting toward the southwest corner of the house near Heltonville where Tad lived. It was a tall tree, at least seventy-five feet high, and it measured thirty inches in diameter at its base.

"It has leaned like that since the windstorm shifted the house off its base and twisted the back barn awry," Tad's pa told him. "It has stood there so long, it seems like a member of the family."

He scanned the tree slowly, from bottom to top, then added, "Some people think we ought to take it down. They think it will fall on the house someday. I know better."

So did Tad.

Two strands of rope hung from a limb on the downside of the tree, cushioning a two-by-eight-inch seat on which Tad and his brother and sisters swung, unafraid their weight might cause the tree to fall. They soared toward the sky, confident on the arm of the tree.

Most youngsters who came to visit soon learned the cedar was safe. They played under it, climbed on it as far as they could walk on the up-side of the trunk, and jumped into the swing as soon as the seat was vacant.

Bugsy was an exception. He was an only child who seldom searched for adventure. The tree looked ominous to him, a thing to be avoided.

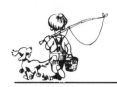

That was an impossibility, he learned one night when he stayed with Tad. A spring storm moved in from the west about midnight, carrying wind gusts that slashed the rain cuttingly against the window panes and caused the big farm house to creak and moan.

Bugsy climbed out of bed, looked out the window at the big cedar, which was weaving back and forth noisily. Bugsy jumped back in bed, telling Tad he expected the tree to crash through the roof and pin them between the branches and the feathered mattress.

When the rain died down, the lightning began, rattling the house from its foundation up. With each stroke of lightning, Bugsy thought the cedar had been hit and its shattered remains would come through the window.

He managed to survive the night.

So did the cedar. It stood firm the next morning, seeming to bow confidentially toward Bugsy when he went to look.

As soon as he finished breakfast, Bugsy ran to the swing under the tree and asked Tad to give him a boost.

The cedar had won another friend.

* * *

Postscript: The house the cedar stood watch over was razed twelve years later. The tree came down then, its mission in life served.

Look Out When High Pockets' About

Youngsters who attended Mundell Church were happy spring had arrived. Warm weather meant they could skinny-dip in the creeks, fish from the banks of streams, bicycle to Heltonville or Norman, play baseball . . . and watch High Pockets drive his 1935 Ford.

High Pockets wasn't the man's real name. The boys called him that because his wide suspenders with the gold-colored snaps pulled his pants almost under his armpits.

He wore a tie on a colored shirt to the rural church and looked uncomfortable most of the time, as all farmers did when they dressed up.

His wife was more fashionable. She wore store-bought clothes, and some of the other women were envious of her appearance.

They appeared to be an odd couple, even though they seemed devoted to each other.

But none of that had anything to do with why the boys at church looked forward to High Pockets' arrival each Sunday in the early 1940s.

"Be ready to run for your lives," one of the youngsters would shout. "Here comes High Pockets."

High Pockets was a good man but a terrible driver, and the boys looked forward to watching him park before church and take off afterwards. He'd try to back up, causing the owners of cars already parked to shake with apoplexy, fearful of what might happen. High Pockets always managed to park after four or five attempts.

He'd keep his foot on the accelerator while the clutch was engaged, causing the motor to race. Then he'd drop his foot from the clutch. The car would jump backwards like it was a descendant of a jackrabbit.

Some of the boys would applaud when he stepped from the car, but High Pockets didn't seem to notice.

After services, the boys would form a circle and wait until High Pockets and his wife decided to leave for home. He'd again race the engine, lift his foot from the clutch, weld both hands to the steering wheel and let the car lurch a few times before turning left on the county road.

The boys again applauded as the dust from High Pockets' car waved goodbye.

High Pockets had entertained the crowd for several Sundays before adults decided it was time to wean the observers from their weekly watch. One of the men walked over to the crowd and informed the boys, "You shouldn't make fun of him. He's a good man, and he has been driving since 1915 and never had an accident."

Tyke looked at the man, grinned and said, "That's because everybody knows by now to keep out of his way."

Tyke's father stormed toward him, his bronzed face reddened by Tyke's remark, and suggested it was time to go home. On the way, he gave a sermon that the preacher would have been glad to hear, except for the swear words. "Only smart alecks make fun of other folks," he said.

Tyke learned later that his friends had received similar rebukes.

The youngsters never again acted like they were entertained by High Pockets. But they sometimes snickered to themselves.

And High Pockets never did learn to drive any better.

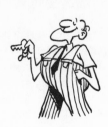

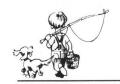

Halloween Remorse
Just Didn't Last

In the light of the day after, Halloween didn't seem as much fun as it did the night before. Moments of merriment, perpetrated with reckless abandon under cover of darkness, surrendered to the empty harshness of reality.

Mischief, even though rarely malicious, carried a price tag payable only with guilty consequences. It was a cost paid by most youths around Heltonville in the 1940s, even though one or two refused to admit they regretted the shenanigans they had committed.

Time, and the reluctance to confess guilt, kept the repentant from helping repair the damage they had wrought. There was school to attend the next day and the first basketball game of the season to be played at night.

Self-reproach came through the day, though. For culprits who rode Bus 7 to school, it came in the morning when they boarded the bus and noticed a farmer, bent and crippled with arthritis, stoop to remove a shattered shock of corn from the gravel road.

The riders had carried it there from his field the night before.

Regret came down the road when a man and his wife herded cattle back in the barn lot. It had seemed harmless, opening the gate as a Halloween prank.

Guilt grew when they saw an elderly widow, bundled against the cold, sweep the remains of bursted pumpkins from her front porch.

And the self-reprehension mounted when they saw bales of hay scattered beside the road. They had been smashed by cars, as the pranksters had hoped. They hadn't considered that someone might have been hurt if the cars had wrecked. They were relieved to know only the hay was harmed.

At school they exchanged stories about the stunts they had pulled off, but the joy of telling failed to meet the anticipation of the night before.

And things grew worse at noon when they walked to the restaurant for lunch. An outhouse they had overturned the night before remained toppled. On their way back to school, they saw the owner and his wife attempt to set the one-holer upright. The youths looked away, to hide their laughter . . . and their shame.

There would be other reminders later in the day to torment their consciences. They would see men remove parts of wagons that had been hoisted to rooftops, women washing soaped windows, clothes lines being restrung, shelled corn being swept from walks.

But it would be nightfall before anyone admitted his regret. That would come as they waited in the dressing room for the reserve game to end and the varsity contest to begin.

Someone would usually say, "I'm never goin' to spend another Halloween wastin' my time creatin' havoc. I could have been home last night restin' up for this game tonight."

The others would agree in unison, "Me, neither."

But their memories were short. They'd carry out their misdeeds the following year and repeat their vows never to do them again.

Lessons sometimes had to be learned over and over when you were young.

Bank of Jars Was Grandma's Wealth

Mrs. J. didn't have much money in the bank, but it didn't bother her a whit. She had a depository that was worth more to her than a fat checking account.

Tad and Tyke, two of her grandsons, learned that one Saturday morning in August when they stopped by to sample the cake, cookies and apple pie they knew she would have made for weekend company.

She served cold milk, whole, with warm wisdom, simple, in addition to dessert, in the kitchen of her farm house east of Heltonville.

"The hot, dry weather has about done-in the garden," she said. "And me, too," she added as an afterthought. She grinned to make sure the boys wouldn't be concerned about her health.

She subconsciously wiped her hands in her apron, poured each of the boys another glass of milk and waved her wrinkled right arm toward the garden.

"I have several bushel baskets of potatoes you can help me carry into the cellar after a while, if you don't mind," she said.

The boys didn't mind. Grandma J. was aging and frail. She had raised four children alone, and years of hard work showed in the stoop of her shoulders and the rivulets in her face.

The least the boys could do for her would be to help her store her potato crop. After a second piece of cake, the boys each grabbed a wire handle on a bushel of spuds and carried the basket to the cellar under Grandma J.'s house.

It was like walking into a Jay C grocery store, except it was cooler than any store. The temperature was between forty and fifty degrees, even though the sun outside already had sent the temperature past eighty.

The boys dumped the potatoes in a bin in the corner. One of them whistled as he turned and saw the rows on rows of canned food that lined the shelves.

"You got enough food here to feed the Fifth Army," he said. "What all you got here, anyhow?"

She smiled the smile of satisfaction. She took as much pride in her cellar

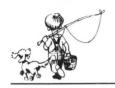

as she did the dinners she served on Sunday.

Her pride was obvious, even to boys. She led them around the big cellar, pointing out Mason, Kerr and Ball jars, some closed with sealing wax, some with zinc caps screwed tight against rubber rings.

"Here are beets, and green beans, corn and tomatoes.

"And here is the fruit—apples, peaches, pears, plums, raspberries, blackberries, gooseberries and cherries.

"And here are the jams and jellies made from grapes, berries and plums, and the preserves, too."

The good things made the boys forget the beets, gooseberries and plums for which they hadn't yet acquired a taste. Tad asked Mrs. J. what she planned to do with all the canned goods. "Ain't no way you can use all this yourself."

She laughed. "Well, I ain't got much money in the bank, so I can't help my kinfolks with cash. But I can see to it none of them ever go hungry."

She thought for a minute, then added, "A good meal can make a person forget how poor he is."

The boys walked out into the bright sunlight and carried the rest of the potatoes into the cellar. When they finished, Mrs. J. asked them to bring a cured ham into the kitchen from the smokehouse: "I'll serve it to you and your folks tomorrow."

The next day she set out a Sunday dinner that couldn't have been bought with all the money in the vaults at Fort Knox.

Mrs. J. was pleased everyone showed up. It made her feel like the richest woman in the world. And she still had enough food in her "bank" for a winter of Sundays to come.

Pride, B'Gosh in His Overalls

Pokey was so excited he didn't even stop to knock. He bounded through the door into the living room, a smile stuck like a decal on his twelve-year-old face.

It was a day or two after Christmas and Tad was eager to hear about the gifts Pokey had received.

With one hand, Pokey caught a peanut Tad tossed to him; with the other hand he held the collar of his mackinaw jacket. Tad knew Pokey had a secret he wouldn't wait to reveal. "Whatcha trying to hide?" he asked.

Pokey unbuttoned the jacket, pulled it off, tossed it on a rocking chair and did a 360-degree turn. He was wearing a new pair of Oshkosh B'Gosh overalls, the envy of every farm boy around Heltonville.

"Got 'em for Christmas," Pokey said, sticking his thumbs under each gallus for emphasis. He walked back and forth in front of the wood stove, the new material swishing with each step he took.

Oshkosh B'Gosh was to overalls in the 1930s and '40s what a Buick was to automobiles.

Tad felt like he was undressed, wearing a pair of Big Mac overalls from the J.C. Penney store in Bedford. Big Macs were OK, but they didn't compare to Oshkosh B'Gosh. The Big Macs had galluses that crossed in the back and two buttons on each side, the top one at belt level.

Pokey's new overalls had a high back that came to the top of his spine. They had four buttons on each side, the top ones under each arm. The buttons held the back and the bib tight, causing him to stand erect.

"Looks 'ke you're in a corset," Tad laughed, trying to hide the hurt he felt for not having a pair, too.

Pokey smiled. "They just feel snug," he answered, jabbing the middle two fingers of his right hand into the loop on the side where a hammer could fit.

The boys shelled a few more peanuts, then decided to go outside to romp around the farm and shoot a few baskets in the barn loft.

Pokey's overalls didn't look new by the time he decided to go home. They were covered with a combination of dirt, dust, hay and other accumulation from the barn.

"Gonna wear your overalls to school when we go back after New Year's?" Tad asked.

Pokey nodded. "After mom washes them," he said.

After the holidays, he showed up at school in the overalls. They were clean and neat and Pokey looked proud as he walked down the hall, until he saw Tad.

Tad was wearing a pair of Oshkosh B'Gosh overalls that hadn't yet been washed. The right back pocket had an outline where the label had been removed.

"I talked about your overalls so much, Dad decided to drive into Bedford and buy me and him both a pair at Keller's store," Tad said.

Pokey feigned a feeling of disgust, frowned and said, "I'll never show you anything else I get new."

Tad knew he was just kidding. Their friendship meant more than even a pair of Oshkosh B'Gosh overalls.

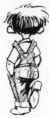

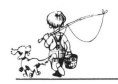

Synthetic Tires
—and Other Sins

Zeke despised phonies, fakes, imitations . . . and synthetic tires. And not necessarily in that order.

Zeke was a dirt farmer who didn't know the meaning of pretense. What you saw in his craggy face was the real Zeke. He made no effort to hide any displeasure, or any happiness, that came his way.

And synthetic tires caused a lot of displeasure to come his way during World War II. Don't get the idea that Zeke was anything less than patriotic. He accepted rationing, used sweetener in his coffee instead of sugar, and, to save gasoline, made only trips that were really necessary.

But that didn't mean he couldn't complain after one of the new synthetic tires he'd just paid a premium price for blew itself to smithereens.

The government turned to synthetic tire production when the Japanese occupied islands in the Pacific that had provided ninety-seven percent of the rubber used in the United States.

The government claimed the synthetic product was better than natural rubber in many respects. But that claim was made by bureaucrats and rubber-company tycoons, who still had access to tires made from pre-war crude rubber.

Zeke bought his first synthetic tires in 1943 and mounted them on the back of his 1937 Buick. The tires looked as good as any others he'd seen. The tread was deep, deep enough, he reasoned, for at least fifteen thousand, maybe twenty thousand miles.

He made a couple of short trips on the tires before he had to drive into Bedford for a piece he needed to fix the mowing machine. It was mid-afternoon and he was in a hurry to get back to finish cutting a field of alfalfa.

The war-time speed limit was thirty-five miles per hour, but Zeke noticed the speedometer was at sixty-five when he passed the Maple Leaf cabins on U.S. 50. It was then he heard a "clap, clap, clap" noise, then a loud "boom." One of the new tires had blown.

He put on a tread-bare spare, drove into Bedford and returned home, more slowly.

A day or two later, he loaded up his family for a trip to the Jackson County Fair at Brownstown. The temperature was in the 90s, hot enough to fry an egg on the concrete pavement of U.S. 50.

The other new synthetic tire blew a half-mile west of Brownstown. Zeke's voice was louder than a carnival barker at the fair. Fortunately, he had managed to replace the spare he'd used a couple days earlier with another old tire.

"Buying them damned fake tires is worse than putting your money in a shell game at the fair," he said as he slammed the trunk lid and got back in the car.

Some of Zeke's neighbors couldn't believe the tires lasted less than a week, but Zeke convinced them after he brought a newspaper clipping to church one Sunday. He read them a report that said the Indiana State Police had tried 158 of the tires and that two-thirds of them had to be replaced before they were driven 1,500 miles.

"The chief difficulty," Zeke read, adjusting his glasses, "is the formation of blisters from the heat generated by even the slightest excess driving speed."

Zeke continued to read, before Clem stopped him, saying, "It says the tires will be replaced if they blow out."

Zeke made a few comments inappropriate for a churchyard, and said, "That's like having a ne'er-do-well write you a bad check to replace one that's done bounced."

He had no choice, though, but to try another pair of synthetic tires. But each time he heard a "clap, clap, clap," he just pulled over to the side of the road, changed the tire and continued to develop his vocabulary.

Twin Ka-booms
Call Off Trade

Some stories are just too good to keep to yourself. That may be why Bill decided to tell one about his father after forty years.

Bill is a nuclear pharmacist at Fort Lauderdale now, but he still remembers his boyhood in Heltonville in the early 1940s. His father, Marshall, was a teacher who loved squirrel-hunting. One of his experiences is described on pages 68-70.

Marshall taught the sixth grade at Heltonville and coached the high school basketball team. He knew when to keep quiet. That's why not many people have heard this story Bill hasn't shared until now.

Marshall hunted with an old twenty-gauge double-barrel shotgun he had traded a bicycle for when he was sixteen. He listened to the taunting at Roberts General Store from his buddies Bish and Bob, who claimed he'd have better luck bagging squirrels if he used a bigger, more powerful twelve-gauge shotgun.

What they said seemed reasonable, but Marshall resisted switching guns for years.

He was having an early breakfast with his wife and Billy one Saturday morning in the fall of 1943 or 1944 when he announced: "A fellow out on Ind. 58 has agreed to trade me an almost new double-barrel twelve-gauge shotgun for my twenty-gauge. We'll stop on the way to town and pick it up."

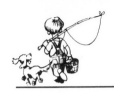

The "we" referred to him and Billy. Mrs. Axsom was skeptical, figuring the deal sounded too good to be true.

But Marshall and Billy made the trade after the man who had the bigger gun said Marshall could return the twelve-gauge, no questions asked, for the twenty-gauge if he wasn't happy.

Marshall and Billy drove out toward Hickory Grove in their 1937 Chevrolet, parked and stepped softly through the woods. After what seemed like hours to Billy, Marshall put his right index finger to his lips, signaling a squirrel had been sighted.

Bill saw the gray sitting on a limb and stuck a finger in each ear while his father took aim. A giant ka-boom! rocked the Henderson Creek hollow. Another ka-boom followed.

The double-barrel blast rocketed Marshall back on top of Billy. Marshall made sure the boy was OK, picked up the shotgun that had gone to the left, then retrieved his Dutch Boy painter's cap from a nearby limb.

As Marshall collected what was left of the squirrel, Billy asked if his dad had pulled both triggers intentionally.

"Just the first. The second was a surprise," Marshall said.

Back in the car, he said, "Well, Billy, I guess we'll stop on the way home and get 'Old Central' back." He called the gun "Old Central" because it had been made by Central Arms Co. in St. Louis.

Billy was happy about his dad's decision, knowing "Old Central" would never react the way the twelve-gauge had.

Later that day, Billy heard his dad ask, "Do we still have any of that Sloan's liniment? Think my shoulder is going to be a little stiff."

In the days that followed, Marshall just shook his head when Bish and Bob talked about their twelve-gauges down at the general store.

"I'm mighty happy with 'Old Central,'" he'd say, never revealing what had happened that Saturday morning.

Billy never forgot that day, though. And "Old Central" is his most prized possession, a reminder of some of his most-treasured memories of his father.

Heroes Got Trimmed at Barber's Court

The courtrooms were barber shops, feed mills, general stores and restaurants. Defendants were referees, coaches and basketball players. Prosecutors were farmers, timbercutters, stonemill workers and loafers.

It was trial by bib overalls.

It made no difference whether the town was Heltonville, Clearspring, Tunnelton, Freetown or other hamlets in Lawrence and Jackson counties.

Only the places and faces were different.

The issue, always the same, revolved around the town's high school basketball game the previous night.

It was the subject on which everyone was an expert. A knowledge of basketball wasn't important. The less one knew about the game, the more he could complain, unrestricted by any semblance to fact. At least, it seemed that way in Heltonville in the 1940s.

Tad and Tyke had no more than entered the barber shop one Saturday when someone complained, between chews of Days Work tobacco, "Hear you fellers lost another game last night."

Before the boys could respond, another man, caressing each side of his overalls between his fingers and thumbs, wondered, "So what else is new?"

Most of the other men in the shop laughed. Neither man had seen the game the night before. The man who was in the chair waited to speak until the barber stopped to whet his razor.

"We don't have good teams like we did back in the late '20s and early '30s. Man, we had some powerhouses then."

The barber had to wait for him to finish yakkin'.

"These kids nowadays don't know how to pass, shoot, dribble or play defense. All they think about are girls, cars and shootin' pool," he went on.

The barber spoke up for the first time. "Don't sound like bad things to think about in your spare time," he said, winking at Tyke.

That didn't stop the Saturday-morning coaches. They complained about the coaching, about the players, about all the good referees having gone to war.

One man said, "Nothing personal, you understand. But, I've seen you guys play. It looks like you try to offset your lack of height by being extra slow. I could go out right now and find syrup running out of sugar trees faster than you move."

One man who had been listening quietly lifted himself up from his seat to act as an attorney for the defense.

"None of you seem to take into consideration the hardship under which this team plays. They've been able to practice only one night a week since the gym burned, and that's at Shawswick. They don't get to play any home games. And some of the best players quit school to join the Navy."

That quieted some of the men. Not the customer in the chair. He just muttered, "Excuses, excuses."

The barber looked at Tad and Tyke and said, "Don't be too concerned about what is said here. Glory would be a dull companion."

That's when Tad said, "Tyke may get some glory in the paper tonight. He scored twelve points last night."

Tyke took on his "aw, shucks!" look, then said, "I just had a good night."

The man in the chair said, "Don't be so humble, Tyke. You're not that good."

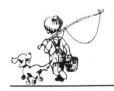

Even Tyke laughed. If his feelings were hurt, he didn't show it.

He and Tad walked toward the door a few minutes later. "See you next week?" the barber asked.

Tad turned and said, "Nope. We're going to spend next Saturday morning at Clearspring. Nobody knows us there, and we can listen to the players up there catch the dickens."

Basketball Brightened Wartime Winters

It is February 25, 1944, a Friday, and the basketball sectionals are being played at sixty-four sites around Indiana.

Some teams already have lost, their dreams of glory gone with the snows of winter. Other teams have yet to play. Their hopes are alive, as fresh as the frost that coats the roofs of barns where basketball goals are hung.

Heltonville will meet Bedford at 7:00 that evening, the final game in the opening round of the ten-team sectional. Heltonville, gymless since the school burned two years earlier, has won but one game. Bedford is big and talented as usual, almost as good as the Stonecutter team that advanced to the state finals the year before.

It has been a busy week for Tad and Tyke and the rest of the Heltonville players. They have washed the laces and removed the smears from their basketball shoes. The barber has trimmed their hair, which they have combed and recombed. And they have thought endlessly about the game.

Their parents don't mind. Basketball is an escape from the darkness of war being waged in southern Europe and in the South Pacific.

School is out for the day so students can attend the two afternoon games. Tad and Tyke have gone to Bedford with their father, who was told by their mother to "buy the boys new trousers so they'll be well-dressed tonight."

They all stop on 15th Street at Sherman-Berner clothiers, where one of the owners says, "So, you're playing Bedford tonight!"

Tad just nods, reflecting his apprehension.

"Well," the haberdasher said, "maybe you can pull off an upset like Mooresville did last night." Martinsville had gone to the semifinals the previous year and many fans thought the Artesians might make it to the state finals this time. Most of the team was back, including Mel Payton, who would later set scoring records at Tulane University, and Hugh Rutledge, who would star for the next four decades as a reporter for *The Indianapolis News*.

The merchant hands Tad the morning paper, folded to the sports section. Mooresville had won, 33-32, beating Martinsville on a one-handed shot by

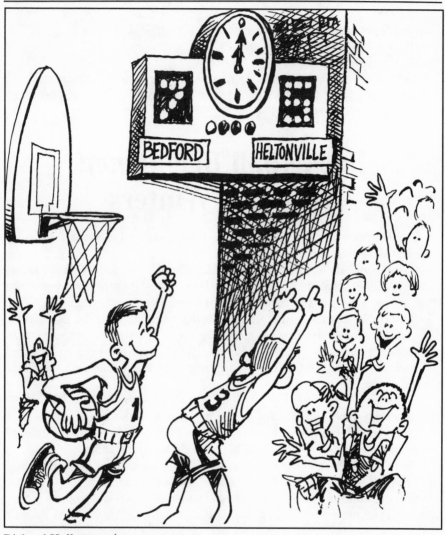

Richard Kellum as time ran out.

Tad reads the paper while his dad pays for the two pairs of pants the merchant had sold while he talked basketball.

Tad and Tyke wear their new duds to the game that night, hanging them carefully on hooks in the gymnasium as they dress for the game. Tyke is calmer than Tad. He's a sophomore, Tad a freshman.

It will be the biggest crowd they have seen. Bedford has maybe 2,500 fans at the game, Heltonville no more than a hundred. The other 1,900 seats are filled with fans backing the underdog Blue Jackets.

Nobody is more surprised than Heltonville coach Marshall Axsom when Heltonville, behind the ball-handling of Junior Norman, plays the Stonecutters

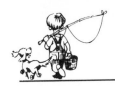

to a 7-5 standoff in the first quarter. It will be the only memorable quarter of the game.

The Mooresville upset of Martinsville will not be repeated. Bedford wins big, 64-21. The Stonecutters will go on to win the sectional and advance to the state semifinals.

Tad and Tyke will go home, to think about next year.

"How'd you do?" their dad asks.

Tyke, not mentioning he'd scored ten points, replies, "Lost."

Tad, who missed a free throw in his only shot, adds, "But we looked good doing it."

It will be 366 days until they will get another shot at a sectional victory.

A List in Time
Might've Saved $7.75

Spring had arrived and only one thing dampened Bogey's thoughts of love. The object of his affection preferred the attention of someone older.

Bogey wasn't easily dissuaded, though. He had pursued the girl's attention, without success, through most of the winter. His persistence was overshadowed only by her resistance.

Maybe that's what caused him to act out of character at a fund-raising event at the school in Heltonville one Friday night in March during World War II.

Among the events was the auction of cakes baked by the girls in the school. The top bidder not only bought the cake, he bought the right to the girl's company while the two of them shared the dessert.

Buyers weren't supposed to know whose cake w ს being auctioned, but Bogey learned, through guile, when to bid. Some of his friends knew, too. That's why they upped the bid each time after Bogey had made an offer. But Bogey fooled them. He kept bidding until the price was higher than the amount of money they had pooled.

The auctioneer stopped and said, "Sold to Bogey for $7.75."

Everyone applauded except the girl who had baked the cake.

Bogey carried the cake to the back of the room. The girl dutifully followed. She sliced the cake and thanked Bogey when he said it was the best he had ever tasted.

But that was about as friendly as she got. She kept telling him about her boyfriend who was in the Navy. She just ignored Bogey when he said he could fill the void in her life until the sailor returned.

And she refused his offer to take her home.

Bogey's friends had drifted down to the pool room by the time he finished the cake. He joined them later. He wished he had gone home instead.

The razzing was unmerciful.

"Must have felt like a big shot, pulling out that check and actin' like you were rich," Chig said.

"The only reason the rest of us didn't get to eat that cake was because we weren't as wealthy as you," Tad said.

Bogey pulled a cue stick from the rack against the wall, eyed down it like he was a pool shark, and said, "I have to confess something.

"If you guys had bid fifty cents more, I wouldn't have been able to write a check. When that check is cashed, I'll have only a quarter left in my account at the Stone City National Bank.

"And I have nothing to show for it, except your amusement."

Chig walked to the pop cooler, pulled out a Royal Crown Cola and handed it to Bogey. "Here's something to wash down your sorrow."

While Bogey sipped the soft drink, his friends ticked off the names of a dozen girls he might like to date.

"Why didn't you guys come up with that list before I spent all my money?" he asked.

Horsing Around
Spoiled an Appetite

Jackie had a sharp wit he kept hidden in the classroom. There was always a chance it might be dulled by overuse.

He saved it for special occasions where it would bring maximum results. He wasn't a ham, but he knew how to play to a crowd.

One of those times came in early April 1944. Spring had come to the hills around Heltonville after a long winter when there were often more reasons to fret than to laugh.

World War II was far from over; young men from the community were being killed in action, and others were still leaving for service. Tires, gasoline, meat, sugar and shoes were rationed. Dark clouds seemed to have no silver linings.

Most of the school had been destroyed by fire, and the war kept it from being rebuilt. The basketball team had practiced at Shawswick once a week and played all its games on the road. It had ended the season with just one victory.

Coach Axsom decided the team deserved a post-season banquet despite the absence of victory. A women's group agreed to serve the meal in the basement of the Christian church.

It was a somewhat formal affair, a bit stuffier than the freshmen were

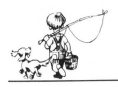

accustomed to. Most of them would have felt more at ease eating raspberries off the briery bushes.

But not Jackie. He sat down next to Loren Raines, the school principal, and started a nonstop conversation. Jackie was undaunted by the fact Raines also was pastor of a church in Bedford.

When Jackie was served, he glanced down at the meat on his plate and mentioned a story he'd read about horse meat being sold as beef. "A lot of people don't know the difference," he said between bites.

Raines looked a little uncomfortable. He tried unsuccessfully to change the subject.

About that time Tad, another freshman, applied pressure on his knife, only to see his piece of meat fly across the table against Raines' arm. The meat had no more than landed when Jackie shouted, "Whoa, you old nag!"

Tad laughed despite his embarrassment. The principal's face turned red, and his Adam's apple bobbed nervously in his throat. He didn't take another bite until pie was served.

Jackie kept talking, eating every bite of his food. "If that was horse meat, it was good," he said, wiping the corners of his mouth with a napkin.

Tad retrieved his meat and sliced it up. Raines watched out of the corner of his eye as Tad chewed and rechewed the meat.

Jackie looked at Tad and said, "It's tough, but good, isn't it?"

Tad nodded, getting into the flow of Jackie's unrehearsed drama.

The principal looked as relieved when the tables were cleared as Jackie did at the end of a school day.

Tad and Jackie never forgot the incident. They quit saying "wait a minute" when one wanted to catch up with the other. Instead, they yelled, "Whoa, you old nag!"

Raines never forgot, either. Which may explain why that was the last banquet the team was served until Jackie and Tad were out of school.

All the Field's a Stage

Bob liked to be the center of attention, even if his stage was a field of clover.

He thought one of his greatest moments in the sun had come one June day in the mid-1940s. He was more excited than usual when he roared up to Tad's house about noon.

Bob was wearing a heavy cardboard hat and a brown shirt with a bandanna tied around the neck. He looked more like a character out of a Jungle Jim movie than a nineteen-year-old farm youth from Heltonville.

"Want to make some money this afternoon?" he asked.

Tad was apprehensive, but he accepted the offer, knowing he could use the money at the July 4 celebration in Freetown.

"Good!" Bob shouted. "Meet me down at the field by Mundell Church at one o'clock. We're going to make hay like you never seen it made before."

Billy was at the field when Tad arrived. Neither knew what to expect when Bob drove up the road, sitting proudly on the seat of a John Deere tractor, the green glistening in the midday sun. The tractor was pulling a new John Deere hay baler.

It was the first pickup baler Tad had seen. The balers he had worked on were stationary and the hay was hauled to them.

"Ever tied wires before?" Bob asked. Tad said, "Not on a baler like this."

"Well, you're going to now," Bob replied. "Billy can punch the wires and you can tie."

Bob started the engine on the baler and climbed back on the tractor. Three or four farmers who had gathered to watch the new baler noticed how important Bob tried to appear.

"He looks like Lindbergh getting ready to take off across the Atlantic," Tad heard one of the spectators say.

Tad thought Bob would drive slowly enough so they'd have time to tie each bale snugly with two strands of wire in figure-eight knots.

Instead, Bob drove the tractor like he was bound for a date. Billy poked the wires through to Tad on the opposite side. Tad tied them as quickly as he could.

Bob not only ignored their shouts to slow down, he didn't even look back.

"Hell with it," Tad said. "I'm going to let some hay spring out the back without getting tied. Maybe that'll get his attention."

It didn't. Bob kept driving. The boys punched and tied, punched and tied, letting hay go unbundled from time to time.

Relief came with Bob's father. He drove his car into the field, looked at the speed Bob was driving and stepped into his path. It was like flagging a freight train.

Bob stopped. "Whatsamatter?" he asked.

"That's the matter," his dad bellowed, pointing to Tad and Billy and the unbaled hay left behind.

"Get off the tractor. I'll show you how to run this thing. But not until you bring these boys a jug of water and let them catch their breath."

The break gave Tad a chance to look at his injuries. The little finger of his right hand was bleeding at the top joint from tugging and knotting the wires.

Bob's dad handed Tad a pair of leather gloves. "These will help," he said.

Then Bob's father climbed up onto the tractor. "What do you want me to do?" Bob asked.

"Just look and listen," his dad said, emphatically.

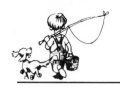

Bob looked and listened the rest of the afternoon, which went much better for Tad and Billy, who kept up at the slower pace.

The next time Billy and Tad worked on the baler, Bob drove again. But this time much more slowly.

* * *

P.S. Automatic twine-tied balers came along later. But the scar remained on Tad's finger.

A Soldier Learns Farming Is Hell

Butch was home on leave after Army Basic and he was proud of his new look. Drill instructors had melted the fat from Butch's body and an inferiority complex from his mind. He looked lean and fit and mean enough to fight a mad bull in a closet.

He strutted, his short sleeves rolled up to his armpits to show his muscles. And he talked about long marches, confidence courses, PT exercises and bayonet training, especially to younger fellows who would have to wait for the joy of military service.

Butch had worked on farms around Heltonville and figured he'd make some extra money while on furlough when Zeke asked if he'd like to help put up a field of hay.

Zeke warned Butch that he might be out of condition for field work since he'd been away for three months.

"Sir," Butch said, "I can handle any job you've got after what I've been through in Basic."

The "sir" came from a habit Butch had picked up from his drill sergeant. Butch figured he would have no trouble outworking Zeke's sons, Tad and Tyke. After all, they were still in their mid-teens and unconditioned to the rigors he had experienced as an Army recruit.

But Butch didn't remember how hard it was to put up hay. Especially in hot weather.

The hay had dried out enough to bale about noon. Zeke drove the tractor while Butch and Tyke picked up the bales and tossed them on the wagon. Tad stacked the hay.

Butch ran between bales as the first wagon was loaded and volunteered to work in the loft when the hay arrived at the barn. He made the work look easy, but his performance changed sharply after the first act. It dipped as the temperature rose.

T'ıe sun boiled down, cooking the stubble and baking Butch. His gait slowed and he stopped from time to time to wipe his brow and put his hands on his knees and breathe deeply.

Tyke and Tad worked at the same pace they had from the start.

Back at the barn, Butch climbed slowly into the loft, which was nearly full of hay harvested earlier in the summer. He stacked bales in a tight spot between the hay and the galvanized roofing that magnified the rays of the sun.

Suddenly, he jumped down, flailing his arms, slapping his hands against his body, stomping his feet and yelling cuss words he'd learned in his Army barracks.

He was being pursued by a swarm of wasps he'd disturbed in their nest between a rafter and the roofing. They attacked him like a volley of mortar shots, finding their mark at least six, maybe seven or eight times.

Zeke, knowing an emergency when he saw one, called a temporary halt and led Butch to the house. Millie, Zeke's wife, applied baking soda to the welts Butch showed her. A couple of stings were in places he preferred to keep private.

Butch was white by that time, the steely look gone from his face. He staggered behind the garage and surrendered his dinner. Zeke had him stretch out in the shade, then placed a folded tarpaulin under his head.

"Let's go to the barn," Zeke told Tad and Tyke. "We'll have to get along without Butch."

He told Millie to keep an eye on Butch: "Make sure he doesn't go into shock."

It was two hours before Butch stirred. Millie wanted to know where he would be sent when he returned to camp.

"I don't know," Butch replied, "but I sure hope it's not to a farm to put up hay."

A Springhouse
and Its Treasures

A springhouse was more than a place to get a cool drink. It was a storehouse, a repository for the pleasant things of summer. Things like muskmelons, watermelons, tomatoes and roasting ears. And cold milk, cream and fresh butter.

Once in a while, a cake was left there for the icing to cool.

The springhouse was nature's refrigeration. It served rural families east of Heltonville until electricity came to the farms in the 1940s.

If buildings could have personalities, the springhouse where Tad lived had one. It was built into a hill over a spring that never stopped flowing, no matter

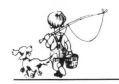

the severity of a drought.

Blocks of soapstone, hand-hewn decades earlier, formed foundation walls. Two basins had been shaped to hold the water. One was big enough for two ten-gallon milk cans, the other, nearer the vein, for drinking water. A ledge wide enough for the corn, tomatoes and other produce was built along the west wall.

A frame building sat atop the foundation. The sides were weather-boarding, painted white. The trim was black, giving the springhouse the same decor as the big farm house atop the hill.

The upper level was used as a milkhouse. A hand-cranked separator centrifugally spun out skimmed milk through one spout, cream through another. The cream was either churned into butter or cooled in the spring for the produce man to pick up later.

Some of the skimmed milk was left in the spring for the boys to drink. Tyke's mother always left a cup for their convenience.

Boys and men would stop at the springhouse on almost any hot day from May through September, but they lingered longer on hot August afternoons when the wind was still, the sun hot and the humidity dripping.

No one ever left a springhouse thirsty . . . or hungry. Watermelons, brought from the sands of White River near Vallonia, had been cooling for days in the spring water. Big red tomatoes, polished to a shine, were in a basket on the ledge.

The tomatoes were offered to anyone who might not like watermelon. There were few takers.

Tad or Tyke or their father didn't need visitors to cut a watermelon. But they felt more comfortable sharing the goodness with others.

One of them would take a big butcher knife, stick it into the side of a striped melon and listen as the rind popped and split, exposing the heart, red and sweet. The melon would be sliced in thick slabs and handed to anyone who awaited the pleasure of the moment. Only the sound of a seed being rifled between teeth interrupted the feast.

One good slice deserved another. One watermelon led to two. One of the hired hands would mention, "Another afternoon like this and you'll be out of melons."

That didn't bother Tad's father. He said, "Reckon that means another trip to the melon fields."

The men tossed the remains of the rinds into a bucket, filled their wooden keg with water and headed back to work, moving even more slowly than they had when they arrived.

But they were smiling the smile of contentment, even though a few more loads of hay waited in the field.

Halloween Chats
Were Non-stop

Conversation seldom paused to catch its breath at Axsom's barber shop in Heltonville. The last Saturday in October 1944 was no exception.

The barber shop that morning was no place for anyone too polite to interrupt another person. The idea was to start talking before someone else finished and to hold the floor as long as possible. There was a lot to talk about.

There was World War II.

The fighting in Europe was going well for the Allies, MacArthur had returned to the Philippines and his Pacific forces were island-hopping their way toward Japan.

Some of the men who had boys in service did most of the talking about the war.

There was the election coming up November 7.

Sharm was a farmer who had grown tired of Franklin Roosevelt. He talked about the possibility of Tom Dewey being able to wrest the White House from "the great white father."

Ralph, a Democrat, said it was no time to change horses in the middle of a stream.

Sharm said, "'Tis if the horses are floundering in the water."

The men talked about the two races for U.S. Senate seats in Indiana that year. Most of them agreed they planned to vote for Bill Jenner, who was a lawyer in Bedford.

Jenner was a Republican who was running against Cornelius O'Brien. The winner was to fill the seat vacant since the death of Frederick Van Nuys.

The men had mixed emotions about who to vote for in the other Senate race, Republican Homer Capehart or Gov. Henry Schricker, but they knew Capehart owned a farm not too far away in Daviess County.

And they argued about how good a job Republican Earl Wilson was doing as the Ninth District representative in Congress. None of them knew much about his opponent, George Elliott of Rising Sun.

They talked, too, without reaching a consensus, about the race for governor between Republican Ralph Gates and Democrat Sam Jackson. "Both good men," Sharm said.

There was the opening of basketball season.

Once the men tired of talking politics, they turned to Tad and Tyke and a couple of other teenagers and asked about the prospects for the basketball season. The team was to open the season the following Friday against Huron.

"Have to be better than last year," Tad said. Everybody in the shop knew the team had won only one game the year before.

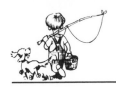

And there was Halloween.

The men told story after story about the pranks they had pulled in Halloweens past, pranks like lifting pieces atop a church and reassembling the running gears of a wagon, turning over outhouses with occupants inside, scaring widows and children, closing off roads.

When they finished recalling those stunts, they turned to Tyke and asked: "Whatta you boys have planned for Halloween?"

Tyke turned to Tad, Jake, and a couple of other teenagers. They all looked at each other.

"Since there ain't nothing left for us to do that's new, we may just stay at home and keep out of trouble," Tyke said.

The men laughed guffaws of doubt. They knew more about the boys' reputation for pranks than they did about the character of candidates running for office.

Time, Not Money, Was Everything

It was May 1945 and jobs off the farm were easy to find. World War II was still under way, and almost every young man around Heltonville had enlisted or been drafted.

Employers hired youngsters they wouldn't have considered under different circumstances.

When Tyke, who was sixteen, learned he could get a job in a limestone quarry, he jumped at the chance to make five to six dollars a day. Billy, Bob, Pokey, Bogey and other fifteen-year-olds took jobs on the railroad for about the same pay.

Tad wanted to join them, but his dad had other plans for him.

"We got fifteen acres of tomatoes to care for, corn and soybeans to cultivate, wheat to combine and hay to harvest," he said, looking ahead to what would be done through the summer.

Tad knew better than to argue. He just sulked for days, waving at his friends when they left for work and returned home.

"Public work," his dad called it. "It ain't all it's cracked up to be. Them boys will find that out sooner or later," he said.

Tad knew his dad meant well. But he would have preferred to be working alongside his friends on the railroad instead of alone in the fields.

Besides, his dad hadn't said what his reward would be for staying home on the farm. He knew there would be some money for him when school started. He just wasn't sure how much he would earn, except for a couple of dollars he was given each weekend.

His friends compared their income each time he saw them. They bragged even more when they started to earn time-and-a-half for overtime.

Tad listened, without saying anything. He was beginning to think his dad was wrong, that Bogey and the others wouldn't become disenchanted with their jobs.

Things began to change after a couple of weeks. The work days grew longer, the sun hotter, their work more demanding. They began to complain about the long hours without a break.

"Me and Dad always stop for a break whenever we want. We don't have any bosses to answer to," Tad told them.

Bogey said, "You don't know how lucky you are. Working on the railroad ain't the same as working for your dad."

"Or working on a siding machine in the stone quarry," Tyke said.

Tad let the comments pass. Tyke kept working at the same quarry hole. He had too much grit to quit.

But the boys who had jobs on the railroad kept having to go farther away from home each day to work. Their hours lengthened as the days grew longer. And their unhappiness grew comparably.

After three weeks, they told Tad they were ready to quit.

"And pass up all the money you're making?" Tad asked.

Bogey said, "Money ain't worth nothing if you're too tired to spend it."

He and the others quit the railroad, telling Tad's father they would be available to help on the farm when needed.

"Me and Tad are doing fine by ourselves right now. We'll come and get you when we need you," Tad's father replied.

Tad was happy. Not because his friends were without jobs, but because his dad had been right.

The Driver Who Expected a Miracle

News Item: Ind. 58 east of Heltonville has reopened following realignment of a stretch of road to eliminate two blind ninety-degree turns through a cut under an abandoned railroad.

* * *

It was a standard warning for every young driver who lived east of Heltonville:

"Be careful when you're going under the trestle."

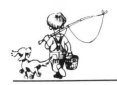

Parents knew the route was an adventure in driving. The drive to Heltonville on Ind. 58 passed through a cut under the Chicago, Milwaukee & St. Paul Railroad trestle. If that wasn't bad enough, the road from the east curved to the left, then back ninety degrees to the north as it approached the cut. The road then turned ninety degrees to the west up a forty-five-degree hill at the exit of the cut.

The cut under the trestle was barely wide enough for one car. Visibility was zero for cars approaching in either direction.

Youngsters like Tyke and Tad were told always to blow the car horn and proceed slowly. If a honk came from the opposite side of the underpass they were told to wait until the other car passed through.

At times, the other car was driven by someone who had been given the same advice. That meant each driver waited and waited before proceeding, usually to meet bumper-to-bumper under the trestle.

The result was the same when each driver honked at the same time, each blast erasing the sound from the other car.

That may have been what happened one fall day when Tyke was driving toward Heltonville. He blew the horn on his dad's 1937 Buick, heard no response and then eased through the underpass. As he exited, another driver started through. The two cars collided.

Tyke wormed out the right side of the Buick. The other driver exited his Chevy the same way.

Tyke, who was sixteen, recognized the other driver. His name was Abner and he was a Bible-quoting, churchgoing middle-aged man who lived at Norman. It was Tyke's intention to accept part of the blame until Abner forgot his religion and started to swear.

He didn't stop until he complained, "And if you had come through here two minutes earlier, this would never have happened."

Tyke, realizing Abner was serious, bit his tongue to keep from laughing, then said, "I'm sorry. I didn't know when you'd be coming through."

Abner's face turned even redder. "Well, you should have," he bellered, the words echoing off the barn roof in the valley.

Once Abner calmed down, he and Tyke examined the two cars. Neither auto needed extensive repairs, but Abner said, "I'll expect you and your dad to pay for having my car fixed."

Tyke explained to his dad, Zeke, what happened and said he'd use the money he'd saved to help repair Abner's car. His dad said, "You'll do no such thing."

Zeke got behind the wheel of the car, told Tyke to climb in and drove to Abner's house. Abner had calmed down and wasn't nearly as vocal with an adult as he had been with Tyke.

He agreed to pay for his own repair, but said, "I hope you tell that boy of yours never to come through the trestle again when I'm on my way home from work."

Tyke laughed as his dad drove off, shaking his head in amazement and muttering about Abner's logic.

Only His Teeth
Were Phony

Zeke never looked in the mirror, except to shave with a straight razor and to comb his thick black hair. There was no pretense about him, no illusion of importance. He wasn't a person who navigated by the star of self-interest.

What you saw was what he was.

The only things false about him were his teeth. And he wore them begrudgingly, to please his wife.

Zeke, of course, farmed and worked at the stonemill in Heltonville at times. Millie insisted Zeke wear his "store-bought choppers," as he called his upper and lower teeth, when he left for work or for town. He usually took the teeth out as soon as he was out of sight, placing them in the glove compartment of his 1937 Buick. He gummed the lunch she had fixed for him, never letting her know the fresh tenderloin strips were difficult to chew.

His charade went on for months, maybe years. It was a secret that might never have been revealed if he hadn't decided to sell the Buick.

The car had served him well through most of World War II. He had paid $300, plus a trade-in, for it in 1940 and added about forty thousand miles to it over the next five years.

He said "sold" when Horace, a storekeeper in Norman, offered him $600 for the car. Horace agreed to let Zeke keep the car until he found another one.

Zeke bought a Chevy sedan for about $450 and had his son Tyke follow him to Norman. Reluctantly, he signed over the Buick to Horace, slowly folded the check and slipped it into the bib pocket of his overalls. He looked like he had lost a friend.

It wasn't until later that he missed his false teeth. He had dressed for church on Sunday morning when Millie noticed his sunken cheeks.

"If you want to be seen with me, you'd better put in your teeth," she said.

"Can't find them," Zeke replied. "And I can't remember where I put them."

Millie stomped into church without waiting for him. Her anger caused Zeke to think about the places he could have left his teeth. It dawned on him during the sermon that they might be in the glove compartment of the Buick.

He tried to locate the Buick the next day.

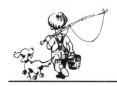

"Done sold that Buick," Horace said, giving Zeke the name of the buyer. Zeke made four, maybe five, trips before finding the new owner at home.

"Mind if I look in the glove compartment?" Zeke asked.

The new owner nodded, waving his arm to grant permission.

The teeth were inside, coated with a film of dust. Zeke held them in the palm of his right hand. "Guess you won't mind if I claim these?"

The man laughed. "Suppose you've missed them."

Zeke patted the left front fender of the Buick.

"Not nearly as much as I miss the car," he said.

Life's Best Things Weren't Expensive

Cecil grew to manhood in the Great Depression, which may explain the sturdiness of his character. Not much seemed to bother him. He kept to himself the things that did.

Like most men of his generation, he learned that happiness was not related to wealth. Other things were more important to him.

Cecil died at the age of seventy, and a lot of people recalled incidents to illustrate the kind of man he was.

Chig remembered the time in the mid-1940s when Cecil operated a garage on a bend where Ind. 58 made double ninety-degree turns at the Chicago, Milwaukee & St. Paul Railroad across from Roberts General Store in Heltonville.

Cecil was there when Chig had his first auto accident, driving a 1934 Chevy into the back of a truck that had stopped, without lights, on U.S. 50 east of Bedford.

It wasn't Chig's fault, but the driver of the truck had no insurance. He offered Chig fifty dollars as a settlement.

The Lawrence County sheriff, who knew the truck driver's reputation, looked at Chig and said, "Take it, son. It's better than nothing."

Chig accepted the fifty dollars and had his car towed to Cecil's garage.

"What will it take to fix it?" Chig asked, knowing he would have to borrow from his dad if the bill ran to more than fifty dollars.

Cecil said, "I don't know, but I'll fix what I can and look in junk yards for the parts I can't repair."

Cecil spent part of ten days repairing the front bumper and replacing both fenders, the radiator and the headlights. Except for a slightly different shade of green paint, the car looked almost as good as it had before the wreck.

"It's ready for you to pick up," Cecil told Chig one day after school.

Chig asked, "What's the damage to my billfold?"

Cecil handed him a bill, scribbled out in grease and lead. Chig looked at the piece of scrap paper with apprehension. Then he grinned. The bill came to $50.10.

"Sorry I couldn't keep it under fifty dollars," Cecil said.

Chig mentioned to a couple of adults he had to pay only $50.10 to have the front end of the car rebuilt.

One of them said, "Cecil's a good man, but he'll never get rich working for nothing."

That Saturday night, Cecil, his wife and their youngsters headed for Bedford with enough money to have a good time.

Cecil might never have been rich, but he knew better how to enjoy life than some of the people who worried about making money.

A Special Friend's Special Courage

Tad, Tyke, Bob, Frank, Cecil and others who grew up with Bob should have been kinder to him when they had the chance.

But they weren't. Maybe it was because they thought complimentary words would have embarrassed him. Chances are they would have.

Or maybe it was because, like most young men, they were reluctant to share their innermost thoughts, even with those whom those thoughts were about.

From the first time they saw him, they remembered him. Chances are they saw him at work at Roberts General Store in Heltonville, his red hair glistening in the April sun.

They didn't pay much attention to his nervous disorder folks called St. Vitus' Dance. He smiled a lot, laughed easily and masked his hardship with his pleasant attitude.

They soon became friends with him and he decided to return to school.

They should have told him it took a special kind of courage for him to go back to school after having been a dropout.

When he graduated in 1946, they should have done more than shake his hand and wish him well. They should have recognized his persistence and shared his sense of accomplishment.

They should have congratulated him when he got a job as the janitor at the school at Heltonville. They were more concerned about him being able to do the job. They shouldn't have been. He did the work as well as anyone could have. But they never told him so.

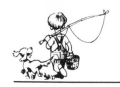

When they offered to help fill the big furnace with shoveled coal, he let them. Reluctantly. He said he was paid to do the work. Not them.

They should have helped him when he ran the restaurant in Heltonville. But they spent too much time in other, less important endeavors. But he managed to run the place anyway, without their help.

They saw him from time to time in the years that followed, joining him for a beer or two as he brought them up-to-date about himself. They never got around to talking about anything really serious, unless you consider basketball, girls who had become women and boys who had grown old, as serious topics.

When he retired after moving on to Bedford Junior High as janitor, they didn't tell him he had earned early retirement. They just toasted his freedom to enjoy the days ahead as he saw fit.

They saw some basketball games with him each season. He enjoyed the sport. They enjoyed his companionship. But they never told him, or, if they did, they didn't remember.

They saw him, for the last time, at the 1988 semistate basketball tournament at Terre Haute. He wouldn't have allowed himself to be seen in the wheelchair if he had felt better.

Even then, he still hadn't lost his sense of humor. He razzed a friend about a girl the man had dated forty years before and recalled the days of their youth together.

Bob Hunter died soon after the semistate. Now it's too late for Tad, Tyke, Bob, Frank, Cecil and the others to tell him all the things they should have.

They should have told him he taught them courage, humor, friendship, persistence, dignity under stress and a lot of other attributes that perhaps have made them all better persons.

They didn't tell him.

But, maybe, he knows, even now, that they considered him a special person.

How a Chevy Drove Him To Abstain

Pokey never hesitated to try something new. Some of the things he attempted turned out well. Some of them went sour.

Pokey had just turned seventeen that August in the mid-1940s when he borrowed money from his dad to buy a car. He acted as chauffeur for anyone who had money to buy gas and a place to go.

He was loafing in town one afternoon when Bogey suggested the two of them drive to watermelon country, buy all the melons they could get in the car and bring them back to sell at a profit.

Pokey said, "Hop in. We're as much as there."

They bought twenty-five to thirty melons in the White River bottom near Medora and drove back to Heltonville, where they offered them for sale under the shade of a tree. Business was good. All the watermelons were sold except one.

"I'll keep this one," Pokey announced.

Bogey wondered why. "You have melons cooling in your spring at home. Why do you want this one?"

He had never seen Bogey drink anything stronger than Nehi soda. Bogey was surprised when Pokey replied:

"Don't want my folks to know I have this one. I've heard you can get a real treat by cutting a plug in a melon, then pouring in a pint of vodka. You then replace the plug and let the alcohol ferment inside the melon. What you then have after a day or two is an exotic drink . . . if the experiment works."

He then opened the trunk lid of his Chevy and placed the melon inside.

Bogey yelled as Pokey drove off, "Let me know when you're ready for a taste test."

Bogey forgot about the melon in the back of Pokey's car. Like a lot of other things, the idea passed from Pokey's mind, too. So did the solitary melon.

August went. September arrived and the weather remained hot, the sun baking the trunk lid day after day.

Pokey, Bogey and a couple of friends were joyriding after school when a tire on Pokey's car went flat. "Good thing I have a spare," he said.

He opened the lid of the trunk and jumped back three paces. His friends fled in another direction, holding their noses as they ran.

They all had trapped skunks and been around farms. An odor worse than any they had ever smelled rose from the trunk of the car and permeated the air

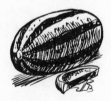

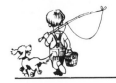

in all directions.

The watermelon had burst as it bounced in the trunks for days-on-days. It had soured, leaving a sickening smell only time would erase.

The boys took turns, no more than a minute each, removing the spare from the trunk. Once the flat was removed, it was tossed inside and the trunk was closed quickly and tightly.

Bogey had wasted no time ribbing Pokey. "Hope you didn't pour good vodka inside the melon."

Pokey's face turned red. "Never got around to it."

Bogey said, "There are a few melons left in the fields. We can still see how vodka watermelon tastes."

Pokey gagged, held his hand over his mouth and said, "I may never eat another melon or taste that first sip of vodka. And I know I'm never going to have the two together."

It was an easy vow to keep as long as he kept the car. The scent reminded him of the pledge each time he opened the trunk.

The School Paper Taught a Lot

Mrs. Barlow hadn't been at Heltonville more than a couple of weeks in September 1946, when she decided the school ought to have a newspaper.

Loren Raines, the principal, agreed to allow the publication when Mrs. Barlow promised any expense could be met by advertising.

She chose the staff for the paper and made selling advertisements seem simple, but then she didn't have to go out and solicit ads. She asked Don, Ralph, Cecil, Bob, Len and a couple of other students to do that.

They readily agreed. They not only thought the job would be easy, they thought they wouldn't have to make up any time they lost from classes.

Cecil and Bob started their ad sales one morning in Bedford, stopping first at the Three Pigs Restaurant, which was just preparing for its grand opening. The manager agreed to buy a small ad, then wrote a check to pay for it to run the entire school year.

The students complimented themselves as they drove downtown from the restaurant on the Northside. "Nothin' to it," one of them told the other.

They made one other quick sale before stopping at the Crowe Furniture Store on the northeast corner of Courthouse Square. That's when they met E.B. Crowe, a former congressman . . . as in the U.S. House of Representatives. He had been retired from Congress in 1940, beaten by Earl Wilson in the Ninth District race.

Cecil and Bob normally would have enjoyed meeting a celebrity of Crowe's stature. But Crowe didn't give them any indication he was enthralled by their appearance at the store, unannounced as it was, for the sole purpose of extracting an account payable.

The students went through their pitch about as skillfully as inexperienced seventeen-year-old salesmen could. E.B. didn't say anything for a while. And a smile was the farthest thing from his face.

He fixed his eyes on Bob, then on Cecil, and said, "Do they mimeograph school papers at county schools so you can read them nowadays? The last time I bought an ad in one of them you couldn't read it."

Bob didn't bat an eye. He stared back at E.B. and said, "You'll be able to read the ad in our paper."

Crowe grumbled, told them what he wanted in the ad, which would be no more than two inches by three inches, grumbled some more, then paid them, suggesting that neither they nor anyone else from the school stop by any more that year for a handout.

The students walked out onto "I" Street. Cecil said, "How do you know he'll be able to read the ad in our paper? We haven't even printed one yet."

Bob said, "You don't think a former United States congressman is going to drive out to Heltonville to pick up a school paper to see if his five-dollar ad can be read, do you?"

Back at school, they told Mrs. Barlow about the incident. She said a few words, some of which were less than complimentary to E.B. Crowe.

"I ought to make you take the money back. If he thinks advertising in the school paper is charity, he doesn't know anything about advertising or charity," she said.

But she decided to keep the money, figuring the paper needed it worse than E.B. Crowe did, which was true.

"By the way," she told Bob and Cecil, "Mr. East wants to see you before you go home."

Mr. East was Irvine East, a teacher who wanted them to be sure they made up the civics assignment they missed that day.

The school paper came out eight or ten times that school year, and the Crowe Furniture Store ad was readable. But just barely.

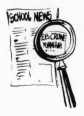

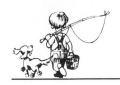
In the Footsteps of the Carpenter

Loren Raines wore a carpenter's apron to some classes and carried a Bible to others.

The hardest thing for students in his shop class was to learn to say "dadgummit," "shucks" or "blast it" when they skinned or smashed a finger. Other words, learned from walls on the outdoor toilet, came to mind more quickly.

Raines was a church minister on Sundays and principal for all twelve grades at Heltonville on weekdays. And he taught woodworking and Bible literature to make sure the township trustee didn't accuse him of loafing on the job.

Some students took both courses in the 1940s. They figured they'd learn how Noah built an ark and how to please the Lord if they ever had to keep one afloat for forty days and forty nights.

When Raines was teaching his Bible class, addressing the assembly of students, or performing his duties as principal, he looked serious, giving an impression that education was a sacred mission, entrusted only to him. It was an impression he may have cultivated to bring dignity and purpose to education.

But that wasn't the real man. Raines had a warm spot inside a false shell which turned to putty when he walked into the basement shop. He removed the coat from one of the light-blue suits he usually wore, hung the apron from his neck and knotted the strings from behind.

The austere look turned soft, the weight fell from his eyelids and a smile grew from the corners of his mouth. His manner was the same, whether it was with seventh graders learning to use a plane or sophomores who had advanced to complicated pieces of furniture.

Students he had scolded minutes earlier for misconduct were praised for squaring a board, for turning rough hardwood lumber into a smooth tabaret, or for refinishing an expensive cherry antique corner cupboard.

An hour in the class seemed no more than ten minutes. While the students cleaned their work areas, Raines removed his apron, adjusted his tie and pulled on his suit coat. His face changed to meet his next assignment.

He walked into the hall and looked in each direction. He was a human caution light, which the students observed as they sped between classes. He walked to his office without smiling, checked to see if there were any phone calls, picked up his Bible and lesson plan and walked briskly to another classroom.

This time he did not remove his coat or change his demeanor. Bible literature was a serious subject, to be taught with decorum.

Maybe that's why, forty years later, Pokey, Bogey, Tad, Tyke, Bob, Jake and his other students still find it easier to smile in their workshops at home than in the sanctuaries of the churches they attend.

A Sackful of Joy for Young Riders

Buck Harrell didn't make much money driving a school bus. Neither did Shorty White, Everett Easton, John Stipp, Gleonard Turpen or Goffria Turpen.

A sign under "Pleasant Run Township" on the sides of each of their buses listed the name of each followed by "owner-operator."

It could also have read "friend-confidante-counselor." The bus drivers were all those things to students who rode their buses over winding, hilly, gravel roads to and from Heltonville each school day in the 1940s.

The drivers maintained order on the buses without making the passengers seem like prisoners. Riders would be safer, the drivers explained, if their chauffeurs could concentrate on driving instead of discipline.

Students responded by keeping the noise level down to a constant clamor.

They didn't expect to be rewarded for their cooperation, but Buck, Everett, Shorty and the other drivers made sure they were on the afternoon when school recessed for the Christmas holidays. The drivers greeted each of their passengers as they bounded onto the bus, carrying presents they'd received in gift exchanges, as well as sacks of candy from their teachers.

The noise level was higher than usual, but the drivers didn't object. They sometimes hummed a Christmas carol as they drove away from the school, knowing the students would follow in song.

The lack of harmony didn't bother them in the least. The noisy excitement of the holiday caromed off the top of the bus, bounced against the sides and roared toward the driver in a crescendo. The drivers smiled and joined in the merriment.

A few of the students eyed the big cardboard boxes the driver had placed to his right at the front of the bus. The mystery of the contents was solved when the first passenger prepared to step off the bus.

"A gift for you," the driver said, ripping open the box and pulling out a brown paper sack.

"And a Merry Christmas," he added. The rider stepped from the bus, already digging through the sack as he turned to wave.

The younger students could only guess what was in the sack. The older ones knew there were peanuts in shells, chocolates with white filling, a Milky

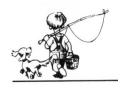

Way or Three Musketeers candy bar, candied orange slices and an apple or tangerine.

Students who wouldn't arrive home until the end of the route sometimes wondered whether there would be any sacks left for them. It was a needless concern. The drivers would have no more forgotten a rider than they would have neglected one of their own children.

The drivers didn't expect any thanks. A few of the students mumbled their gratitude as they left the bus. Others just took the sacks and jumped off the bus, forgetting their manners in the excitement of the moment.

But words weren't needed. The appreciation showed in the youngsters' facial expressions.

Buck, Everett, Shorty, Goffria, Gleonard and John could have put to other uses the money they spent on the students. But nothing they could have bought would have brought them as much pleasure as giving a sackful of joy.

Give 'Em Hell Harry
Had the Last Laugh

Nothing is certain in politics. Clarence learned that in 1948 and his friends have never let him forget it.

Make that tormentors. Friends may not be quite accurate.

Clarence rode from Heltonville to work at the General Motors plant in Bedford in the late 1940s with Dale and Slim. Dale and Slim leaned toward Democrats in most elections, or that's the impression they left with Clarence. That may have been to agitate him.

Clarence had a low appreciation for Democrats. In fact, he had no tolerance at all for some of them. Especially for President Harry Truman.

Clarence's blood boiled each workday as he, Dale and Slim drove past a big billboard that faced them as they rounded a curve on Ind. 58 east of Bedford. An oversized picture of President Truman smiled down at them with a message urging their support.

Dale and Slim returned Truman's smile each day, adding words of encouragement. Truman didn't hear the messages, but Clarence did. He reacted with some choice words of his own, some of which would have been new even to Truman, who wasn't known for his refined language.

Clarence's comments grew harsher as the election neared. And each day he would remind Dale and Slim of the polls which showed Republican challengers Tom Dewey with a big edge over Truman. Clarence, like most other Republicans, was certain Truman would be ousted from office.

The three men drove toward Bedford as usual Election Day. Dale mentioned as they passed the billboard that Truman was still looking good.

"The [expletive deleted] won't be smiling tomorrow," Clarence said, mentioning something about Truman's ancestry. He repeated the comment on the way home that day.

Truman overcame an early Dewey lead that night and scored one of the biggest upsets ever in presidential politics.

Dale and Slim agreed before they picked up Clarence the next morning to ignore the election results on the way to work.

Clarence looked downcast as he got in the car, expecting continual harassment enroute to Bedford. Dale and Slim greeted him, but said no more.

Clarence fidgeted in his seat, waiting for the taunting to begin. He waited in silence until the men were three or four miles from Bedford, when he almost begged: "Well, somebody say something!"

His companions ignored his plea until they reached the billboard. They stopped the car at the big sign. Slim rolled down the window, took a long look and said: "I'll be darned. Ol' Harry is still smiling. Good for him."

Slim and Dale said later they could almost see the smoke coming from Clarence's ears.

Clarence didn't calm down until the billboard was changed a week or so later.

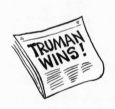

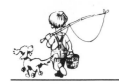

Dads Knew You
Had To Take Falls

To Tad, Tyke, Billy, Ray, Pokey and Bogey, he was "Dad" or "Pa."

Not one of them called him "Father." "Father" seemed too austere, too formal. Only youngsters from rich families or characters in books addressed their dads as "father" in the 1930s and '40s.

Farm boys had a special rapport with their dads, maybe because they had grown up at their dads' side. They had learned to walk, their hands in their dad's, in barnlots, stumbling at first, falling at times.

Their dads, fearing they might raise momma's boys, gave their sons little comfort when they slipped or fell. The boys learned that life, while mostly beautiful, can at times be ugly.

Dads explained to their sons that all things that grow eventually die, that time is short and that some effort should be expended each day toward pursuit of a purpose.

The boys were taught to be stewards of the soil, that the earth is a precious thing to be cultivated and not captivated. They were told to be kind to animals that could not care for themselves.

They learned to be on time, to do an honest day's work for an honest dollar and to work even when they didn't feel like it.

They learned to plow, first behind a team of horses, later at the wheel of a tractor. They learned to plant and to harvest, to raise crops and, when the work was done, to raise a bit of cane, too.

They learned how to sip a bottle of pop and have a good time in the company of men at the general stores, grain elevators and barber shops around Heltonville and Norman.

They learned the art of spinning yarns and telling stories, but more importantly they learned how to listen.

They learned that dads could be as gentle as the morning dew or as rough as barbed wire. Dads could accept the mistakes of youth, but never carelessness, unconcern or laziness.

Farm dads would swear when things didn't go right in the tool shed or in the field. But they never cursed in the presence of women, and their sons dared not, either.

Dads conversed more with their sons than with their daughters. It wasn't because they liked the boys more. They just felt more at ease talking about things their sons needed to know.

Sometimes in groups, when dads thought their sons weren't listening, they'd wonder to each other how their sons might turn out when they became adults.

Some of them lived long enough to find out; some didn't.

Those who did are mostly gone now.

And nobody misses them more than their sons.

Now, forty or so years later, they think of their dads and recapture a moment they shared as father and son.

In the video of their minds, they can relive their time together.

There are memories time cannot erase.

And as their thoughts fade back to the immediacy of the moment, the sons can almost hear their dads whisper:

"Sure you can't stay and talk a while longer?"

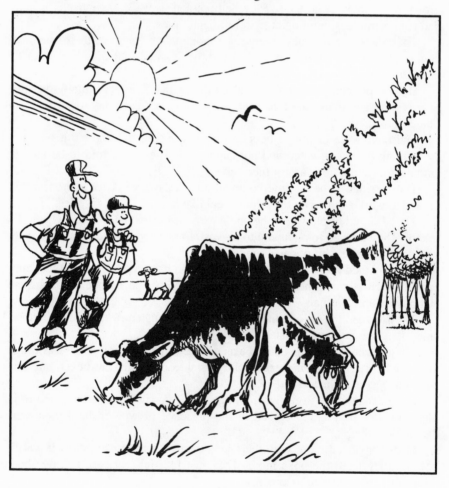

Index

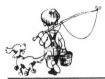

The Author

Wendell Trogdon grew up on a farm near Heltonville in Southern Indiana and has retained his love of small towns and country life. That love is reflected in his award-winning column for *The Indianapolis News*, "Those Were the Days," which has appeared weekly since 1975.

A graduate of Franklin College and a U.S. Army veteran, the author began his career in journalism at the Logansport *Pharos-Tribune*. Since joining *The News* in 1957, he he has been a reporter, suburban editor, news editor and assistant managing editor. He is also the author of "Quips," a front-page feature which has appeared daily in *The News* since 1974.

A basketball fan since even before playing for the Heltonville high school squad, he is the author of two books on Indiana high school basketball: *No Harm, No Foul* and *Basket Cases*.

He and his wife, Fabian, live in Mooresville, Indiana. They have three grown daughters, Tamara, Deanna and Jenell.

THE ARTIST

Gary Varvel was born the same year Wendell Trogdon began working at *The Indianapolis News*. The artist's own career at *The News* began in 1978. As the newspaper's chief artist, he has illustrated the daily "Quips" column and feature stories and has designed section covers.

A graduate of Danville (Indiana) High School, he attended The Herron School of Art while cartooning for the *Danville Gazette*. He later worked as production manager and editorial cartoonist at *The County Courier* in Brownsburg.

He lives near Avon, Indiana, with his wife, Carol, and their two small children, Ashley and Brett.